IMPORTANT: Read these instructions *BEFORE* proceeding!

Enclosed with your course book, you will find the FasTrax® answer sheet. Use this form to answer all the final exam questions that appear in this course book. If you are completing more than one course, be sure to write your answers on the appropriate answer sheet. Full instructions and complete grading details are printed on the FasTrax instruction sheet, also enclosed with your order. Please review them before starting. *If you are mailing your answer sheet(s) to Western Schools, we recommend you make a copy as a backup.*

ABOUT THIS COURSE

A Pretest is provided with each course to test your current knowledge base regarding the subject matter contained within this course. Your Final Exam is a multiple choice examination. **You will find the exam questions at the end of each chapter.**

In the event the course has less than 100 questions, leave the remaining answer boxes on the FasTrax answer sheet blank. **Use a <u>black</u> pen to fill in your answer sheet.**

A PASSING SCORE

You must score 70% or better in order to pass this course and receive your Certificate of Completion. Should you fail to achieve the required score, we will send you an additional FasTrax answer sheet so that you may make a second attempt to pass the course. Western Schools will allow you three chances to pass the same course...*at no extra charge!* After three failed attempts to pass the same course, your file will be closed.

RECORDING YOUR HOURS

Please monitor the time it takes to complete this course using the handy log sheet on the other side of this page. See below for transferring study hours to the course evaluation.

COURSE EVALUATIONS

In this course book, you will find a short evaluation about the course you are soon to complete. This information is vital to providing Western Schools with feedback on this course. The course evaluation answer section is in the lower right hand corner of the FasTrax answer sheet marked "Evaluation," with answers marked 1–20. Your answers are important to us; please take a few minutes to complete the evaluation.

On the back of the FasTrax instruction sheet, there is additional space to make any comments about the course, the school, and suggested new curriculum. Please mail the FasTrax instruction sheet, with your comments, back to Western Schools in the envelope provided with your course order.

TRANSFERRING STUDY TIME

Upon completion of the course, transfer the total study time from your log sheet to question 20 in the course evaluation. The answers will be in ranges; please choose the proper hour range that best represents your study time. You **MUST** log your study time under question 20 on the course evaluation.

EXTENSIONS

You have two (2) years from the date of enrollment to complete this course. A six (6) month extension may be purchased. If after 30 months from the original enrollment date you do not complete the course, *your file will be closed and no certificate can be issued.*

CHANGE OF ADDRESS?

In the event you have moved during the completion of this course, please call our student services department at 1-800-618-1670, and we will update your file.

A GUARANTEE TO WHICH YOU'LL GIVE HIGH HONORS

If any continuing education course fails to meet your expectations or if you are not satisfied in any manner, for any reason, you may return it for an exchange or a refund (less shipping and handling) within 30 days. Software, video, and audio courses must be returned unopened.

Thank you for enrolling at Western Schools!

WESTERN SCHOOLS
P.O. Box 1930
Brockton, MA 02303
(800) 438-8888
www.westernschools.com

Documentation for Nurses

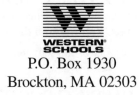

WESTERN® SCHOOLS
P.O. Box 1930
Brockton, MA 02303

Please use this log to total the number of hours you spend reading the text and taking the final examination.

Date	Hours Spent
_____	_____
_____	_____
_____	_____
_____	_____
_____	_____
_____	_____
_____	_____
_____	_____
_____	_____
_____	_____
_____	_____
_____	_____
_____	_____

TOTAL [   ]

Please log your study hours with submission of your final exam. To log your study time, fill in the appropriate circle under question 20 of the FasTrax® answer sheet under the "Evaluation" section.

Documentation for Nurses

D0126381

Instructions: Mark your answers to the following questions with a black pen on the "Evaluation" section of your FasTrax® answer sheet provided with this course. You should not return this sheet.

Please use the scale below to rate how well the course content met the educational objectives.

A	Agree Strongly	C	Disagree Somewhat
B	Agree Somewhat	D	Disagree Strongly

After completing this course, I am able to

1. Identify the importance and purpose of complete documentation in the medical record.

2. Identify professional and regulatory requirements for documenting patient care.

3. Discuss different nursing documentation methods and cite the advantages and disadvantages of each method.

4. Discuss the move toward computerized nursing documentation and describe at least three requirements necessary when using computerized nursing documentation.

5. Describe charting techniques and strategies to improve documentation.

6. Use the nursing process to improve sound documentation.

7. Discuss charting practices that decrease liability risk.

8. Discuss personal professional liability insurance and the steps to take when preparing for the defense of a malpractice lawsuit.

9. Describe specific nursing practices that could lead to documentation disasters and potential lawsuits.

10. Describe documentation methods used in specific departments.

11. Discuss the legal importance of and nursing responsibilities involved with informed consent and describe the importance of the Patient Care Partnership.

12. Determine situations that require incident reports and explain the purpose of these reports.

13. Discuss how advanced practitioners differ from other nurses and how nurse practitioners document management of patient care.

14. The content of this course was relevant to the objectives.

15. This offering met my professional education needs.

16. The objectives met the overall purpose/goal of the course.

17. The course was generally well written and the subject matter was thoroughly explained. (If no, please explain on the back of the FasTrax instruction sheet.)

18. The content of this course was appropriate for home study.

19. The final examination was well written and at an appropriate level for the content of the course.

20. **PLEASE LOG YOUR STUDY HOURS WITH SUBMISSION OF YOUR FINAL EXAM.**
    Please choose the response that best represents the total study hours it took to complete this 24-hour course.

    A. Less than 20 hours

    B. 20–23 hours

    C. 24–27 hours

    D. Greater than 27 hours

CONTENTS

FIGURES AND TABLES

Chapter 11

Chapter 12

Chapter 13

PRETEST

1. Begin this course by taking the pretest. Circle the answers to the questions on this page, or write the answers on a separate sheet of paper. Do not log answers to the pretest questions on the FasTrax test sheet included with the course.

2. Compare your answers to the PRETEST KEY located in the back of the book. The pretest answer key indicates the course chapter where the content of that question is discussed. Make note of the questions you missed, so that you can focus on those areas as you complete the course.

3. Complete the course by reading each chapter and completing the exam questions at the end of the chapter. Answers to these exam questions should be logged on the FasTrax test sheet included with the course.

1. Documentation is a critical factor in patient care because it

    a. provides proof of care, evaluates patient outcomes, and is used as evidence of care in legal cases.

    b. provides conflict of interest, does not take much time, and has no relationship to care provided.

    c. can be done by anyone providing care to a patient and has no legal ramifications.

    d. has no significance, can be anything, and is not based on regulations.

2. Mr. Jones is admitted for regulation of his insulin. Forms that might be found in his chart include

    a. nursing initial assessment form and vital signs graphic sheet.

    b. birth certificate and patient education record.

    c. delivery records and anesthesia assessment.

    d. consent form and passport picture.

3. The Joint Commission on Accreditation of Healthcare Organizations (JCAHO)

    a. publishes the "Accreditation Manual for Hospitals" quarterly journal.

    b. publishes a manual as the basis for the Joint Commission's evaluations.

    c. publishes a manual to be used by physicians to determine if nurses are following appropriate standards.

    d. is a publishing company specializing in nursing tests and manuals.

4. Nursing standards of professional performance

    a. are based on physician activities such as quality assurance.

    b. are described in terms of the highest level of reasonable care.

    c. apply only to registered nurses in educational settings.

    d. are described in terms of minimal requirements for nursing activities.

5. The oldest and least-accepted method of documentation today is

   a. SOAP format.

   b. APIE format.

   c. narrative notes.

   d. Charting by Exception (CBE) format.

6. If you forgot to put a checkmark in the box on a flow sheet next to the words "Breakfast Given," then legally, the patient

   a. was not given breakfast.

   b. only ate 50% of his breakfast.

   c. received breakfast but ate nothing.

   d. refused breakfast.

7. Computerized nursing documentation

   a. decreases patient confidentiality and allows access by everyone.

   b. is less accurate and more costly and requires more time.

   c. is a less efficient method of communicating and requires major applications.

   d. allows easier access to patient information and is more legible.

8. Each time you make an entry in a medical record, you should include the

   a. date the patient was admitted.

   b. time and day of the week only.

   c. date, the time, and your name and title.

   d. doctor's name and patient's birth date.

9. The Health Insurance Portability and Accountability Act was designed to

   a. cause patient information to be shared with research institutions.

   b. prevent patients from accessing their medical records.

   c. improve health care delivery and promote privacy of patient's health information.

   d. not affect nurses when it is implemented in the future.

10. A well-documented patient record provides

    a. gaps in care provided to a patient.

    b. written evidence that minimal standards of care have been met.

    c. oral communication of essential facts.

    d. support for the theory that patients are experts about their own care.

11. A key issue in many malpractice cases is

    a. failure to document.

    b. documentation of too much information.

    c. documentation of direct patient statements.

    d. the CBE method of documentation.

12. The doctrine of *respondeat superior*

    a. prevents a hospital from being liable for the actions of its employees.

    b. requires a hospital to be at fault.

    c. provides that a hospital is responsible whether or not the employee is named.

    d. makes the hospital liable for independent contractors.

13. The policy that covers a claim when a nurse no longer carries liability insurance is called a claims

    a. bought policy.

    b. made policy.

    c. occurred policy.

    d. brought policy.

14. In determining whether a nurse has been negligent, the nurse's care will be compared with

    a. what an educated layperson would do in the same or a similar situation.

    b. what a medical student with similar experiences would do in the same or a similar situation.

    c. what a reasonable and prudent nurse would do in the same or a similar situation.

    d. what a nurse who functions as a risk manager would do in the same or a similar situation.

15. When correcting a documentation error, the nurse should

    a. use correction fluid to cover the mistake.

    b. throw the original page away.

    c. erase the statement or mark it out to obliterate it.

    d. draw one line through the entry, write "ME" above the original words, and initial and date the entry.

16. Specialty areas in an institution may require special forms to provide adequate care for patients. These forms are normally developed through use of

    a. JCAHO and Emergency Medical Treatment and Active Labor Act regulations.

    b. specialty organization guidelines.

    c. diagnosis related groups and American Medical Association standards.

    d. quality assurance requirements.

17. A patient's informed consent to treatment may be obtained by

    a. a physician or an advanced practice nurse.

    b. a nurse.

    c. either a nurse or physician.

    d. the attorney for the institution.

18. When charting an incident such as a patient fall, you should

    a. describe the incident factually in the chart but not mention an incident report.

    b. indicate in the notes that the incident is described in full in the attached incident report.

    c. be sure to note that you were not the one who left the side rail down that caused the fall.

    d. have the patient checked out medically but not chart the incident unless an injury occurred.

19. For the jurors in a malpractice case, the best evidence of what really happened is usually considered to come from

    a. the defendant.

    b. the plaintiff.

    c. an expert witness.

    d. the medical record.

20. Hospital privileges for an advanced practice nurse are

    a. determined by a designated hospital committee consisting of medical staff or hospital management.

    b. determined by federal legislation.

    c. determined by state legislation.

    d. not essential for an independent advanced practice nurse to function within a hospital.

INTRODUCTION

Nursing documentation is a critical component of nursing practice. Inadequate or poor documentation may result in the appearance of malpractice, negligence, fraud, or abuse. Documentation allows nurses to protect their careers by bringing together the best available facts about nursing diagnoses, interventions, and outcomes regarding the care provided to their clients. The purpose of this course is to provide information to help nurses explore the professional and regulatory requirements of documentation; to review documentation processes and systems; to be aware of the impact of nursing documentation on patient care, the nursing career, and reimbursement; and to learn steps to avoid litigation.

The course is geared toward the general undergraduate staff nurse; however, any nurse would benefit from reviewing the information. The chapters addressing legal aspects, preparation for deposition or trial, and documentation disasters provide nurses at any educational level with helpful information. Chapter 13 addresses information about advanced practice nurse documentation and requirements. This chapter is included to illustrate similarities and differences between undergraduate nursing documentation and advanced practice nursing documentation. Undergraduate nurses should find this chapter informative in regard to requirements that may assist them in deciding whether to further their education.

The goal of this book is to provide a general review of documentation, present tips for improving documentation, inform nurses about the preparation for depositions and trials, and encourage nurses to document in order to prepare for and protect themselves against lawsuits.

Note: Sample documents throughout this course book have been reduced in size to fit the pages of this book. The original forms varied in size.

CHAPTER 1

PURPOSE OF DOCUMENTATION

CHAPTER OBJECTIVE

After completing this chapter, the reader will be able to identify the importance and purpose of complete documentation in the medical record.

LEARNING OBJECTIVES

After studying this chapter, the reader will be able to

1. explain the beginning of documentation and its evolution.

2. identify purposes of a health care record.

3. specify ten records one might find in a patient's medical chart.

4. indicate forms specifically used by nurses in documenting patient care.

5. identify trends in nursing documentation.

INTRODUCTION

Accurate documentation of patient symptoms and observations is critical to proper treatment and recovery. Starting on the first day of nursing school, students are advised about the requirements for complete and proper documentation. However, documentation still becomes somewhat burdensome and time-consuming. Nurses commonly experience conflict between time spent caring for patients and time needed to accurately record what care was pro-vided and patient responses to treatment. When time is limited, nursing care may take priority and what is documented may not tell the whole story.

EVOLUTION OF DOCUMENTATION

Documentation is a vital part of nursing prac-tice. It has been defined as "anything written or printed that is relied on as a record of proof for authorized persons" (Daniels, 1997, p. 181). It is the recording of pertinent patient data in a clinical record. Good documentation reflects quality of care and evidence of each health care team member's accountability in providing care. Written communi-cation must contain (a) appropriate language and terminology; (b) correct grammar, spelling, and punctuation; and (c) logical organization. Nursing documentation is not a new requirement; however, it has become increasingly important in determining the quality and cost of patient care.

Documentation has been considered important since the days of Florence Nightingale. In her *Notes on Nursing*, Nightingale indicated nurses need to record the care provided to patients. Most of the documentation during Nightingale's time was used for communication of medical orders and not to observe, assess, or evaluate patient status. Today, documentation is one of the most critical skills nurses perform. Many nurses approach documenta-tion as a chore; however, one's entire nursing career could depend on the accuracy and completeness of the charting that has or has not been done.

Nursing documentation was not always thought of as a critical part of patient care. In 1951, the Joint Commission on Accreditation of Healthcare Organizations (JCAHO) was established and promoted formalization of nursing standards, which provided a method by which nursing care could be evaluated. Prior to that time, nursing notes were removed from a patient's chart and destroyed when a patient was discharged. Hospitals are now required by JCAHO to establish quality improvement programs to conduct objective, ongoing reviews of patient care. JCAHO has standards in regard to patient records, including information that must be present in the record. JCAHO requires institutions to establish quality care and methods to monitor policies and practice. Nurses must be aware that JCAHO regulations require completion of the patient's records within 30 days following discharge. The medical records department may ask nurses to remind physicians to complete their records.

In the early 1970s, nursing documentation was finally considered an important and legal part of a patient's chart. With the development of diagnosis related groups (DRGs), nursing documentation became an important component in determining monetary reimbursement for care. DRGs provide a method for classifying patients into categories based on age, diagnosis, and treatment requirements. It is the basis for the U.S. Department of Health and Human Services' prospective payment system. The federal Centers for Medicare & Medicaid Services (CMS) (previously Health Care Financing Administration [HCFA]) requires every patient be classified into one or more of about 500 DRGs. This is necessary for reimbursement for services provided. The CMS also sets a length of stay for each DRG, and documentation must be provided if a patient remains hospitalized beyond the established time. The key source of information for determining the patient's course of treatment and the correct DRG assignment is the medical record. Because of this reimbursement method, poor documentation may create financial disaster for a hospital. If quality care is provided for fewer expenses than allotted by the DRG, the hospital is allowed to keep the difference, thus realizing a profit.

The North American Nursing Diagnosis Association (NANDA) is an organization involved in developing and promoting the use of nursing diagnoses. The organization formed in 1973 and since 1975 has continued to develop and refine nursing diagnoses. The diagnoses define problems nurses are able to treat because they are qualified to do so. They assist nurses with assessing patients' biophysical, psychosocial, psychological, environmental, learning, and discharge planning needs. Newly developed components of NANDA address patient strengths as well as problems and also address the move toward wellness.

Even though NANDA is not a regulating body, many admission assessment forms are based on nursing diagnoses. After completing an admission assessment, the nurse selects the appropriate choice from the list of accepted nursing diagnoses to identify actual and potential problems. The identified problems can assist the nurse to develop nursing diagnoses and a plan of care.

The plan of care should guide patient care and documentation in the medical record. Once the plan of care is established, it needs to be regularly reviewed and updated. When a patient's record is reviewed, the identified nursing diagnoses, interventions, and outcomes should be compared to the documentation in the nursing notes. This comparison can be used to determine whether the patient's highest priority problems were identified and whether the nursing interventions were effective. Other parts of the patient's record may also be reviewed to verify that the nurse carried out the plan of care.

Documentation is the very core of nursing. Nurse practice acts and professional standards require nursing documentation and specify the patient's needs that guide the documentation. Through documentation, changes in a patient's condition can be tracked, decisions about the patient's needs can be made and recorded, and continuity of care can be ensured. Good charting saves time, effort, and money. Effective documentation is a systematic, timely, accurate, well-written account of nursing care provided for patients. It must comply with standards established by regulatory and accrediting organizations, insurance companies, and the institution. What is charted may be examined by many reviewers, including accrediting, certifying, and licensing organizations; quality improvement professionals; Medicare and insurance company reviewers; researchers; and, in some cases, attorneys and judges. Therefore, nursing documentation is a critical part of the complete medical record.

PURPOSE OF MEDICAL RECORDS

A medical record is a valuable source of data used by all members of a health care team. Its purposes are to serve as a planning tool for patient care; to record the course of a patient's treatment and changes in medical condition; to document communication between all health care team members; to protect the legal interests of the patient, the organization, and health care providers; to provide a database for use in statistical reporting, continuing education, and research; and to provide information necessary for third-party billing and regulatory agencies. The medical record must be accurate, complete, current, readily accessible, and systematically organized.

Nursing documentation communicates a patient's assessment to other health care providers and team members. Professional responsibility and accountability are the most important reasons for accurate documentation. Nurses are managing patients with increased complex problems that require increased technology and equipment for care. Documentation is part of a nurse's overall responsibility for patient care because it facilitates care, enhances continuity of care, and helps coordinate treatment and evaluation of the patient. Documentation allows a nurse to take credit for care provided, the patient's response, and actions taken. Documentation must clearly communicate the nurse's judgment and evaluation of a patient's status. The patient's medical record should provide information about a specific situation or illness and the events that occurred during the situation.

Another reason for accurate and complete nursing documentation is that it may be used in malpractice cases. The patient's record is considered a legal document that can be used as evidence in a legal action. When a patient makes an accusation of negligence or malpractice against a health care provider, the record becomes a major source of information about the care that the patient received. Many lawsuits are won or lost by the amount of or lack of nursing documentation. Nursing documentation provides critical evidence about whether a standard of care was met. The patient's chart is the best evidence of what happened to the patient; it becomes the witness that never lies and never dies. Accurate, timely, and complete charting helps track quality patient care and protects nurses, physicians, and the hospital from litigation.

The patient's chart is used for auditing and for quality assurance. It helps organizations review and evaluate the quality of care given in an institution. Hospital accreditation is partially based on nursing documentation. The documentation must meet current requirements and demonstrate compliance with standards. Current JCAHO standards direct all health care facilities to establish policies about the frequency of documentation and necessary types of documentation. Professional organizations and regulatory agencies require that documentation include initial and ongoing assessments, any variations from the assessment, patient teaching, response to treatment or therapy, and relevant statements made by the patient and the family.

Managed care has evolved and necessitated the need to document accurate care for cost containment. Documentation of care helps organizations receive reimbursement from third-party payers, including private insurance companies and government sources of reimbursement, such as Medicare and Medicaid. The complexity of patient problems and the intensity of patient needs must be documented to ensure complete reimbursement. Each patient's record must provide the DRG code and documentation of appropriate care to facilitate the receipt of appropriate payment.

A patient's chart may also be used for education and research. Data gathered from medical records of patients may yield a variety of research studies. Students use medical records as educational tools. Patient records provide a comprehensive view of specific patients, their health problems, their medical treatments, nursing interventions, and the response to treatment interventions. Medical records help students understand patients' individual experiences with specific health problems.

COMMON NURSING FORMS

Each patient's medical record may include a number of specific forms, some of which are listed in Table 1-1. Although this table is not all-inclusive, it does provide a good representation of forms commonly found in medical records. Forms allow for quick, easy, and comprehensive documentation, and they are more accessible than long, detailed progress notes. Nurses are the primary people documenting on these forms. Discussion of some common nursing forms follows.

TABLE 1-1: COMMON FORMS THAT MAY BE FOUND IN A PATIENT'S CHART

Medical records vary by institution and the services provided. All records should contain some or all of the following basic information, if applicable to the patient:

- Patient identification and demographic data
- Informed consent for treatment and procedures
- Medical history, physical, and diagnosis
- Initial nursing admission assessment
- Anesthesia assessment
- Nursing diagnosis or problems
- Nursing or multidisciplinary care plan
- Record of nursing treatments and evaluations
- Diagnostic and therapeutic orders
- Health care providers' progress notes
- Medication and treatment records
- Results of diagnostic studies
- Operative reports
- Delivery records
- Nurses' notes of nursing observations
- Vital sign graphs or records
- Consultation notes and reports
- Reports from other disciplines (social services and recreational, occupational, and activity therapy)
- Physical therapy reports
- Nutritional notes and reports
- Fluid intake and output charts
- Patient education
- Discharge plan and summary

(Daniels, 1997; Pozgar, 2002)

Nursing History Forms

The nursing history form, or admission assessment form, must be completed by a registered nurse within a specified time frame from the time of a patient's admission, usually within 24 hours. The form contains basic biographical data such as the patient's age; method of admission; physician; the admitting medical diagnosis or chief complaint; a brief medical-surgical history, including medication and drug allergies; the patient's perceptions about illness or hospitalization; and a review of health risk factors. A nursing physical assessment of all body systems may also be included on the form or on a different form.

The data collected serves as a baseline with which changes in the patient's status may be compared. Baseline data is very important. The exact form may differ by institution and is dependent upon standards of practice and the institution's nursing care philosophy. A sample nursing history form is found in Figure 1-1 on pages 6 to 8.

Graphic Sheets and Flow Sheets

Graphic sheets and flow sheets allow nurses to readily see and assess changes in patient status. They provide a quick, efficient method to record information about vital signs and routine patient care. When a significant change is observed, the nurse may further document the assessment, intervention, and evaluation of that change in a narrative or progress note. The graphic sheet or flow sheet provides a quick, easy reference that all health care team members can use in assessing a patient's status. A sample graphic flow sheet is found in Figure 1-2 on page 9.

Nursing Kardex

Daily patient care is commonly recorded on a flip-over card that is kept in a portable index file or notebook at the nurses' station. Most Kardex forms have an activity and treatment section with a nursing care plan section. Referral to the Kardex throughout the shift helps a nurse organize information and plan care. The up-to-date Kardex reduces the need for continual referral to the patient's chart for routine information. Depending on the institution's requirements, the Kardex may become part of the patient's permanent record. The Kardex provides the nurse an opportunity to communicate useful information to the nursing team about a patient's

unique needs. A sample Kardex form appears in Figure 1-3 on pages 10 and 11.

Even though the Kardex is helpful, it does have disadvantages. Access is limited to nurses and does not allow space for writing an extensive plan for multiple complex patient problems. In such instances, the nurse should consult the care plan. Another disadvantage is that the Kardex may not be updated routinely and thus a nurse may miss a current or active order.

24-Hour Patient Care Records and Acuity Charting System

Twenty-four hour patient care records eliminate unnecessary record-keeping. Accurate assessment information is documented on a flow sheet in checklist format. The form is the basis for the acuity charting system, which requires nurses to document interventions used to identify patient acuity. The acuity rating compares patients with one another and provides a system for determining staffing patterns. See Figure 1-4 on pages 12 to 14 for an example of a 24-hour patient care record.

Standardized Care Plans

Standardized care plans have simplified nursing documentation by providing preprinted, established guidelines to be used for patient care for specific problems. After the initial nursing assessment is completed, the nurse selects the appropriate standardized care plan and individualizes it to meet the patient's specific needs. Many standardized care plans provide spaces for writing specific outcomes of care and recording the dates by which the outcomes should be achieved. A major advantage is that specific standards of care have been established and can easily be adapted to specific patients. The educational needs of the patient can easily be identified and addressed. Standardized care plans improve continuity of care and decrease documentation time.

A major disadvantage of standardized care plans is the risk of not taking the time to individualize the

text continues on page 10

FIGURE 1-1: SAMPLE NURSING HISTORY FORM (1 OF 3)

WELLSTAR
Health System

ADULT ADMISSION
DATABASE

☐ KENNESTONE   ☐ DOUGLAS
☐ COBB   ☐ WINDY HILL
☐ PAULDING

If patient is 17 or under, use the Pediatric Database **Form initiated by (Unit Name)** _____ Date: _____ Time: _____	

ADMISSION DATA: ☐ Patient ☐ Family ☐ Other: Emergency Contact/Phone#

REASON FOR ADMISSION:

VITAL SIGNS: Ht. _____ Wt. _____ ☐ Actual ☐ Stated   Temperature _____ ☐ Tympanic ☐ Oral ☐ Axillary ☐ Rectal
Pulse _____ Respirations _____ Blood Pressure _____   Fetal Heart Tones _____

ALLERGIES: ☐ Y ☐ N   Type Reaction: ☐ Drug ☐ X-ray dye ☐ Food Ⓟ Latex   **Allergy Band applied**   ☐ Yes
List: _____   **Identification Band applied**   ☐ Yes

ADVANCED DIRECTIVES/PATIENT RIGHTS/RELIGIOUS/SPIRITUAL/CULTURAL:

Have you completed a written document, such as a Living Will, that tells us what you would want in terms of your future healthcare? ☐ Yes ☐ No

If no: Provide written information; consult Social Services if further info requested. Ⓢ

If yes: Copy on chart ☐ Y ☐ N If copy not on chart: 1. Refer all inpatients to Social Services Ⓢ *"Need copy of advance directive"*

2. Document content per patient/family: _____

Do you have any questions regarding your rights and responsibilities as a patient? ☐ Y ☐ N (If yes, review with patient/family)

Are there any special considerations/needs related to your religious/cultural/spiritual beliefs (such as blood transfusions, dietary restrictions, etc.)?

Are there any spiritual practices that are important to you? _____

Would you like for us to contact your church or someone from Pastoral Services for you? Ⓒ Y ☐ N

If yes, contact name _____ Date/time contacted _____

COMMUNICATIONS: English ☐ Y ☐ N   If no, language spoken _____ Interpreter: ☐ Y ☐ N
Speech: ☐ Clear ☐ Slurred ☐ Mute ☐ Aphasic ☐ Other _____
Vision: ☐ Normal ☐ Blind ☐ Contact(s) ☐ Glasses ☐ Lens Implant   Hearing: ☐ Normal ☐ Deaf ☐ Hard/Hearing ☐ Hearing aid

LEARNING ASSESSMENT: How do you best learn? ☐ Video ☐ Verbal ☐ Written ☐ Demo ☐ Other _____
Identified barriers to learning: ☐ None ☐ Emotional ☐ Physical ☐ Cognitive

HABITS/HISTORY: Tobacco: ☐ Never ☐ Stopped date _____ _____ packs/day _____ years
Alcohol: ☐ Never ☐ Stopped date _____ If yes, when was last drink _____ Recreational Drugs: ☐ Y ☐ N Type/amt. _____

Medications Taken at Home: (Include prescription drugs, aspirin, eye drops, inhalers, birth control, over the counter, herbal medications, natural therapies, complementary therapies, dietary supplements and vitamins) Ⓟ **Coumadin** Ⓟ **TPN**

Home Medications	Dose	Freq	Route	Last Dose	Home Medications	Dose	Freq	Route	Last Dose

Medicines: ☐ None brought ☐ Sent Home ☐ Pharmacy ☐ Insulin Pump ☐ Pain Control Pump
☐ Other _____ ☐ Exceptions _____

Prior Hospitalizations, Surgeries, Invasive Diagnostic testing, etc.:

Describe: _____ Date: _____ Describe: _____ Date: _____

Describe: _____ Date: _____ Describe: _____ Date: _____

Describe: _____ Date: _____ Describe: _____ Date: _____

SIGNATURE: **RN/LPN**   **DATE:**   **TIME:**

FIGURE 1-1: SAMPLE NURSING HISTORY FORM (2 OF 3)

WELLSTAR
Health System

☐ KENNESTONE   ☐ DOUGLAS
☐ COBB   ☐ WINDY HILL
☐ PAULDING

**ADULT ADMISSION
DATABASE – Page 2**

PAST MEDICAL HISTORY/REVIEW OF SYSTEMS: Check all that apply

Anesthesia: ☐ Malignant hyperthermia ☐ Self ☐ Family Member _____ ☐ Complications _____ ☐ Other _____

Cardiovascular: ☐ Abnormal EKG/When? _____ ☐ Heart Attack/When? _____ ☐ Angina/Chest Pain ☐ CVA/TIA/When? _____
☐ Slow/Rapid/Irregular pulse (which) ☐ Congestive Heart Failure ☐ Mitral Valve Prolapse ☐ High Blood Pressure
☐ Pacemaker ☐ Aneurysm ☐ Heart Murmur ☐ Bleeding or Clotting Problems

Endocrine: ☐ Diabetes Mellitus ☐ Cirrhosis ☐ Pancreatitis ☐ Hepatitis ☐ Hyper/Hypo Thyroidism ☐ Other _____

Eyes: ☐ Eye Glasses ☐ Contact Lenses ☐ Glaucoma

Gastrointestinal: ☐ Hiatal Hernia ☐ Bleeding Ulcers ☐ Rectal Bleeding ☐ Reflux ☐ Crohns/Ulcerative Colitis ☐ Colostomy, etc. ☐ Heart Burn

Kidney & Bladder: ☐ Kidney Stones ☐ Kidney Failure ☐ Dialysis ☐ Kidney Transplant ☐ Prostate Problems ☐ Urinary Tract Infection

Lung: ☐ Abnormal CXR ☐ Collapsed Lung ☐ Chronic Lung Disease ☐ Lung Cancer ☐ Emphysema ☐ Bronchitis ☐ TB
☐ Chronic Cough ☐ Excessive Sputum ☐ Asthma (last attack _____) ☐ Wheezing   SOB: ☐ @/Rest ☐ after activity

Neurologic: ☐ Epilepsy (last attack _____) ☐ Paralysis ☐ Muscle Weakness ☐ Muscle Disease ☐ Nerve Injury
☐ Parkinson's ☐ Migraine Headaches ☐ Spinal Meningitis

OB/Gyn: ☐ Last Menstrual Period _____ ☐ Female Problems ☐ Currently Pregnant ☐ Problems with Childbirth

Orthopedic: ☐ Neck/Back Pain ☐ Arthritis ☐ Other _____

Teeth: ☐ Dentures/Bridges ☐ Loose Teeth ☐ Caps or Crowns ☐ Gum Disease ☐ Bleeding

---

ADMISSION PAIN ASSESSMENT

Is patient able to give self-report of pain? If no, complete assessment with significant other.	☐ Y ☐ N
Does patient have any ongoing pain problems?	☐ Y ☐ N
Does patient have pain now?	☐ Y ☐ N
Did patient take medication for pain prior to admission? (if yes, list under medication history)	☐ Y ☐ N
Does patient use alternative treatments for pain?	☐ Y ☐ N

Mark location(s) of pain body figure with a "P"

Current pain intensity: (Circle)   0 1 2 3 4 5 6 7 8 9 10

Average/usual pain intensity: (Circle)   0 1 2 3 4 5 6 7 8 9 10

Pain scale used: ☐ 0-10 numbers/faces scale   ☐ 0-10 behavior scale

Pain quality: ☐ Throbbing ☐ Sharp ☐ Pressure ☐ Dull ☐ Burning
☐ Cramping ☐ Tender ☐ Aching ☐ Other _____

Onset/Duration: Time of onset _____ ☐ Constant ☐ Intermittent

Pain worsens during: ☐ Day ☐ Night ☐ Activity/movement ☐ Other

Comfort/function goal: (Circle)   0 1 2 3 4 5 6 7 8 9 10

Additional Comments:

Front   Back

Mark figure above for location(s) of pain and skin condition

FALL RISK ASSESSMENT: (Circle points)   Age > 65: 10   Unsteady gait: 20   Disoriented: 10   Recent falls (past 3 months): 20

*Fall Prevention Protocol   Dementia or Psychosis: 10   Incontinent/Diurectics: 10   Sedatives or Antipsychotics: 10

Further function assess Rehab Services: ☐ Yes ☐ No   * Implement > 18 y.o. & score > 40 (See nurses notes)   *Score:

BRADEN CHART   ☐ Examined ☐ Verbal

SKIN: Surface Intact ☐ Y ☐ N   ☐ Warm ☐ Dry ☐ Pink ☐ Cool ☐ Moist ☐ Mottled ☐ Cyanosis   **RISK:** 15-16 Low

A – Abrasion   Amp – Amputation   B – Burn   Br – Bruises   D – Decubitus   Dr – Drain   E – Erythema   13-14 Mod
I – Incision   J – Jaundice   L – Laceration   Lc – Lice   O – Ostomy   P – Pin   R – Rash   < 11 High
S – Scar   V – Vascular Access   W – Wound   Points ↓

Sensory Perceptions	1 Completely Limited	2 Very Limited	3 Slightly Limited	4 No Impairment	
Moisture	1 Completely Moist	2 Very Moist	3 Occasionally Moist	4 Rarely Moist	
Activity	1 Bedfast	2 Chairfast	3 Walks Occasionally	4 Walks Frequently	
Mobility	1 Completely Immobile	2 Very Limited	3 Slightly Impaired	4 No Limitations	
Nutrition	1 Very Poor	2 Probably Inadequate	3 Adequate	4 Excellent	
Friction & Shear	1 Problem	2 Potential Problem	3 No Apparent Problem		
				Ⓦ Score < 16	Total Score

SIGNATURE: **RN/LPN**   **DATE:**   **TIME:**

FIGURE 1-1: SAMPLE NURSING HISTORY FORM (3 OF 3)

WELLSTAR
Health System

**ADULT ADMISSION
DATABASE – Page 3**

☐ KENNESTONE   ☐ DOUGLAS
☐ COBB   ☐ WINDY HILL
☐ PAULDING

PHYSICAL ASSESSMENT – Complete for: Peri-Op, Behavioral Health, Women's Unit, Invasive, Central Clinical Admissions

Operative/invasive site has been confirmed and verified: Site location _____ ☐ Right ☐ Left ☐ Bilateral ☐ N/A
PATT ☐ Y ☐ N _____ RN   **Day of Procedure** ☐ Y ☐ N _____ RN

COGNITIVE/NEURO: Oriented to: ☐ Person ☐ Place ☐ Time   ☐ Decreased LOC
Behavioral: ☐ Alert ☐ Anxious ☐ Angry ☐ Drowsy ☐ Cooperative ☐ Lethargic ☐ Confused ☐ Combative

GASTROINTESTINAL: ☐ Ostomy Site _____
Abdomen: ☐ Soft ☐ Firm ☐ Flat ☐ Distended ☐ Tender   Bowel Sounds: ☐ Present ☐ Absent ☐ Hypo ☐ Hyper

GENITOURINARY: Voiding without difficulty: ☐ Y ☐ N   Toileting: ☐ Self ☐ Min ☐ Max
☐ Cloudy ☐ Concentrated ☐ Incontinence ☐ Distended Bladder ☐ Catheter ☐ Frequency ☐ Other _____

NUTRITION:
I do not always have enough money to buy the food I need ☐ Yes ☐ No
Without wanting to, I have lost or gained ten pounds in the past six months ☐ Yes ☐ No
I am on a special diet and do not understand the diet ☐ Yes ☐ No
I eat fewer than two meals per day ☐ Yes ☐ No
Nutrition Resource Sheet given   Initials _____

RESPIRATORY: ☐ Normal ☐ Labored ☐ Shallow ☐ Wheezing ☐ Productive Cough _____ ☐ O₂ at home ___ L/min ☐ Trach
Breath Sounds (RT): ☐ Clear ☐ ↓'d ☐ Absent ☐ Congested   Breath Sounds (LT): ☐ Clear ☐ ↓'d ☐ Absent ☐ Congested

PRE-PROCEDURE PLAN OF CARE: (check all that apply) ☐ assess current understanding of procedure ☐ provide pre/post op teaching
☐ Keep side rails up ☐ provide aseptic environment ☐ provide privacy during prep ☐ limit traffic ☐ limit physical exposure except as required
☐ provide warm blankets ☐ confirm patient identity and allergy ☐ keep family informed of progress ☐ N/A ☐ Other: _____

SIGNATURE: RN/LPN   DATE: TIME:

ADMITTED FROM: ☐ EC ☐ Home ☐ Admissions ☐ MD Office ☐ PACU ☐ OR VIA: ☐ WC ☐ Stretcher ☐ Bed ☐ Other
UNIT ORIENTATION: ☐ Patient ☐ SO ☐ N/A ☐ Chaplain Service ☐ Visitation Policy ☐ Intercom ☐ Bathroom
☐ Bed/Door Labeled ☐ Bed Rails ☐ Shower ☐ Smoking Policy ☐ TV/Phone Valuables: ☐ Yes ☐ No Given to:
Recent change in activity status: [RS] Yes ☐ No

NUTRITION STATUS: Diet at home _____ [ND] Newly Diagnosed Diabetic [D] Limited Diabetic Education [D] No Home Glucose Monitoring
Alterations: [N] Difficulty Swallowing [N] Tube Feeding _____ ☐ Nausea & Vomiting ☐ Eating Disorder ☐ Ulcer
☐ Hiatal Hernia [N] Unable to eat for > 3 days [N] Recent Weight Loss > 10%/3 mos. [N] Recent Weight Gain > 10%/3 mos.
☐ Nutrition Resource Sheet given 23° patient   Initials _____

IMMUNIZATIONS: ☐ Flu ☐ TB ☐ Hepatitis ☐ Pneumonia

[B] Home medical equipment will be used during hospital stay. Notify Biomed prior to use of home equipment.

Notify: By computer or phone within 24 hours of admission to unit

	Initiated By	Date/Time			Initiated By	Date/Time
Wind Ostomy Continency Nurse	(w)		/	Pastoral Care	(C)	/
Food and Nutrition	(N)		/	Social Services	(S)	/
Diabetic Education	(D)		/	Pharmacy	(P)	/
Respiratory Therapy	(R)		/	Biomed	(B)	/
Discharge Planning	(DP)		/	*Rehab Services	(RS)	/
				*MD order PT, OT, ST		/

Outpatient Care Management Patient: ☐ NA ☐ Unknown ☐ CHF ☐ Asthma ☐ COPD ☐ Diabetes ☐ Other
DISCHARGE PLAN: Probable Disposition ☐ Home: _____ ☐ Other: _____
Home Health Service: ☐ Y ☐ N Agency _____ ☐ Hospice Phone: _____ Equipment: _____
Discharge to: [DP] Home [DP] Nursing Home [DP] Personal Care Home ☐ Other _____
     Rehab ☐ LTAC [DP] Subacute [DP] IRU ☐ Other _____
Primary Care Giver/Emergency Contact: _____ Relationship: _____ Phone: _____
SIGNATURE: RN/LPN   DATE: TIME:

Nursing Notes:

_____

_____

_____

_____

FIGURE 1-2: SAMPLE GRAPHIC FLOW SHEET

St. Joseph Hospital
Augusta, Georgia

**INTAKE/OUTPUT
and GRAPHIC RECORD**

ROOM #

Date																									

Weight	kg	kg	kg	kg

Hosp./P.O. Day	HD. ____/POD ___	HD. _____/POD ____	HD. ____/POD ___	HD. ____/POD____

Hour of Day	08 12 16 20 24 04	08 12 16 20 24 04	08 12 16 20 24 04	08 12 16 20 24 04

TEMPERATURE

C	F
40	104°
39⁴	103°
38⁸	102°
38³	101°
37⁷	100°
37²	99°
98⁶°	98°
36⁶	98°
36¹	97°
35⁵	96°

Pulse Oximetry				
PULSE				
RESP.				
BP				

Shift	D	E	N	TOTAL	D	E	N	TOTAL	D	E	N	TOTAL	D	E	N	TOTAL
INTAKE: Oral																
IV																
Minibottles																
Blood																
Hyperal /Lipids																
Other _____																
SHIFT INTAKE																
24 HR. INTAKE																
OUTPUT: Voided																
Catheter _____																
Emesis																
Stool																
Other _____																
SHIFT OUTPUT																
24 HR. OUTPUT																
Time																
RN Signature/Title																

Reprinted with the permission of St. Joseph Hospital, Augusta, GA.

plan of care. In addition, plans must be formally updated and kept current and the costs of printing and storing the forms may become problematic. Standardized care plans are not designed to replace the nurse's professional judgment and decision-making process. See Figure 1-5 on pages 15 and 16 for an example of a standardized care plan.

Medication Administration Record

The medication administration record (MAR) provides a list of the patient's medications, dosages, routes, and times for administration, and it includes spaces for indications by the nurse if the medication has been given. Accurate documentation is crucial so that patients receive the appropriate drug, dose, and route of administration. If a patient refuses a drug or is off the unit for a specific diagnostic reason, the nurse should document in the nurses' notes the reason the medication was not given. Some notation (such as an asterisk or the space circled) is made on the MAR to indicate that the medication was not given. See Figure 1-6 on pages 17 and 18 for a sample MAR.

Discharge Summary Form

To insure that the patient's discharge results in desirable outcomes, discharge planning begins at admission. These outcomes may be documented on the discharge summary form. Revisions to the care plan provide evidence of patient and family involvement in the discharge-planning process. Discharge summary forms make the summary concise and informative. A copy of the form is usually sent home with the patient. The form may include information about the patient; identification of possible problems; names and phone numbers of people to contact if problems or questions arise; teaching, activity, diet, medication, wound care, and special instructions; and the date and time of the next physician's visit. The information provides for continuity of self-care upon discharge. See Figure 1-7 on page 19 for an example of a discharge summary form.

FIGURE 1-3: SAMPLE KARDEX FORM (1 OF 2)

MENTAL STATUS		PATIENT TREATMENT PLAN - FFCB		VITAL SIGNS:
☐ Alert ☐ Lethargic ☐ Oriented ☐ Comatose ☐ Confused ☐ Sedated ☐ Other: ____		ST. JOSEPH HOSPITAL - AUGUSTA, GEORGIA ALLERGIES: _____		Freq: _____ NSDO/Epid:_____ FHR _____ ADMISSION BASELINE V.S: T P Wt.

ACTIVITY:
☐ Up ad lib
☐ Ambulate ____day
☐ Up with Assist
☐ Up in chair ____day
☐ BRP Only
☐ Bedrest

☐ Daily Weights

BLADDER:
☐ Continent
☐ Incontinent
☐ Up to Bathroom
☐ BSC
☐ Bedpan
☐ Ostomy
☐ Foley _____
☐ Cath _____

BOWEL:
☐ Continent
☐ Incontinent
☐ Up to Bathroom
☐ BSC
☐ Bedpan
☐ Ostomy
☐ Enema: ☐ Fleets____
                  ☐ SSE____
☐ Oil Retention ____

R   BP   Ht.
Other _____

INTAKE & OUTPUT
☐ Q8H ☐ Q4H ☐ Q2H ☐ Q1H
☐   IVs ☐ Foley ☐ Other ____

FEEDINGS _____ Freq ____
☐   Mother _____
☐   Staff _____
☐   Gavage _____
☐   Breast Pump _____
DIET _____

AM/PM CARE: SPEC. NEEDS
☐ Self   ☐ Turn q2H
☐ Assist   ☐ Traction
☐ Total   ☐ Glasses
☐ Shower   ☐ Hearing Aid
☐ Pericare   ☐ TDD
☐ Other _____
            BABY:
☐ Initial
☐ Demo
☐ Sponge

Form #1900025-11/93 Phoenix-Commercial Printers

OTHER: _____
_____
_____
_____

CODE STATUS _____

RESPIRATORY THERAPY

☐ TC / DB _____

☐ INC. Spirometer _____
_____

Oxygen _____ L/Min
       via: _____

☐ IPPB

☐ Dietary consult _____
☐ Force Fluids   ☐ Salt Sub
          SUPPLEMENTS:
☐ Fruit basket   ☐ Snacks
          GUEST MEAL
☐ B'fast ☐ Lunch ☐ Supper

FIGURE 1-3: SAMPLE KARDEX FORM (2 OF 2)

ANCILLARY REFERRALS NEEDED
- ☐ Social Work
- ☐ Home Health Care
- ☐ Pastoral Care
- ☐ Dietary
- ☐ Speech Therapy
- ☐ Physical Therapy
- ☐ O/T
- ☐ Diabetic Educator
- ☐ Other: _____

PATIENT/FAMILY TEACHING NEEDS

_____

_____

_____

_____

_____

_____

_____

CIRCUMCISION: Date: _____
- ☐ Gomco
- ☐ Plastibell
- ☐ Mogen
- ☐ Vaseline
- ☐ H2O2
- ☐ Other _____

HIGH RISK FALL LABEL

DISCHARGE NEEDS:
- ☐ Home Health Care
- ☐ New Arrival Program Member
- ☐ Short Stay / 24 hr. stay
- ☐ 23 Hr. Observation
- ☐ Dressing Supplies
- ☐ Diabetic Supplies
- ☐ Personal Care Assistance
- ☐ Assistance with Household Tasks
- ☐ Other: _____

IF EMERGENCY NOTIFY:
Name: _____
Relation: _____
Phone: _____

VALUABLES: ☐ To Home
☐ To Safe

MEDICATION:
☐ To Home
☐ To Pharmacy

EPIDURAL CATH LABEL

LABORATORY Date Due		DAILY LABS Date Due		RADIOLOGY Date Due		TREATMENTS	Freq Times
☐ Met Screen:		☐ Blood Glucose:				☐ Dressing Chg.	
☐ Chemstrip:						☐ Sitz Bath/Hygienique	
						☐ Heat Lamp/Peri Light	
						☐ Cold Pack	
						☐ Other	
		Date Due	EKG/ECHO				
Date Due	MISC			CONSULTING PHYS:			
		AIRBORNE PRECAUTIONS: Reason:		Religion: Annointed:			

Room #	Adm. Date	Age	DOB	MR#	ACCT #	OLD RECORD ☐ To Floor ☐ Microfilm	☐ C/Section ☐ NSVD	Date	Time	☐ Male	☐ Female

Name	Diagnosis	Physician	Pediatrician	Blood Type Mother: Baby:	Rh Coombs	Wt: Length: Apgar:

Reprinted with the permission of St. Joseph Hospital, Augusta, GA.

FIGURE 1-4: SAMPLE 24-HOUR PATIENT CARE RECORD (1 OF 3)

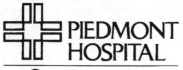

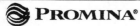

MED-SURG 24 HOUR RECORD

DATE _____

	Normal Parameters	Time:	Time:	Time:
Nervous System	Alert, oriented to person, place, time; follows commands; verbalization clear, understandable; equal movement and symmetry of strength of all extremities. Pupils equal and react briskly to light; eyes open spontaneously.	WITHIN NORMAL ❏ Pupil size: R _____ L _____ Not checked ❏ Eyes open to: Speech ❏ Pain ❏ None ❏ Verbal response: Confused ❏ Inappropriate ❏ Incomprehensible ❏ Slurred ❏ Aphasic ❏ None ❏ Best motor response: Localizes to pain ❏ Flexes to pain ❏ Extends to pain ❏ None ❏ See nursing notes ❏	WITHIN NORMAL ❏ Pupil size: R _____ L _____ Not checked ❏ Eyes open to: Speech ❏ Pain ❏ None ❏ Verbal response: Confused ❏ Inappropriate ❏ Incomprehensible ❏ Slurred ❏ Aphasic ❏ None ❏ Best motor response: Localizes to pain ❏ Flexes to pain ❏ Extends to pain ❏ None ❏ See nursing notes ❏	WITHIN NORMAL ❏ Pupil size: R _____ L _____ Not checked ❏ Eyes open to: Speech ❏ Pain ❏ None ❏ Verbal response: Confused ❏ Inappropriate ❏ Incomprehensible ❏ Slurred ❏ Aphasic ❏ None ❏ Best motor response: Localizes to pain ❏ Flexes to pain ❏ Extends to pain ❏ None ❏ See nursing notes ❏
Respiratory	Respirations 12-24 per minute at rest; even; no distress. Symmetrical chest expansion; breath sounds clear bilaterally; no abnormal breath sounds. No dyspnea, or dyspnea that is managed effectively.	WITHIN NORMAL ❏ Irregular ❏ Labored ❏ Shallow ❏ Asymmetrical ❏ Cough ❏ Trach ❏ Secretions ❏ Describe: _____ Crackles ❏ Rhonchi ❏ Wheezes ❏ Location _____ 02 _____ L/min via NC ❏ VM ❏ NRB ❏ Chest tube R ❏ L ❏ Leak ❏ Suction _____ Drainage _____ See nursing notes ❏	WITHIN NORMAL ❏ Irregular ❏ Labored ❏ Shallow ❏ Asymmetrical ❏ Cough ❏ Trach ❏ Secretions ❏ Describe: _____ Crackles ❏ Rhonchi ❏ Wheezes ❏ Location _____ 02 _____ L/min via NC ❏ VM ❏ NRB ❏ Chest tube R ❏ L ❏ Leak ❏ Suction _____ Drainage _____ See nursing notes ❏	WITHIN NORMAL ❏ Irregular ❏ Labored ❏ Shallow ❏ Asymmetrical ❏ Cough ❏ Trach ❏ Secretions ❏ Describe: _____ Crackles ❏ Rhonchi ❏ Wheezes ❏ Location _____ 02 _____ L/min via NC ❏ VM ❏ NRB ❏ Chest tube R ❏ L ❏ Leak ❏ Suction _____ Drainage _____ See nursing notes ❏
Cardiovascular	Regular apical /radial pulse 60-100 beats per minute, normal sinus rhythm (rhythm checked in selected areas). No paresthesia. Peripheral pulses 2+ palpable and equal bilaterally. Capillary refill <3 seconds. Neck veins flat at 45° if checked. No edema. No calf pain.	WITHIN NORMAL ❏ Radial/apical pulse: _____ Irregular ❏ Rhythm _____ Capillary refill sluggish ❏ Neck veins not checked ❏ or _____ Edema: 1+ ❏ 2+ ❏ 3+ ❏ Pitting ❏ Non-pitting ❏ Location _____ LT / RT: DP, PT, Radial — 0 = absent, 1+ = weak, 3+ = bounding See nursing notes ❏	WITHIN NORMAL ❏ Radial/apical pulse: _____ Irregular ❏ Rhythm _____ Capillary refill sluggish ❏ Neck veins not checked ❏ or _____ Edema: 1+ ❏ 2+ ❏ 3+ ❏ Pitting ❏ Non-pitting ❏ Location _____ LT / RT: DP, PT, Radial — 0 = absent, 1+ = weak, 3+ = bounding See nursing notes ❏	WITHIN NORMAL ❏ Radial/apical pulse: _____ Irregular ❏ Rhythm _____ Capillary refill sluggish ❏ Neck veins not checked ❏ or _____ Edema: 1+ ❏ 2+ ❏ 3+ ❏ Pitting ❏ Non-pitting ❏ Location _____ LT / RT: DP, PT, Radial — 0 = absent, 1+ = weak, 3+ = bounding See nursing notes ❏
Pain	Pain-free, or pain that is managed effectively. Scale 0 = No Pain 10 = Worst Pain imaginable	Pain score _____ /10 Description: See nursing notes ❏	Pain score _____ /10 Description: See nursing notes ❏	Pain score _____ /10 Description: See nursing notes ❏

FIGURE 1-4: SAMPLE 24-HOUR PATIENT CARE RECORD (2 OF 3)

	Normal Parameters	Time:	Time:	Time:
GI	Abdomen soft, non-tender. Active bowel sounds all 4 quadrants. No nausea, vomiting, diarrhea, constipation. Stool soft, formed, brown.	**WITHIN NORMAL** ❏ Abdomen: Tender ❏ Distended ❏ Ascites ❏ Bowel sounds: Absent ❏ Hypoactive ❏ Hyperactive ❏ Ileostomy/Colostomy ❏ Stool _____ Feeding tube _____ Gravity ❏ Suction ❏ Drainage tube ❏ Drainage _____ See nursing notes ❏	**WITHIN NORMAL** ❏ Abdomen: Tender ❏ Distended ❏ Ascites ❏ Bowel sounds: Absent ❏ Hypoactive ❏ Hyperactive ❏ Ileostomy/Colostomy ❏ Stool _____ Feeding tube _____ Gravity ❏ Suction ❏ Drainage tube ❏ Drainage _____ See nursing notes ❏	**WITHIN NORMAL** ❏ Abdomen: Tender ❏ Distended ❏ Ascites ❏ Bowel sounds: Absent ❏ Hypoactive ❏ Hyperactive ❏ Ileostomy/Colostomy ❏ Stool _____ Feeding tube _____ Gravity ❏ Suction ❏ Drainage tube ❏ Drainage _____ See nursing notes ❏
GU	Voiding without difficulty. Bladder not distended after voiding. Urine clear and yellow to amber. Absence of vaginal or penile discharge or swelling.	**WITHIN NORMAL** ❏ Has not voided ❏ Foley ❏ Odor ❏ Incontinent ❏ Urine color/character Other ❏ _____ See nursing notes ❏	**WITHIN NORMAL** ❏ Has not voided ❏ Foley ❏ Odor ❏ Incontinent ❏ Urine color/character Other ❏ _____ See nursing notes ❏	**WITHIN NORMAL** ❏ Has not voided ❏ Foley ❏ Odor ❏ Incontinent ❏ Urine color/character Other ❏ _____ See nursing notes ❏
Musculoskeletal/Skin	Skin warm, dry, intact; turgor elastic; color within patient norm; mucous membranes moist and intact. Functional ROM of all joints; absence of joint swelling, tenderness. No muscle weakness; steady sitting balance; steady gait. Braden score >16 or careplan reflects interventions. Date____Score____	**WITHIN NORMAL** ❏ ROM limited ❏ Location Gait unsteady ❏ Weakness ❏ Needs assistance with ADL ❏ Joint swelling ❏ Location Temp: Cool ❏ Diaphoretic ❏ Hot ❏ Turgo: Loose ❏ Tight ❏ Color: Pale ❏ Flushed ❏ Cyanotic ❏ Jaundiced ❏ Oral mucosa: Dry ❏ Cracked ❏ Ulcerations ❏ Other: See nursing notes ❏	**WITHIN NORMAL** ❏ ROM limited ❏ Location Gait unsteady ❏ Weakness ❏ Needs assistance with ADL ❏ Joint swelling ❏ Location Temp: Cool ❏ Diaphoretic ❏ Hot ❏ Turgo: Loose ❏ Tight ❏ Color: Pale ❏ Flushed ❏ Cyanotic ❏ Jaundiced ❏ Oral mucosa: Dry ❏ Cracked ❏ Ulcerations ❏ Other: See nursing notes ❏	**WITHIN NORMAL** ❏ ROM limited ❏ Location Gait unsteady ❏ Weakness ❏ Needs assistance with ADL ❏ Joint swelling ❏ Location Temp: Cool ❏ Diaphoretic ❏ Hot ❏ Turgo: Loose ❏ Tight ❏ Color: Pale ❏ Flushed ❏ Cyanotic ❏ Jaundiced ❏ Oral mucosa: Dry ❏ Cracked ❏ Ulcerations ❏ Other: See nursing notes ❏
Surgical Incisions/DSGs	Dressings dry and intact. No evidence of redness, increased temperature or tenderness in surrounding tissues or incision site. Wound edges approximated; no drainage. Staples, steri-strips, sutures intact.	#1 Site: _____ Dressing: Bandaid ❏ Staples ❏ Sutures ❏ Strips ❏ None ❏ Changed ❏ **WNL** ❏ Appearance: #2 Site: _____ Dressing: Bandaid ❏ Staples ❏ Sutures ❏ Strips ❏ None ❏ Changed ❏ **WNL** ❏ Appearance: #3 Site: _____ Dressing: Bandaid ❏ Staples ❏ Sutures ❏ Strips ❏ None ❏ Changed ❏ **WNL** ❏ Appearance: See nursing notes ❏	#1 Site: _____ Dressing: Bandaid ❏ Staples ❏ Sutures ❏ Strips ❏ None ❏ Changed ❏ **WNL** ❏ Appearance: #2 Site: _____ Dressing: Bandaid ❏ Staples ❏ Sutures ❏ Strips ❏ None ❏ Changed ❏ **WNL** ❏ Appearance: #3 Site: _____ Dressing: Bandaid ❏ Staples ❏ Sutures ❏ Strips ❏ None ❏ Changed ❏ **WNL** ❏ Appearance: See nursing notes ❏	#1 Site: _____ Dressing: Bandaid ❏ Staples ❏ Sutures ❏ Strips ❏ None ❏ Changed ❏ **WNL** ❏ Appearance: #2 Site: _____ Dressing: Bandaid ❏ Staples ❏ Sutures ❏ Strips ❏ None ❏ Changed ❏ **WNL** ❏ Appearance: #3 Site: _____ Dressing: Bandaid ❏ Staples ❏ Sutures ❏ Strips ❏ None ❏ Changed ❏ **WNL** ❏ Appearance: See nursing notes ❏

FIGURE 1-4: SAMPLE 24-HOUR PATIENT CARE RECORD (3 OF 3)

	Shift Summary	Time:	Time:	Time:
IV Sites	**NORMAL PARAMETERS:** Insertion sites and/or surrounding area free of redness, tenderness, swelling, drainage. IV line(s) are functioning as expected. Dressing clean, dry, secure.	#1 Site _____ **WNL** ❏ Condition _____ Dressing change ❏ Tubing change ❏ #2 Site _____ **WNL** ❏ Condition _____ Dressing change ❏ Tubing change ❏ See nursing notes ❏ #IV pumps ___	#1 Site _____ **WNL** ❏ Condition _____ Dressing change ❏ Tubing change ❏ #2 Site _____ **WNL** ❏ Condition _____ Dressing change ❏ Tubing change ❏ See nursing notes ❏ #IV pumps ___	#1 Site _____ **WNL** ❏ Condition _____ Dressing change ❏ Tubing change ❏ #2 Site _____ **WNL** ❏ Condition _____ Dressing change ❏ Tubing change ❏ See nursing notes ❏ #IV pumps ___
Activity		Up ad lib ❏ Bed Rest ❏ BRP self ❏ Assist ❏ #____ Dangle Self ❏ Assist ❏ Chair Self ❏ Assist ❏ Ambulate Self ❏ Assist ❏ Room ❏ Hall ❏ Tolerance _____ TCDB q ___H Self ❏ Assist ❏ See nursing notes ❏	Up ad lib ❏ Bed Rest ❏ BRP self ❏ Assist ❏ #____ Dangle Self ❏ Assist ❏ Chair Self ❏ Assist ❏ Ambulate Self ❏ Assist ❏ Room ❏ Hall ❏ Tolerance _____ TCDB q ___H Self ❏ Assist ❏ See nursing notes ❏	Up ad lib ❏ Bed Rest ❏ BRP self ❏ Assist ❏ #____ Dangle Self ❏ Assist ❏ Chair Self ❏ Assist ❏ Ambulate Self ❏ Assist ❏ Room ❏ Hall ❏ Tolerance _____ TCDB q ___H Self ❏ Assist ❏ See nursing notes ❏
Hygiene		Bath Complete ❏ Partial ❏ Shower ❏ Refused ❏ Self ❏ Assist ❏ Mouth Care q ___ H Self ❏ Assist ❏ See nursing notes ❏	Bath Complete ❏ Partial ❏ Shower ❏ Refused ❏ Self ❏ Assist ❏ Mouth Care q ___ H Self ❏ Assist ❏ See nursing notes ❏	Bath Complete ❏ Partial ❏ Shower ❏ Refused ❏ Self ❏ Assist ❏ Mouth Care q ___ H Self ❏ Assist ❏ See nursing notes ❏
Nutrition	Diet _____ _____	Tube feeding ❏ Residual _____ NPO ❏ Self ❏ Assist ❏ Feed Pt. ❏ B'fast All ❏ <1/2 ❏ > 1/2 ❏ Lunch All ❏ <1/2 ❏ > 1/2 ❏ See nursing notes ❏	Tube feeding ❏ Residual _____ NPO ❏ Self ❏ Assist ❏ Feed Pt. ❏ Supper All ❏ <1/2 ❏ > 1/2 ❏ HS snack ❏ See nursing notes ❏	Tube feeding ❏ Residual _____ NPO after MN ❏ Reason _____ See nursing notes ❏
Safety	Bed in low position; call light within reach	ID Band on ❏ Siderails _____ Rounds Q _____ H and PRN Restraint/protective device type _____ Sitter ❏ Family at bedside ❏ See nursing notes ❏	ID Band on ❏ Siderails _____ Rounds Q _____ H and PRN Restraint/protective device type _____ Sitter ❏ Family at bedside ❏ See nursing notes ❏	ID Band on ❏ Siderails _____ Rounds Q _____ H and PRN Restraint/protective device type _____ Sitter ❏ Family at bedside ❏ See nursing notes ❏
	Isolation - Type			
Other	Equipment, treatments, physician notification, etc.			
	CP Signature			
	RN Signature			
	RN Signature			

FIGURE 1-5: SAMPLE STANDARDIZED CARE PLAN (1 OF 2)

Interdisciplinary Plan of Care

Problem	Desired Outcome	Patient Specific Problem (Date each entry)	Plan (Date each entry)	Outcome Status
Pain	1. Pain is controlled with medication and/or comfort measures 2. Pain free with medication and/or comfort measures			
Nutrition Hydration Elimination	1. Adequate nutrition status 2. Intake meets nutrition needs 3. Adequate elimination status			
Mobility, Safety and Self Care	1. Dependent, does not participate 2. Requires assistive person and device 3. Requires assistive person 4. Independent with assistive device 5. Completely independent			

Patient Stamp Plate

Initials/Signatures:

Outcome Status Key:
− Deteriorated   M Maintaining
+ Progressing Toward Outcome   ✓ Outcome Met

FIGURE 1-5: SAMPLE STANDARDIZED CARE PLAN (2 OF 2)

Problem	Desired Outcome	Patient Specific Problem (Date each entry)	Plan (Date each entry)	Outcome Status
Supportive Care	1. Patient and family are coping appropriately. 2. Spiritual needs addressed 3. Issues of crisis and loss addressed			
Tissue Perfusion/ Oxygenation	1. Vital signs within normal limits and/or at baseline 2. Pulses improved or at baseline 3. Extremities warm and normal color 4. Patent airway 5. Adequate ventilation 6. Level of consciousness within normal limits for patient 7. Skin Integrity maintained			
Infection	1. Afebrile 2. Incision clean, warm, dry and no signs of redness 3. Infection control measures initiated 4. No purulent secretions 5. WBC's normalizing			
Communication	1. Oriented to environment and condition 2. Hears spoken language 3. Understands instructions 4. Expresses needs and emotions			
Discharge Planning	1. Identify discharge needs and support systems 2. Collaborate with team 3. Patient and Family agree to plan of care ☐			

Saint Joseph's Hospital of Atlanta
MRC approved 8/10/99

Patient name _____ MR# _____

Reprinted with the permission of St. Joseph's Hospital, Atlanta, GA.

FIGURE 1-6: SAMPLE MEDICATION ADMINISTRATION RECORD (1 OF 2)

Department of Nursing
MEDICATION RECORD FORM

REGULARLY SCHEDULED DOSES

INSTRUCTIONS: Make First Entry on
Day of Week That Medication is Started

Identify All Initials On Reverse Side

ALLERGIES: _____

_____

START EXPIRE	MEDICATION Dose,Route	Date: SUN.	Date: MON.	Date: TUES.	Date: WED.	Date: THURS.	Date: FRI.	Date: SAT.

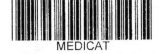

MEDICAT

FIGURE 1-6: SAMPLE MEDICATION ADMINISTRATION RECORD (2 OF 2)

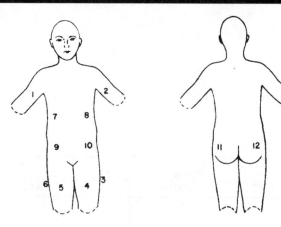

Identify Injection Site with circled
Code Number

e.g. ④ = Anterior Left Thigh

NOTE: 7, 8, 9, 10 are for
subcutaneous injections only.

1. Right Deltoid	4. Ant. Left Thigh	7. Right Upper Quadrant	10. Left Lower Quadrant
2. Left Deltoid	5. Ant. Right Thigh	8. Left Upper Quadrant	11. Left Gluteal Area
3. Lat. Left Thigh	6. Lat. Right Thigh	9. Right Lower Quadrant	12. Right Gluteal Area

FULL NAME OF NURSE	INITIALS	TITLE

Reprinted with the permission of Medical College of Georgia Children's Medical Center, Augusta, GA.

FIGURE 1-7: SAMPLE DISCHARGE SUMMARY FORM

ST. JOSEPH HOSPITAL
Augusta, Georgia

Patient Discharge Instruction

Room #

Date: _____ Time Discharged: _____ Ambulatory   W/C   Stretcher | Accompanied By: _____

Discharged/Transferred to: Home   Other   Name of Facility: _____

Transportation: Car   Ambulance | Left AMA: Yes No | Expired: Yes No | Funeral Home: _____

Pronounced Dead: Time: _____ By Dr.: _____ | Autopsy: Yes No | Autopsy Forms/Permits Signed: Yes No

LEVEL OF INDEPENDENCE:
☐ Self Care   ☐ Partial Assistance   ☐ Maximum Assistance   Support services at home: _____
Care Needs after D/C: _____
_____

Discharged with: ☐ Glasses/contacts   ☐ Dentures   ☐ Meds from pharmacy   ☐ Valuables
☐ Hearing/speech aid   ☐ Other: _____

PATIENT/RESPONSIBLE PERSON INSTRUCTED ON FOLLOWING WITH RETURN DEMONSTRATION AS NECESSARY

1. Medications/Prescriptions:

Name	Dose	Freq.	Name	Dose	Freq.	PMI Sheet Given	
						Yes	No
						Yes	No
						Yes	No
						Yes	No
						Yes	No
						Yes	No
						Yes	No

2. Diet: Type: _____   Instructions: _____

3. Printed Instructions Given: Yes   No   Type: _____

4. Activity: ☐ Up as Desired   ☐ Walking   ☐ Do Not Lift   ☐ Bath/Shower
☐ Use Walker   ☐ Driver   ☐ Do Not Climb Stairs   ☐ Other: _____
☐ Use Crutches   ☐ Do Not Bend   ☐ Sexual Activity _____

5. Treatments: ☐ Cold/Heat   ☐ Sitz Bath   ☐ Foley Care | *6. Equipment/Supplies:*
☐ Dressing Change   ☐ Pericare/Light   ☐ Ostomy Care
☐ TED Hose   ☐ Cast Care   ☐ Bladder Instr.
☐ J-Vac   ☐ Circ. Check   ☐ Bowel Instr.

Problems to Report to Physician: ☐ Bleeding   ☐ Fever (   )   ☐ Difficulty Breathing
☐ Unrelieved Pain   ☐ Nausea/Vomiting   ☐ Redness at Operative Site

Comments: _____

Agency to provide services at home: _____ Phone: _____

Your hospital Social Worker is: _____ Phone: _____

Appointment with Dr.: _____ Date: _____ Time: _____

These instructions have been reviewed/read to me and I understand them.

Signature _____ Relationship _____

Nurse Signature: _____ Hospital Phone Number and Unit Extension _____

Reprinted with the permission of St. Joseph Hospital, Augusta, GA.

TRENDS IN CHARTING

In the past, documentation was process-oriented and emphasized tasks performed by health care providers. Today, increased consumer awareness, increased acuity of the patient, and increased emphasis on health care outcomes has created the need for changes in nursing documentation. Consumers expect nurses to be knowledgeable, competent, and caring while providing high-quality, highly technical care. This care must be recorded in the patient's chart. Complex health problems, decreased lengths of stay, and increased patient acuity require documentation systems that reflect safe, efficient, and effective care.

Significant trends in documenting patient care have been observed. Trends include changes in traditional care planning and efforts to meet the need for increased documentation and improved communication while making charting less time consuming. Beginning in the 1990s, handwritten care plans were replaced with standardized care plans that require individualization to meet specific patient needs. Another trend at that time was the use of critical pathways, or care maps.

Increasing documentation efficiency is another trend. Methods have been developed to reduce the amount of time required for nursing documentation. Emphasis is being placed on documenting patient care outcomes, especially those that influence discharge planning. Trends aimed at improving communication through documentation involve using nursing diagnoses. A shift is also occurring from narrative and problem-oriented documentation to Focus charting and charting by exception. Furthermore, computerized documentation is becoming the primary means of documenting care in the 21st century. Some of these trends will be discussed in more detail throughout this course.

CONCLUSION

Nursing documentation is a critical component of nursing practice. It allows nurses to protect their careers by bringing together the best available evidence about nursing diagnoses, interventions, and outcomes about the care provided. It also protects nurses from inaccurate claims of malpractice and negligence.

The purpose of this course is to provide information to help nurses explore the professional and regulatory requirements for the documentation process; review documentation processes and systems; be aware of the impact of nursing documentation on patient care, the nursing career, and reimbursement; and learn steps to avoid litigation.

Nursing documentation methods must change to keep pace with rapid changes in the health care system. Patient outcomes are the latest trend for documenting patient care. The transition to outcome charting is not easy. It is now critical for nurses to document nursing judgments rather than tasks. Different forms used for nursing documentation vary from institution to institution. Representative forms a nurse may encounter were presented in this chapter. There are numerous charting methods that help nurses document outcomes and communicate complete, accurate, and clearly understood health care interventions and will be discussed further in the course.

EXAM QUESTIONS

CHAPTER 1
Questions 1-6

1. Documentation is a critical factor in patient care because it

   a. encourages lawsuits and disciplinary actions.

   b. provides the patient with a method to record his or her care.

   c. provides proof of the type of care rendered.

   d. underwrites the cost of patient care.

2. Nursing documentation is thought to have begun with the need for nurses to record their actions initiated by

   a. Virginia Henderson.

   b. JCAHO.

   c. Florence Nightingale.

   d. DRGs.

3. The purpose of a medical record is to

   a. serve as a planning tool for patient care.

   b. serve as a method to blame others for not providing appropriate care.

   c. collect data against insurance claims.

   d. increase nurses' work by requiring nonsense notes.

4. When reviewing Mr. Jim Jones medical record, a nurse would probably find which of the following forms?

   a. Medical history, operative report, and delivery record

   b. Physical therapy report, PAP smear report, and graphic record

   c. Medication record, nurses notes, and patient education

   d. Consultation notes, progress notes, and birth weight record

5. Effective documentation encompasses

   a. entries into patient records to show lack of the need for care.

   b. entries of nursing activities performed on behalf of the patient.

   c. oral communication of nonessential facts given during the shift report.

   d. scratch notes that can be discarded once the patient is discharged.

6. Increased consumer awareness, increased acuity of the patient, and increased emphasis on health care outcomes has created the need for such changes in nursing documentation as

   a. increased length of stay.

   b. continued use of handwritten care plans.

   c. reintroduction of the exclusive use of narrative notes.

   d. increased documentation efficiency.

CHAPTER 2

REGULATORS AND REGULATIONS

CHAPTER OBJECTIVE

After completing this chapter, the reader will be able to identify professional and regulatory requirements for documenting patient care.

LEARNING OBJECTIVES

After studying this chapter, the reader will be able to

1. indicate Joint Commission on Accreditation of Healthcare Organizations standards related to proper documentation.

2. specify the relationship of diagnosis related groups to patient documentation and reimbursement.

3. explain nursing standards and their implications for documentation.

4. state the relationship between nurse practice acts and documentation.

5. describe the relationship between state and federal regulations and documentation.

6. describe the relationship between agency policies and nursing documentation.

INTRODUCTION

Nursing documentation of patient care and patient responses to that care is essential for effective communication between health care providers. As mentioned in Chapter 1, Florence Nightingale viewed documentation as a vital part of professional practice. Nightingale stressed the need for documentation so that data could be collected for better understanding of the management of patient care.

In the 1930s, Virginia Henderson promoted the use of written care plans to communicate patient care information. The use of written care plans continues today; however, care plans may not be considered part of patients' permanent records. Institutions have developed standardized care plans to make nursing documentation easier. The standardized care plan must be individualized for each patient. Numerous regulators and regulations govern the nursing documentation process. The regulators and regulations that will be discussed in this chapter include the Joint Commission on Accreditation of Healthcare Organizations (JCAHO), diagnosis related groups (DRGs), the U.S. Food and Drug Administration (FDA), nursing standards, nurse practice acts, state and federal regulations, specialty organizations, and agency policies and practices.

JOINT COMMISSION ON ACCREDITATION OF HEALTHCARE ORGANIZATIONS

The formation of JCAHO in 1951 led to the formalization of nursing standards. JCAHO uses nursing documentation as a way to evaluate nursing care. JCAHO standards direct all health care facilities to establish policies about the frequency and documentation of patient assessment. The commission is beginning to define outcome indicators to use in determining a health system's performance. These indicators may be used to compare health care institutions within a given community. Both high and low acuity patients are measured so that outcomes reflect the institution's overall patient population. The indicators serve as a grading system to help determine which institutions provide better care.

JCAHO, along with the federal Centers for Medicare and Medicaid Services (CMS) (previously Health Care Financing Administration [HCFA]), requires that documentation include initial and ongoing assessments, any variations in patient status, patient teaching, response to therapy, and relevant statements made by the patient. Accreditation given by JCAHO or the American Osteopathic Association (for osteopathic hospitals) is a voluntary process that most hospitals seek. Adherence to the accreditation standards is not legally mandated, but submitting to the accreditation process proves the intent of the institution to provide quality care.

Recently, JCAHO published a second edition of *A Practical Guide to Documentation in Behavioral Health Care*. This guide provides information on improving documentation practices in behavioral health organizations. In the guide, documentation is broken down into three sections:

1. the process and structure of care, including data collection and action planning

2. the process and structure of screening and assessment, addressing how to collect and analyze data efficiently

3. the process and structure of treatment and care planning, looking at care and discharge planning, care plan reviews, and progress notes.

DIAGNOSIS RELATED GROUPS

In 1970, DRGs moved nursing documentation forward as a way to determine monetary reimbursement for care. In 1983, implementation of the DRG reimbursement system for Medicare patients brought major changes in patient care. Hospitals were paid a predetermined amount for patient care based on Medicare-assigned DRGs and were forced to find ways to shorten patients' hospital stays. As a result, early discharge of patients led to the growth of home health care for follow-up.

The CMS, created in 1977 (as HCFA), is authorized to administer and enforce Medicare and Medicaid programs within the DRG parameters. Hospitals and other health care providers must meet standards established by the CMS before they can be reimbursed for treating Medicare patients. CMS form 485 is a physician's plan of care for a Medicare patient and must be completed and filed for the patient to receive home health care. The form lists physician's orders for treatment by skilled services, medications, and the patient's functional limitations and permitted activities. The patient must have physician certification that he or she is confined to his or her home. The physician and the home health agency both complete the form. After it is signed and dated by both parties, it is then submitted for reimbursement.

The nurse's role in this process involves making sure the form is completed and signed by the physician. It would be wise for the nurse to document in the nursing notes that the form was signed and forwarded to the proper authorities.

U.S. FOOD AND DRUG ADMINISTRATION

The FDA has taken an active role in establishing standards for computerized documentation, especially with regard to medications. Even though their guidelines are geared toward pharmacists, they also have implications for nursing. In 2002, the FDA released an updated version of its ongoing series *Guides for Electronic Records, Signatures, and Maintenance*. The guide provides specific information about key principles and practices, addresses frequently asked questions, and describes two examples of approaches for maintaining electronic patient records. As most health care organizations and institutions move toward electronic documentation and record-keeping, it is imperative that they meet standards and guidelines laid out by accrediting and regulatory agencies.

NURSING STANDARDS

Standards are considered the minimal requirements for nursing activities. They are not absolute because they depend on subjective determinations about what describes minimum acceptable behaviors. If nurses do not perform duties within accepted standards of care, they may put themselves in jeopardy of legal actions and may put their patients at risk for harm or injury. Therefore, when a nurse's conduct is alleged to be negligent and a patient is injured, the nurse's conduct is compared with that of other ordinary, reasonable, and prudent nurses with the same level of education in the same or similar circumstances.

In 1955, the American Nurses Association (ANA) published an official definition of nursing practice; however, it did not address nursing documentation.

Likewise, the 1965 revision, which presented a fuller definition of nursing as an independent profession, did not specifically address documentation. The 1980 ANA policy statement and the 1991 *Standards of Clinical Practice* (ANA, 1991b) mandated accurate data collection and proper documentation.

In 1985, the ANA established that the role of nursing documentation include stating a plan of care and that each nurse should follow that plan. The ANA emphasized that each nurse is responsible for data collection and assessment of patients' health statuses. The nurse determines the nursing care plan, which is directed toward designated goals. Evaluation of the effectiveness of the nursing care is recorded, and reassessment and revisions to the plan of care are a major nursing role.

The ANA has a new brochure, *Principles for Documentation* (ANA, 2003), that can be used to assist in nursing documentation. The guide includes policy statements, principles, and recommendations to assist nurses with documenting details in patient charts that aid compliance with institutional and regulatory requirements. It also includes other information about how to remain in compliance with institutional regulatory requirements.

The guide is based on the 2001 edition of the ANA's *Code of Ethics for Nurses with Interpretive Statements* and the 1998 edition of the *Standards of Clinical Nursing Practice (2nd ed.)*. The principles are based also on standards set forth by state and federal regulatory agencies, the Centers for Medicare and Medicaid Services (CMS), and accrediting organizations, such as JCAHO and the National Committee for Quality Assurance.

The ANA also has established the Nursing Information & Data Set Evaluation Center (NIDSEC). The purpose of this center is twofold: to develop and disseminate standards pertaining to information systems that support the documentation of nursing practice and to evaluate voluntarily submitted information systems against these standards. The need for an evaluation center arose out of a need for standards pertaining to nursing data and information systems. Standards have been developed to evaluate the completeness, accuracy, and appropriateness of nursing data sets. JCAHO standards provided the model used for establishing the system. Further information about the NIDSEC may be obtained by contacting the ANA.

STATE AND FEDERAL REGULATIONS

Nurse practice acts are statutory laws created by state elected legislative bodies. These statutory acts describe and define the legal boundaries of nursing practice within each state. Each state has the authority and power to regulate health care providers. Individual nurse practice acts address documentation requirements and specify how, when, and by whom charting should be done.

Nurse Practice Acts

Nurse practice acts are designed to protect the public, guide scope-of-practice issues, and define and set standards for nursing practice. All 50 state legislatures, the District of Columbia, and five U.S. territories have passed nurse practice acts that define the scope of nursing practice and the framework within which nurses must practice. These acts are the most definitive legal statutes and legislative acts regulating nursing practice.

The ANA and the National Council of State Boards of Nursing (NCSBN) have developed and published models to serve as guides for individual state boards to develop and revise their respective nurse practice acts.

Most state nurse practice acts reflect the writings and guidelines of the ANA. Nurse practice acts also set educational requirements for nurses, distinguish between nursing and medical practice, and define nursing practice. Although the definitions of nursing and its scope of practice are often similar, differences exist from state to state. Therefore, each nurse is

responsible for knowing the scope of practice in the state or jurisdiction in which he or she practices.

Nursing Licensure

The board of nurse examiners (BNE) for each state regulates nursing practice within the state by establishing licensure based on an established minimal level of competency to protect the public. The BNE of each state develops rules and regulations to clarify the state's nurse practice act and to regulate nursing practice. They have the authority to:

- prescribe regulations establishing educational requirements and admission standards for licensure of nurses and, in some states, for advanced practice nurses

- delineate the tasks that nurses and advanced practice nurses are permitted to carry out, either independently or in collaboration with physicians

- establish criteria and administrative processes for disciplining nurses, usually with authority to impose appropriate penalties.

The predominant model in the United States is that nurses are licensed in the state in which they practice. Nurses who hold dual or more licenses have successfully passed the licensure exam in one state and applied and paid for reciprocity, or licensure without examination, in one or more other states. In 1997, the NCSBN approved the concept of initiating and implementing multistate licensure for registered nurses (RNs).

Telehealth and telemedicine allows nurses to practice in states in which they are not licensed. The issue of practicing without a license becomes an issue for nurses working in areas for underserved patients. According to the terms of the compact proposed by the NCSBN, nursing licensure is issued by the state in which the nurse resides. Any state entering into the compact may grant a multistate privilege for a nurse to practice outside his or her state of residence; however, the nurse is held accountable for complying with all laws governing nursing practice in the state in which the patient is located. Although the remote state (compact state) may discontinue the multistate privilege, the state of residence (home state) retains authority to take disciplinary action against the holder of the license.

Multistate Licensure

Multistate licensure is a system of licensure by which a nurse can hold a single license that permits practice in more than one state. A mutual recognition model is one in which the nurse is held accountable for the nursing practice laws and other regulations in the state where the nurse provides services. It allows a nurse who is licensed under multistate licensure to practice (whether physically or electronically) in a state that has adopted the interstate compact. An interstate compact is an agreement (legislatively placed) between two or more states, in this case to remedy the problem of nurses wanting multistate licensure. In March of 1998, Utah became the first state to adopt the NCSBN compact language in its state legislature and to enact the mutual recognition RN licensure model. In April of 2003, 20 other states had compact legislation enacted with pending dates for implementation (ANA, 1998; NCSBN, 2003). Many other states have legislation accepted or pending.

Health care facilities (such as hospitals, skilled nursing facilities, intermediate nursing facilities, and managed care institutions) must obtain state and often federal licenses before they become operational. Several states have passed legislation or developed regulations requiring hospitals to have risk management programs. The mandate focuses on patient safety rather than on fire prevention, equipment maintenance, or security. Risk management programs evaluate nursing documentation for signs of quality control and adherence to institutional policies and procedures.

Legislation and rules that affect risk management may be created at city and county levels. City and county legislative bodies commonly adopt or adapt federal and state requirements. For example, a county water department may set standards for use of purification chemicals. Building codes, fire safety regulations, and occupancy permits are yet another example of local government regulations. These city and county regulations could dictate specific requirements that need to be documented.

Americans with Disabilities Act

An example of a federal statute enacted by the U.S. Congress is the Americans with Disabilities Act (ADA), which made physical barriers and discrimination bias against any disabled person illegal. The ADA discusses the rights of disabled people. HIV-positive patients are considered disabled under this act. It outlines how both patients and/or healthcare providers with HIV should be treated. Also included is information about how to handle healthcare providers who are unwilling to care for HIV-positive patients. In 1990, the ADA stated that an infected person could not be discriminated against based on fear of contagiousness. Coworkers who refuse to work with HIV-positive people can leave companies open to indirect charges of discrimination. Confidential information about infectious diseases must be carefully documented and protected.

Nurses must be concerned with balancing their own rights with protecting patients' rights. Both parties are afforded protection against discrimination and protection of privacy by federal and state laws. Careful documentation is required to meet the need to care for patients yet protect patient privacy. Nurses are encouraged to review institutional policies with regard to documentation in cases of infectious disease.

Legislation enacted by the US Congress sets guidelines that all people within the various states and jurisdictions must follow. When state legislatures enact laws, they cannot conflict with federal statutes.

SPECIALTY ORGANIZATIONS

Because hospitals are still organized around specialty services, many national professional organizations provide additional documentation guidelines and standards of practice. These guidelines tend to be more stringent than federal and state regulations. Specific criteria for documentation in specialty areas are addressed by the professional organization's criteria. Standards of professional performance are described in terms of competency, not reasonable care. Nurses are encouraged to contact professional organizations for guidelines and policies for proper documentation in a specific specialty area of practice. Several specialty organizations are listed in Table 2-1 on page 29.

AGENCY POLICIES AND PRACTICES

Administrative policies and rules of hospitals and other institutions are another source of professional standards. Failure to abide by a facility's policies and procedures may be evidence of a lack of ordinary and prudent care. Internal standards established by individual health care facilities are frequently more specifically defined than external standards. Many facilities adopt, adapt, and individualize federal, state, and professional standards. Internal standards may be higher or more stringent than external standards but are never lower. If an internal standard at a facility is higher than the minimum standard, the institution will be held accountable to the higher internal standard. Most institutions have specific requirements about the frequency of documentation, the type of documentation, and even the level of education necessary for completion of some of the forms in a patient's record.

CONCLUSION

Nurses must understand the regulations and regulators of nursing documentation, their legal limits, and the influence that regulations and regulators have on daily practice. This knowledge, along with good judgment and sound decision making, ensures safe and appropriate nursing practice and documentation of care provided.

TABLE 2-1: NATIONAL NURSING SPECIALTY ORGANIZATIONS

Academy of Medical-Surgical Nurses (AMSN)

Air & Surface Transport Nurses Association

American Academy of Ambulatory Care Nurses (AAACN)

American Association of Critical-Care Nurses (AACN)

American Association of Diabetes Educators (AADE)

American Association of Legal Nurse Consultants (AALNC)

American Association of Neuroscience Nurses (AANN)

American Association of Nurse Anesthetists (AANA)

American Association of Nurse Life Care Planners (AANLCP)

American Association of Occupational Health Nurses (AAOHN)

American Association of Spinal Cord Injury Nurses (AASCIN)

American College of Nurse-Midwives (ACNM)

American Holistic Nurses Association (AHNA)

American Long-Term & Subacute Nurses Association

American Nephrology Nurses' Association (ANNA)

American Nursing Informatics Association (ANIA)

American Organization of Nurse Executives (AONE)

American Psychiatric Nurses Association (APNA)

American Radiological Nurses Association (ARNA)

American Society for Long-Term Care Nurses

American Society of Ophthalmic Registered Nurses, (ASORN)

American Society for Pain Management Nursing (ASPMN)

American Society of PeriAnesthesia Nurses (ASPAN)

American Society of Plastic and Reconstructive Surgical Nurses (ASPRSN)

American Urological Association Allied (AUAA)

Association of Nurses in AIDS Care (ANAC)

Association of Operating Room Nurses (AORN)

Association of Pediatric Oncology Nursing (APON)

Association of Peri-Operative Registered Nurses

Association for Professionals in Infection Control and Epidemiology (APIC)

Association of Rehabilitation Nurses (ARN)

Association of Women's Health, Obstetric, and Neonatal Nurses (AWHONN)

Case Management Society of America (CMSA)

Dermatology Nurses Association (DNA)

Emergency Nurses Association (ENA)

Endocrine Nurses Society (ENS)

Home Healthcare Nurses Association (HHNA)

Hospice & Palliative Nurses Association (HPNA)

International Nurses Society on Addictions (IntNSA)

International Society of Nurses in Genetics (ISONG)

International Transplant Nurses Society (ITNS)

Infusion Nurses Society (INS)

League of Intravenous Therapy Education (LITE)

National Association of Clinical Nurse Specialists (NACNS)

National Association of Hispanic Nurses (NAHN)

National Association of Neonatal Nurses (NANN)

National Association of Nurse Massage Therapists (NANMT)

National Association of Nurse Practitioners in Reproductive Health (NANPRH)

National Association of Orthopaedic Nurses (NAON)

National Association of Pediatric Nurse Associates and Practitioners (NAPNAP)

National Association of School Nurses (NASN)

National Black Nurses Association (NBNA)

National Council of State Boards of Nursing (NCSBN)

National Federation of Licensed Practical Nurses (NFLPN)

National Federation for Specialty Nursing Organizations (NFSNO)

National Gerontological Nursing Association (NGNA)

National League for Nursing (NLN)

National Nurses Society on Addictions (NNSA)

National Nursing Staff Development Organization (NNSDO)

National Organization for Associate Degree Nursing (NOADN)

National Student Nurses' Association (NSNA)

Oncology Nursing Society (ONS)

Sigma Theta Tau International Honor Society of Nursing

Society of Gastroenterology Nurses and Associates (SGNA)

Society of Otorhinolaryngology and Head-Neck Nurses (SOHN)

Society of Urologic Nurses and Associates (SUNA)

Society for Vascular Nursing (SVN)

Transcultural Nursing Society (TCNS)

Wound, Ostomy, and Continence Nurses Society (WOCN)

(Aiken, 2003; Aiken & Catalano, 1994)

EXAM QUESTIONS

CHAPTER 2
Questions 7-15

7. JCAHO

    a. publishes a manual to be used by physicians to determine if nurses are following appropriate standards.

    b. requires that documentation include initial and ongoing assessments.

    c. determines the amount of payment based on Medicare-assigned DRGs.

    d. lays out the details of the NIDSEC.

8. A hospital bill payable by Medicare differs from payment by other insurance coverage in that the

    a. Medicare pays the hospital the same amount as all other insurance payors.

    b. hospital receives payment according to a DRG assigned by the hospital.

    c. hospital receives payment according to a DRG assigned by Medicare.

    d. DRG is not subject to review or involved in any payment system.

9. Nursing standards of care are the basis for nursing practice and are considered to be

    a. rules that apply only to physicians and institutions.

    b. the minimal requirements for nursing practice.

    c. nonvariable in regard to the level of practice they dictate.

    d. used only by nurses who work in hospitals in the southern and western United States.

10. The ANA has established the Nursing and Data Set Evaluation Center (NIDSEC) to

    a. provide a listing of all licensed nurses in the United States.

    b. describe and define how each state regulates health care providers.

    c. establish standards for computerized documentation of medication administration.

    d. develop and disseminate documentation standards and to evalutate information against standards.

11. Documentation is regulated by nurse practice acts, which are designed to

    a. protect the public, guide scope of practice, and define nursing practice standards.

    b. apply only to RNs who supervise students in educational settings.

    c. include technical standards for specific procedures and treatments.

    d. regulate the practice and privileges only of specialists such as certified nurse anesthetists.

12. Each state has statutory acts that describe and define legal nursing licensure and practice. The purpose(s) of licensing professional nurses is to

 a. establish the highest level of competency required of a nurse.

 b. regulate and restrict nursing practice to hospital jobs.

 c. generate state revenue and regulate nursing practice.

 d. establish a minimal level of competency and protect the public.

13. Jane RN passed her nursing exam in Texas (home state) and is practicing in Utah (compact state). She knows that as she documents,

 a. Texas has no authority to take disciplinary action against her documentation methods.

 b. she must have a Utah (home state) nurse co-sign her nursing documentation.

 c. she must comply with all Utah laws governing nursing practice and documentation.

 d. she cannot document nursing care in Utah until she passes another exam.

14. Many national professional organizations provide additional guidelines and standards of practice that

 a. tend to be more stringent than federal and state regulations.

 b. replace all other rules and regulations.

 c. have no bearing on any procedures or guidelines established by an institution.

 d. replace nursing licensure and guide documentation.

15. If an internal institutional standard is higher than the federal or state standard the

 a. federal standard still takes priority over all accountability.

 b. institution is held accountable to the higher internal standard.

 c. institution does not have to work as hard to meet JCAHO standards.

 d. institution has determined the federal and state standards to be inferior.

CHAPTER 3

TYPES OF DOCUMENTATION

CHAPTER OBJECTIVE

After completing this chapter, the reader will be able to discuss different nursing documentation methods and cite the advantages and disadvantages of each method.

LEARNING OBJECTIVES

After studying this chapter, the reader will be able to

1. describe available methods of nursing documentation.

2. specify the advantages and disadvantages of each method.

3. select examples of each method of charting that are available in institutions.

4. identify general considerations when selecting a documentation system.

INTRODUCTION

Although some nurses approach documentation as a chore, one's entire nursing career could depend on the accuracy and completeness of charting. Patient care documentation is a concern for all patient care managers, executives, staff developers, and educators who must ensure that standards are met and documentation is complete. Patient care providers know charting is something they must do,

but they often leave documentation to the last minute; thus, it may not always clearly reflect the total picture of patient care.

Every day, nurses are faced with the challenge of caring for complex, acutely ill patients and their families in addition to trying to manage time for documenting the care provided. Over the years, numerous documentation methods have evolved. Methods to decrease the amount of time required for documentation have been developed and implemented in a variety of settings. Institutions may adopt certain methods for documentation and may even modify methods to fit their specific needs.

This chapter discusses commonly used methods of documentation that hospitals and health care settings have adopted for their specific needs. In addition, other documentation systems are presented.

NARRATIVE NOTES

Narrative-style nursing documentation, also called *narrative notes,* is one of the oldest methods of nursing documentation. It is a diary or story format in simple paragraph form used to describe the patient's status and the interventions, treatments, and patient responses that have occurred during the shift. It is frequently used in acute, long-term, ambulatory, and home care settings. Before the development of flow sheets, this was the only method used for documenting nursing care. However, narrative notes may become lengthy and time consuming because nurses may tend to ramble, and routine care and normal assessment findings are reported along with significant findings and identified problems. It is often difficult to discover the most important information because there is no single, correct order in which to chart patient events. Although narrative notes are still one of the most commonly used documentation methods, they are seldom the primary method of documentation and are often used with flow sheets.

Narrative charting is easy to use in emergency situations in which a simple chronological order is needed. Well-written narrative notes can be an excellent record of what happened during the patient's time under a nurse's care. However, narrative documentation is now considered to be the least desirable format of nursing documentation because information is often scattered throughout the record, they lack structure and chronological information, and they tend to ramble. Very few institutions rely on narrative nursing notes; most have adopted other methods of documentation that save time and avoid duplication of information. A sample of a narrative note is found in Table 3-1.

TABLE 3-1: NARRATIVE NOTE

6/16/03. 10:45 AM. Patient found sitting on floor next to bed. States he does not know how he got there. VS = BP 142/89; P 76; R 20. Oriented to time and place. Appears in no distress. J. Double, orderly, called to assist getting patient into chair. Patient able to move all extremities and stood up by own efforts. Orderly assisted patient to bathroom. Voided approximately 250 cc clear, pale yellow urine. Returned to chair by himself. No bruising, redness, or abrasions noted to hips or legs. Dr. Jones notified of patient's condition and assessment. No new orders received. Call light within reach. Patient instructed to call for assistance with ambulation.

_____ J. Falls, RN

Advantages of Narrative Notes

There are several advantages of well-written narrative nursing notes:

- Because they are the oldest documentation method, most nurses are familiar with them.

- The method is flexible and can be used in many clinical settings.

- Narrative charting paints a picture of patient care provided over an extended period.

- Narrative documentation can easily be combined with other documentation methods, such as flow sheets.

Disadvantages of Narrative Notes

There are also disadvantages to narrative documentation:

- Narrative notes tend to be subjective and lack evidence of the nursing analysis and critical decision making.

- Narrative notes often lack structure, may be disorganized, and lack continuity.

- They may be task-oriented, with little or no emphasis on evaluation.

- Tracking problems and following the patient's progress may be difficult because various health care providers chart about the same event on different shifts or days.

PROBLEM-ORIENTED CHARTING

Charting with the problem-oriented medical record (POMR) system places emphasis on patient problems. This method is frequently used in acute, long-term, and home health care. Dr. Lawrence Weed developed the system in the late 1960s to improve documentation of patients problems in clinical settings (Tiller, 1994). A POMR record consists of baseline data, a problem list, a plan of care for each problem, progress notes, and a discharge summary.

Database. The database is the foundation for identifying patient problems. It involves collecting information at the time of admission or initial contact with the patient. The database helps prioritize needs and develop the plan of care. The database should be active and updated as necessary to ensure continuity of care.

Plan of Care. The care plan is developed from the problem list. Nurses usually include nursing diagnoses, expected outcomes, and interventions in their care plans.

Progress Notes. The progress of patient's status is monitored and documented in the patient's record. The problems are addressed following certain formats. If the institution uses an integrated medical record, all health care providers (nurses, physicians, and others) document on the same progress record.

Discharge Summary. At discharge, a summary should address each problem and how each problem was or was not met. A detailed note should be written for problems not met. This is especially helpful for communicating information to other hospitals, home health providers, referral agencies, and the patient.

Methods used for documenting with the POMR system are based on processes similar to the nursing process. The two most commonly used systems are SOAP(IER) and (A)PIE.

SOAP(IER) Notes

Physicians and nurse practitioners commonly use SOAP notes as their method of documentation. These notes are intended to improve the quality and continuity of patient services by enhancing communication between health care providers and to assist with better recall of details about each patient. The system helps identify, prioritize, and track patient problems so they can be addressed in a timely and systematic manner. It provides an ongoing assessment of patient progress and response to interventions.

SOAP notes provide a problem-solving structure for the health care provider. Because SOAP notes require adequate documentation to verify interventions, they help to organize the health care provider's thought process about the patient and to assist in planning quality care. Usually, a complete SOAP note is written on every shift for all unresolved problems or whenever the patient's condition changes. Some institutions have expanded SOAP to the SOAPIER format. The expansion still incorporates all the steps of the nursing process.

The following acronyms explain the SOAP and the SOAPIER charting methods:

S = Subjective data (what the patient says)

O = Objective data (what is observed or measured)

A = Assessment (nursing diagnosis)

P = Plan (short- and long-term plans)

I = Intervention (nursing action)

E = Evaluation (assessment of interventions)

R = Revisions (changes to plan of care).

An example of a SOAPIER note is displayed in Table 3-2.

Advantages of SOAP Notes

One of the major advantages of the SOAP method of documentation is that it promotes interdisciplinary collaboration. Here are some other advantages:

- It is well structured and adds consistency to the documentation of patient care.

- It follows the nursing process.

- Problems are easily tracked and monitored.

- It can easily be used with standardized care plans.

Disadvantages of SOAP Notes

Disadvantages of SOAP documentation are listed here:

- It emphasizes the chronology of problems rather than their priorities and may become repetitious and time-consuming if assessments and

TABLE 3-2: SOAPIER NOTE

6/17/03
8:00 AM

     S: Patient stated, "I feel dizzy when I move from the chair to the bed."

     O: Patient had unsteady gait and held the chair, bedside table, and bed when moving. BP 160/100, P 98, R 24, shallow. Neuro check within normal limits.

     A: High risk for injury due to sensory and motor deficit.

     P: Assist patient with all ambulation. Instruct to use call bell and call for assistance when getting out of bed.

     I: Call Dr. Smith to report findings and assessment. Repeat neuro checks in 30 minutes. No new orders received.

8:45   E: Resting in bed. BP 140/86, P 72, R 18. Neuro exam within normal limits. Reassess in 1 hour. Patient constantly calls for assistance. Still experiencing dizziness with walking.

     R: High risk for fall due to sensory and motor instability.

                                               C. Nurse, RN

implications apply to more than one problem.

- The charting requires a rethinking of process and a need to identify what information applies to each part of the format.

- Redundancy may occur between the problem list and the care plan.

- It is not the most efficient method of documentation because each problem requires a SOAP note.

- The integrated progress note method has met resistance from health care providers.

- SOAP documentation does not lend itself to settings where there is rapid patient turnover or emergency situations.

(A)PIE Charting

The PIE method of charting was developed in 1984 at a hospital in North Carolina (Tiller, 1994). It is similar to SOAP; however, it is based specifically on the nursing process. PIE charting simplifies daily documentation by eliminating the care plan and including an ongoing plan of care. With this system, nurses and physicians document on separate forms. Some institutions have modified the PIE system by adding an assessment component (A) to the beginning of the process. The system then becomes APIE.

The APIE acronym stands for:

A = Assessment (objective and subjective information)

P = Problem (nursing diagnosis)

I = Intervention (what the nurse did to correct, improve, or change the problem)

E = Evaluation (subjective and objective results of intervention).

APIE charting is composed of a patient care flow sheet and progress notes.

Patient Care Flow Sheet

The daily flow sheet consists of a 24-hour list of specific assessment criteria in the areas of human needs. Vital signs and routine components of care are normally listed. Any deviations from normal are noted, usually with an asterisk (*), and the deviation is addressed in the nursing progress notes.

Progress Notes

Following the initial assessment, a specific problem list is developed or a standardized problem list for specific diseases or systems is used, and problems are documented in the progress notes.

North America Nursing Diagnosis Association (NANDA) nursing diagnoses should be used for identification of the problem. Each problem is numbered, usually by priority, and reference to the problem number is made in the progress notes rather than rewriting the stated problem. An example APIE note is displayed in Table 3-3.

TABLE 3-3: APIE NOTE
6/17/03
9:00 AM
A: Assessment completed. See flow sheet. Patient twisting in bed. Frowning. P #1: Pain at incision site related to Cesarean section yesterday.
9:15 AM
I, P#1: Medicated for pain as ordered. See MAR.
10:30 AM
E, P#1: Patient sleeping quietly in bed.
S. Que, RN

Advantages of APIE Charting

There are several advantages of APIE charting:

- APIE charting simplifies the documentation process by using a flow sheet to reduce redundancy in charting.

- It eliminates the care plan because the progress notes become the plan of care.

- Because the use of nursing diagnoses is emphasized, APIE charting reflects part of the nursing process.

- Each problem is identified, addressed, and evaluated each shift.

- It lends itself well to primary nursing and can be used in acute care settings where a patient's condition changes quickly.

- APIE charting enhances professional credibility by improving nursing notes and identifying specific nursing interventions.

Disadvantages of APIE Charting

Like all methods, APIE charting also has some disadvantages.

- With the elimination of a plan of care, some outcomes may not be addressed.

- All nurses must understand the process and be able to use the same level of sophistication and knowledge to identify problems and interventions.

- The plan of care becomes the responsibility of the registered nurse (RN).

- The staff mix must be assessed to determine if the system is appropriate.

- The requirement to chart problems every 8 and 24 hours can create lengthy documents, especially if the patient has many problems.

FOCUS CHARTING

Focus charting is a documentation system frequently used in acute and long-term care settings that is consistent with the Joint Commission on Accreditation of Healthcare Organizations (JCAHO) requirements for documenting patient responses and outcomes. Hospital staff nurses in Minneapolis who expressed frustration with the SOAP method of charting developed the system in 1981 (Tiller, 1994). The Focus charting format allows documentation of any patient situation and includes data, action, and response (DAR) for each identified concern. It is not necessary to have each component of the DAR in each charting entry; however, the use of all three components helps promote optimum documentation.

Focus charting (see Table 3-4) moves away from charting only problems to identifying patient concerns. These concerns do not have to be worded in nursing diagnosis terminology. The focus may be a sign or symptom, a condition, a nursing diagnosis, a behavior, a significant event, or an acute change in a patient's condition.

TABLE 3-4: FOCUS CHARTING

Date	Time	Focus	Progress Notes
6/18/03	1430	Pain	D: Patient complaining of pain at incision site.
			A: Patient repositioned and supported with pillows. Morphine 10 mg IM given in rt. gluteus.
	1530		R: Patient states he "feels better." Pain decreased and he has been able to sleep.
			J. Good, RN

Advantages of Focus Notes

Focus notes allow for flexibility in documentation, with the following advantages:

- Focus charting provides structure for the progress notes.

- The method promotes the nursing process.

- It increases the ease with which information can be located.

- Nurses are encouraged to broaden their thinking and to use critical thinking to include any patient concern, not just problem areas.

- Focus charting is easily understood and may be adapted to most health care settings.

Disadvantages of Focus Notes

There are also disadvantages to using Focus notes:

- Monitoring is necessary or Focus notes may become narrative notes lacking documentation of patient responses to interventions.

- They require nurses to change their thinking process and evaluate patient's progress toward outcomes and document the response.

- They may be difficult to construct and may lack accuracy and logical judgment.

CHARTING BY EXCEPTION

Charting by exception (CBE) has become a very popular method of documentation. Hospital staff nurses in Wisconsin developed the process in 1983 (Tiller, 1994). The motivation behind the system came from trying to overcome documentation problems by making normal findings and routine care more obvious. It was a shorthand method based on clearly defined standards of practice and predetermined criteria for nursing assessments and interventions. The process greatly reduces the time required for documentation, updating the information, and making patient status readily available.

Standard assessments are arranged in a flow sheet format. Predefined normal findings and interventions are integrated into the form. Each institution must have their predefined normal findings on file, and each nurse must follow the standards established for "normal." The nurse need only document significant findings or exceptions to the predefined norms. A narrative note is written when the standardized statement on the form is not met. The assumption with CBE is that all standards are met with a normal or expected response unless otherwise documented. Changes in patient status are easy to track because that is the only time additional notes are written.

The CBE system uses the following or similar symbols on the flow sheet:

√   The assessment was completed and no abnormal findings were noted.

*   Significant abnormal findings are present and are described in a narrative note.

→   The patient's status remains unchanged from the previous entry.

The CBE system uses standards of practice that apply to all clinical areas as well as to areas specific to specialty units. Protocols define the nursing interventions concerned with an expected clinical course for a specific patient population. The nurse is still required to complete a nursing admission physical assessment and use standard individualized care plans. Narrative notes or SOAP(IER) notes may be used to document exceptions. A sample CBE form is found in Figure 3-1.

Advantages of CBE Documentation

CBE documentation decreases charting time and also has the following advantages:

- Current data and assessments are kept at the patient's bedside.

FIGURE 3-1: SAMPLE CBE FORM (1 OF 2)

Multidisciplinary Action Plan	POINT OF SERVICE (POS) 0-2 Hours DATE: _____	OBSERVATION STATUS 3-23 Hours DATE: _____	ADMISSION Inpatient Day 1 DATE: _____
Consults	Spiritual Care PRN	Spiritual Care PRN	Spiritual Care PRN MDs PRN based on comorbidities Assess community resources (see day 4)
Tests	EKG Chem 24 PT, PTT CBC W/diff **Cardiac Screen**	**EKG @ 6th hr** _____ **& 12th hr** _____ EKG prn with cp - notify MD of cp. **Cardiac screen @ 6th hr** _____ **& 12th hr** _____ Cardiac testing after 12th hr: CATH _____ Nuc. Studies _____ Other _____ PTT per heparin protocol if on IV heparin	**EKG @ 6th hr** _____ **& 12th hr** ____(if not in c.o.u.) EKG prn with cp - notify MD of cp. **Cardiac screen @ 6th hr** _____ **& 12th hr** _____ If not drawn in c.o.u. Cardiac testing after 12th hr: CATH _____ Nuc. Studies _____ Other _____ PTT per heparin protocol if on IV heparin
Treatments	VS Q4H and PRN with cp (notify MD of cp) Supplemental 0₂ PRN _____ Cardiac monitor Peripheral INT (prefer #18g. Catheter in left hand/arm). I&O	**Admit to C.O.U.** VS Q4H and PRN with cp (notify MD of cp) Supplemental 0₂ PRN _____ Cardiac monitor Peripheral INT (prefer #18g. Catheter in left hand/arm). I&O q shift If adm. BS> 200, accuchecks AC & HS x 2. Notify MD if remains elevated _____ _____	**Admit to C.C.U. if tests positive** VS Q4H and PRN with cp (notify MD of cp) Supplemental 0₂ PRN _____ Cardiac monitor Peripheral INT (prefer #18g. Catheter in left hand/arm). I&O q shift If adm. BS> 200, accuchecks AC & HS x 2. Notify MD if remains elevated _____ _____
Medications	**ASA 325mg po** Nitrates PRN Narcotics/Analgesics PRN GI meds PRN Anticoagulants/Antiplatelets PRN	**ASA 325 mg po (if not on POS)** Nitrates PRN Narcotics/Analgesics PRN GI meds PRN Anticoagulants/Antiplatelets PRN Home meds as ordered	**ASA 325 mg po (if not on POS)** Nitrates PRN Narcotics/Analgesics PRN GI meds PRN Anticoagulants/Antiplatelets PRN Consider Beta Blockers Consider Calcium Blockers
Diet	NPO	NPO until hour 6 Card. Screen results known then clear liquid if no diag. tests scheduled; adv to cardiac diet. Other:	NPO until hour 6 Card. Screen results known then clear liquid if no diag. tests scheduled; adv to cardiac diet. Other:
Activity /Safety	Bedrest Bleeding Prec. if on anticoagulants Ambulate with assistance if being discharged from ED	BR with BRP Bleeding Prec. if on anticoagulants Ambulate with assist. if being discharged from C.O.U.	BR with BRP Bleeding Prec. if on anticoagulants
Teaching	Orient to unit; Explain all procedures Pt. to report significant S/S PRN **P/F**	Orient to unit; Explain all procedures Pt. to report significant S/S PRN **P/F**	Orient to unit; Explain all procedures Pt. to report significant S/S PRN **P/F** Complete Adv. Directives per protocol Begin cardiac teaching **P/F**
Discharge Planning	DC home if tests neg. & cond. stable Admit to C.O.U. if tests neg. & cond. stable Admit to inpt if tests positive	**Complete Adm-Hx Assessment form** **Initiate DC plan screening tool** DC home if tests neg./cond. stable Use DC instruction form for outpt referrals Admit to inpt if tests positive	**Complete Adm-Hx Assessment form if not done in C.O.U.** **Initiate DC plan screening tool if not done in C.O.U.** Access support systems
Shift/Time			
Neuro			
CV			
Resp			
GI			
GU			
Integ			
Musculoskel			
Psych/Social			
Pain			
Surgical Dressing			
Incision/Wound			
IV/Epidural			
Reproductive			
Neurovascular			
Neuro Checks			
Safety Level			
Equipment			
Initials			

FIGURE 3-1: SAMPLE CBE FORM (2 OF 2)

Multidisciplinary Action Plan	Inpatient Day 2 DATE: _____	Inpatient Day 3 DATE: _____	Inpatient Day 4 DATE: _____
Consults	Spiritual Care PRN MDs PRN based on comorbidities **Patient Education** **Dietary** Soc. Serv. PRN	Spiritual Care PRN MDs PRN based on comorbidities **Case Mgr. if no scheduled discharge date on or before Day 4**	Outpatient referrals (ck all that apply) Outpatient card. Rehab.____ Smoking Cess.___ Dietary ___ Heart school ___ Stress Mgt_____ Diabetes mgt_____ Parish nurse _____ MDs _____ Family CPR classes _____
Tests	EKG (early AM) _____		
Treatments	**Transfer to telemetry if in critical care** VS Q4H and PRN with cp (notify MD of cp) Supplemental 0₂ PRN _____ Cardiac monitor Peripheral INT I&O q shift	VS Q4H and PRN with cp (notify MD of cp) Room Air Cardiac monitor Peripheral INT I&O q shift	VS Q4H and PRN with cp (notify MD of cp) Room Air Cardiac monitor - remove telemetry pack prior to D/C Peripheral INT - remove IV catheter prior to D/C I&O q shift
Medications	**ASA 325mg po QD** Meds as ordered from Day 1 Other: B-blocker Anticoagulant Ca++ blocker Antiplatelet ACE-1 GI Meds Nitrates	**ASA 325mg po QD** Meds as ordered from Day 2 Other: B-blocker Anticoagulant Ca++ blocker Antiplatelet ACE-1 GI Meds Nitrates	**ASA 325mg po QD** Meds as ordered from Day 3 Other: B-blocker Anticoagulant Ca++ blocker Antiplatelet ACE-1 GI Meds Nitrates
Diet	Cardiac Diet Other _____	Cardiac Diet Other _____	Cardiac Diet Other _____
Activity /Safety	May shower if able to walk 5 minutes (=3 laps) Ambulate in hall TID as tolerated OOB to chair as tolerated	May shower if able to walk 5 minutes (=3 laps) Ambulate in hall QID as tolerated OOB to chair as tolerated	May shower if able to walk 5 minutes (=3 laps) Ambulate in hall QID as tolerated OOB to chair as tolerated
Teaching	MI teaching content **P/F** CAD risk factors **P/F** **Angina/use of NTG P/F** Diet **P/F** Medications **P/F**	Same as Day 2 **Angina/use of NTG P/F; plus** Discharge advice **P/F** ADL's **P/F** Home walk protocol **P/F**	Reinforce/Review individual teaching plan (include outpatient referrals/follow up as listed in Consults Day 4.) **P/F**
Discharge Planning	DC home if neg. for MI w/outpt referrals as ordered (See Consults Day 4). Misogram to SS for psychosocial/financial assessments; MD order and misogram to SS for Home Health/DME needs.	Same as Day 2	D/C home with appropriate outpatient referrals (see Consults above). Use DC Instruction form.

Shift/Time						
Neuro						
CV						
Resp						
GI						
GU						
Integ						
Musculoskel						
Psych/Social						
Pain						
Surgical Dressing						
Incision/Wound						
IV/Epidural						
Reproductive						
Neurovascular						
Neuro Checks						
Safety Level						
Equipment						
Initials						

Assessment Key:
✔ = abbreviated normal
✔C = comprehensive normal
✳ = comprehensive abnormal, see progress record
➡ = continued comprehensive abnormal
D = deferred

Teaching Key: P - Patient
F - Family

Method Codes: A-audiovisual, **C**-CCTV, **D**-demonstration, **E**-explanation, **G**-group class, **H**-handout, **I**-Initiated, **P**-practice, **R**-reinforce

Patient Name_____ MR# _____

- All data are immediately recorded on flow sheet, thus eliminating the need to make notes.

- Guidelines for CBE charting are printed on the back of the form.

- Trends in patient status are easy to follow.

- Normal findings are clearly defined, so that everyone knows what constitutes a normal finding.

- Repetitive charting of routine care is eliminated.

Disadvantages of CBE Documentation

The following are disadvantages of the CBE system:

- There is duplication of charting with the system because nursing diagnoses are written on both the problem list and the care plan.

- The system was developed for use with an all-RN staff.

- The system requires a major change in an institution's documentation system when implemented.

- Reimbursement may be compromised by the CBE system until it becomes more widely accepted.

- The legal system is suspect of the lack of documentation used with this system.

- Every section must have a documented response or it could be interpreted as having not been done. This could be construed as not meeting the minimal standard of care.

CLINICAL PATHWAYS

Clinical pathways, also known as critical or care pathways, define a patient's progress through a managed care situation within a given time frame, determined by the allocated length of stay for a given diagnosis related group (DRG). Pathways are an abstract or theoretical representation of predicted progress based on known probabilities toward predetermined outcomes for patients who are receiving a specified, time-limited program of care.

In the mid-1950s, the critical pathway method was first used in an oil and chemical refinery. The earliest documentation of use in health care was in the mid-1980s, when the care path concept was adapted to review delivery of care at the New England Medical Center in Boston. In health care, the process is a multidisciplinary mechanism for predicting the problems, interventions, and expected outcomes for a specific disease process across the continuum of care (Tiller, 1994).

No matter what definition is used, pathways contain the same key elements. They promote the coordination of patient care delivery for a specific subset of patients through the use of a standardized, interdisciplinary process. Interventions are predictably sequenced, based on a timeline of either time or outcomes. They are directed at achieving specific patient outcomes within a specified time period.

In some institutions, a clinical pathway is given to each patient on admission. This form lists in lay terms what the patient may expect on each day of his or her hospitalization. The patient is encouraged to write questions or comments that need clarification from the physician or nurse. Discharge instructions are found on the last page, which are later individualized by the RN and sent home with the patient.

All health care providers use one critical pathway as a monitoring and documentation tool. Documentation tools can be developed that incorporate the pathways, thus eliminating other nursing documentation forms and reducing duplication and time required for charting. Frequently, checklists are used and the CBE method incorporated. The most common format is set up in a grid. The time frame normally is placed across the top of the page, and events, treatments, and outcomes are listed down the left side of the page.

When positive or negative variances (changes from the expected) occur, they should be noted and additional documentation added. In addition, the variance needs to be justified or actions taken to rectify the variance. Variances and corrective actions are documented and analyzed by the multidisciplinary team so they can further improve care and make changes to the clinical pathway as needed. See Figure 3-2 on pages 43-56 for an example of a clinical pathway.

Advantages of Clinical Pathways

The following are advantages of using clinical pathways for documenting patient care:

- Continuity of care is easily communicated.

- Novice health care providers are given a structure within which to provide care.

- Patients are integral to the planning process.

- The entire health care team is involved in all phases of patient care.

- Discharge planning and teaching begin very early in the patient's care process.

- A creative critical decision-making process is encouraged, which leads to better patient outcomes.

Disadvantages of Clinical Pathways

The following disadvantages may be present with the use of clinical pathways:

- The use of standardized plans inhibits nurses' identification of unique, individualized therapies.

- Plans must be routinely updated to ensure that they are current and appropriate.

- Large numbers of plans take up storage room and may be costly to print.

- The facility's staff mix must be acknowledged.

- Patient assessment, decision making, and evaluation remain the responsibilities of the RN.

- The knowledge and skills of the majority of the staff must be considered.

- Noncompliance with the system may reflect the lack of knowledge and skills of the staff.

OTHER METHODS OF DOCUMENTATION

Other methods of nursing documentation are also available. Many methods have been developed for specific use within units or institutions. Most of the methods are adaptations or variations of Focus charting and CBE.

CORE

CORE charting focuses on the nursing process, the core of nursing documentation. The method consists of a database (D), plan of action (A), and evaluation (E). The major advantages of CORE are that the method incorporates the entire nursing process into one system. It groups nursing diagnoses and functional status assessments together, and it promotes concise documentation with minimal repetition. The disadvantages of CORE are that the method does not always present information chronologically and nursing notes may not always relate to the plan of care.

FACT

The FACT system incorporates elements of CBE. This method consists of flow sheets for specific services (F); assessment (A); concise, integrated progress notes and flow sheets (C); and timely entries recorded when care is given (T). The method can easily be adapted to computer systems and is outcome oriented. Advantages of the method are that it:

- eliminates duplication

- encourages consistent language and structure

- permits immediate recording of current data

- is readily accessible at the patient's bedside

- eliminates the need for different forms.

Disadvantages of the FACT documentation method are that the narrative notes may be too brief, nurse perspective may be overlooked, and the nursing process framework may be difficult to identify.

text continues on page 57

FIGURE 3-2: SAMPLE CLINICAL PATHWAY FORM (1 OF 14)

EMORY HEALTHCARE
EMORY HOSPITALS

Carotid Endarterectomy
Clinical Pathway

Initiated by______________ Date ___/___/___ Time ________

Medicare LOS 6.6 days
Target LOS 4 days

Patient Problem	Intermediate Care Discharge Criteria	Date Achieved Signature	Discharge Outcomes	Date Achieved Signature
Self care deficit	Able to transfer from bed to chair with minimal assistance	Date: ___/___/___ ________ Signature	Able to tolerate adequate oral foods and fluids	Date: ___/___/___ ________ Signature
Pain	Pain controlled with oral or IM analgesics	Date: ___/___/___ ________ Signature	Pain controlled with oral analgesics	Date: ___/___/___ ________ Signature
Knowledge deficit	Verbalizes knowledge of procedure	Date: ___/___/___ ________ Signature	Verbalizes knowledge of: 1. Wound care 2. Activity progression 3. Diet 4. Signs of possible complications 5. Meds 6. Follow-up care 7. Risk factor modification	Date: ___/___/___ ________ Signature
Potential for complications	**Neurological:** Stability as indicated by non-fluctuating neurological state **Cardiovascular:** Hypo or hypertension not requiring vasoactive IV drips **Respiratory:** Airway patency	Date: ___/___/___ ________ Signature	**Neurological:** Stable neuro state **Cardiovascular:** Stable status and BP well controlled on po meds if indicated **Respiratory:** Airway patency **Infection:** No evidence of clinical wound infection	Date: ___/___/___ ________ Signature

04ClinPath024 7/96
Developed by an interdisciplinary Task Force led by Tina J. Davidson, R.N., M.S.N. Page 1 of 14 7467

FIGURE 3-2: SAMPLE CLINICAL PATHWAY FORM (2 OF 14)

Patient Assessment
Vascular Surgery

Standard (If standard not met explain in space provided or in Narrative Notes)	Date ___/___/___ Time _____	Date ___/___/___ Time _____	Date ___/___/___ Time _____
Cardiovascular	Rhythm: ☐ Regular ☐ Irregular Telemetry: ☐ Yes ☐ No Rhythm _____ Ectopy _____ Specific Pulse Checks:	Rhythm: ☐ Regular ☐ Irregular Telemetry: ☐ Yes ☐ No Rhythm _____ Ectopy _____ Specific Pulse Checks:	Rhythm: ☐ Regular ☐ Irregular Telemetry: ☐ Yes ☐ No Rhythm _____ Ectopy _____ Specific Pulse Checks:
	DP PT Radial R L Key: + Present, - Absent, Dop-Doppler	DP PT Radial R L Key: + Present, - Absent, Dop-Doppler	DP PT Radial R L Key: + Present, - Absent, Dop-Doppler
Respiratory -Regular & unlabored -No cough -Lung sounds clear bilaterally -On room air	☐ Meets Standard O₂ _____	☐ Meets Standard O₂ _____	☐ Meets Standard O₂ _____
Gastrointestinal -Soft & non-distended -Bowel sounds present	☐ Meets Standard BM within last 8h? ☐ Yes ☐ No	☐ Meets Standard BM within last 8h? ☐ Yes ☐ No	☐ Meets Standard BM within last 8h? ☐ Yes ☐ No
Neuromuscular/Safety -Alert & oriented -Speech clear & coherent -Moves all 4 extremities equally -Hand grasps strong & equal -Gait steady -Swallows without difficulty	☐ Meets Standard	☐ Meets Standard	☐ Meets Standard
Skin -Warm, dry & intact -Color normal	☐ Meets Standard	☐ Meets Standard	☐ Meets Standard
Surgical wound	☐ N/A	☐ N/A	☐ N/A
Urinary -Voiding, continent -Clear, yellow urine	☐ Meets Standard	☐ Meets Standard	☐ Meets Standard
Drainage tubes (describe)	☐ N/A	☐ N/A	☐ N/A
Peripheral Edema -Absent	☐ Meets Standard	☐ Meets Standard	☐ Meets Standard
IV Therapy -No redness -No swelling/tenderness -Site and tubing < 72h old	☐ N/A ☐ Meets Standard Site _____ Fluid _____	☐ N/A ☐ Meets Standard Site _____ Fluid _____	☐ N/A ☐ Meets Standard Site _____ Fluid _____
Special Equipment (describe)			
Discomfort (describe)			
Signature/Title			

FIGURE 3-2: SAMPLE CLINICAL PATHWAY FORM (3 OF 14)

Inter-disciplinary ActionPlan	Arteriogram Pre Arteriogram □ AM Admit □ Ambulatory	Initials N|D|E	Date: __/__/__ Post Arteriogram	Initials N|D|E	Time	Interdisciplinary Progress Notes
Consults	Anesthesiology Case manager					
Tests	Arteriogram BCP I & II Hematology profile CXR EKG UA with micro		Results on chart			
Treatments						
Medication reminders			Identify and continue usual medications Start ASA 325mg q day			
Nutrition	Clear liquids prior to arteriogram		General diet NPO after MN except meds			
Activity/ Safety	Up ad lib ♦ Risk Management protocol □ Yes □ No Implemented @ ___ Visually checked q 2 h♦ Bed in low position and locked Call light in reach Siderails up x 2♦ ID armband on patient		Bedrest x 6h then out of bed with assistance only ♦ Risk Management protocol □ Yes □ No Implemented @ ___ Visually checked q 2 h♦ Bed in low position and locked Call light in reach Side rails up x 2♦ ID armband on patient			
Assessment			Vital signs per post arteriogram orders, then q 4h (see flow sheet p. 6)			
Patient/ family education	Informed consent Video "Your Surgical Experience" Review Lay Pathway					
Discharge planning	Initial assessment of financial capability for obtaining medication & supplies		Complete pre-op screening activities			

Expected Outcome	Outcome Met?	Initials	Reason outcome not achieved (circle one)	If outcome not met, record intervention(s) Continue to address until outcome is achieved
Anesthesiology preop assessment completed	□ Yes □ No		a. Anesthesiologist unavailable b. Other (Specify) ___	

♦ Reflects changes if Risk Management protocol implemented.

Initials/Signature   Initials/Signature   Initials/Signature

____/_____   ____/_____   ____/_____

____/_____   ____/_____   ____/_____

FIGURE 3-2: SAMPLE CLINICAL PATHWAY FORM (4 OF 14)

Patient Assessment
Vascular Surgery

Standard (If standard not met explain in space provided or in Narrative Notes)	Date ___/___/___ Time _____	Date ___/___/___ Time _____	Date ___/___/___ Time _____
Cardiovascular	Rhythm: ☐ Regular ☐ Irregular Telemetry: ☐ Yes ☐ No Rhythm _____ Ectopy _____ Specific Pulse Checks: (DP / PT / Radial — R, L) Key: + Present, - Absent, Dop-Doppler	Rhythm: ☐ Regular ☐ Irregular Telemetry: ☐ Yes ☐ No Rhythm _____ Ectopy _____ Specific Pulse Checks: (DP / PT / Radial — R, L) Key: + Present, - Absent, Dop-Doppler	Rhythm: ☐ Regular ☐ Irregular Telemetry: ☐ Yes ☐ No Rhythm _____ Ectopy _____ Specific Pulse Checks: (DP / PT / Radial — R, L) Key: + Present, - Absent, Dop-Doppler
Respiratory -Regular & unlabored -No cough -Lung sounds clear bilaterally -On room air	☐ Meets Standard O_2 _____	☐ Meets Standard O_2 _____	☐ Meets Standard O_2 _____
Gastrointestinal -Soft & non-distended -Bowel sounds present	☐ Meets Standard BM within last 8h? ☐ Yes ☐ No	☐ Meets Standard BM within last 8h? ☐ Yes ☐ No	☐ Meets Standard BM within last 8h? ☐ Yes ☐ No
Neuromuscular/Safety -Alert & oriented -Speech clear & coherent -Moves all 4 extremities equally -Hand grasps strong & equal -Gait steady -Swallows without difficulty	☐ Meets Standard	☐ Meets Standard	☐ Meets Standard
Skin -Warm, dry & intact -Color normal	☐ Meets Standard	☐ Meets Standard	☐ Meets Standard
Surgical wound	☐ N/A	☐ N/A	☐ N/A
Urinary -Voiding, continent -Clear, yellow urine	☐ Meets Standard	☐ Meets Standard	☐ Meets Standard
Drainage tubes (describe)	☐ N/A	☐ N/A	☐ N/A
Peripheral Edema -Absent	☐ Meets Standard	☐ Meets Standard	☐ Meets Standard
IV Therapy -No redness -No swelling/tenderness -Site and tubing < 72h old	☐ N/A ☐ Meets Standard Site _____ Fluid _____	☐ N/A ☐ Meets Standard Site _____ Fluid _____	☐ N/A ☐ Meets Standard Site _____ Fluid _____
Special Equipment (describe)			
Discomfort (describe)			
Signature/Title			

FIGURE 3-2: SAMPLE CLINICAL PATHWAY FORM (5 OF 14)

Inter-disciplinary ActionPlan	Day of Surgery Pre-op	Initials N|D|E	Date: __/__/__ Post-op	Initials N|D|E	Time	Interdisciplinary Progress Notes
Consults			Case manager			
Tests			Results on chart			
Treatments			O2 at ____ liters per NC to keep sat ≥ 95% IVF			
Medication reminders	Anesthesia pre-ops Antibiotic: _____		MSO4 IV prn pain Nitroprusside gtt, Nitroglycerine gtt, or Phenylephrine gtt to control BP Oxycodone Acetaminophen Metoclopramide Antibiotic: _____ x _____ doses			
Nutrition	NPO		Sips of full liquids			
Activity/ Safety	◆ *Risk Management protocol* ☐ Yes ☐ No Implemented @ ____ Visually checked q 2 h◆ Bed in low position and locked Call light in reach Side rails up x 2◆ ID armband on patient		Bedrest with head of bed at 30 degrees Turn, cough & deep breathe q 2h Notify physician if patient is unable to void. Male patient may stand to void if BP stable. ◆ *Risk Management protocol* ☐ Yes ☐ No Implemented @ ____ Visually checked q 2 h◆ Bed in low position and locked Call light in reach Side rails up x 2◆ ID armband on patient			
Assessment	Complete pre-op checklist		VS q 30 mins x 2, then hourly Neuro checks q 30 mins x 2, then q 1h I & O q 2h Continuous pulse oximetry & arterial line monitoring Telemetry			
Patient/ family education			Orient patient and family to intermediate care unit			
Discharge planning						

Expected Outcome	Outcome Met?	Initials	Reason outcome not achieved *(circle one)*	If outcome not met, record intervention(s) *Continue to address until outcome is achieved*
Patient will be able to void spontaneously	☐ Yes ☐ No		a. b. c.	

◆ Reflects changes if Risk Management protocol implemented.

Initials/Signature

____/_____

____/_____

Initials/Signature

____/_____

____/_____

Initials/Signature

____/_____

____/_____

FIGURE 3-2: SAMPLE CLINICAL PATHWAY FORM (6 OF 14)

Post Arteriogram Assessment

Date: ____/____/____

BP q 1h x 5; Check puncture site and distal pulses q 30mins. x 4; q 60mins. x 3; then q 4h

Time	BP	*DP	*PT	*Radial	Puncture site: _____

*Distal pulses 0 + = no pulse 1 + = weak 2 + = normal 3 + = bounding D = doppler only

Intermediate Care Assessment

Date: ____/____/____

BP, P, R and Neuro checks q 30mins. x 2 then hourly until the am of POD 1; Temp q 4h

Time	Art. BP	Cuff BP	P	R	Temp	Neuro Checks*	Pulse Oximetry	Drips (gtts/dose)	Comments

*Neuro standard defined as alert & oriented, clear speech, equal hand grasps, moves all four extremities equally.

FIGURE 3-2: SAMPLE CLINICAL PATHWAY FORM (7 OF 14)

Date & Time	Interdisciplinary Progress Notes

FIGURE 3-2: SAMPLE CLINICAL PATHWAY FORM (7 OF 14)

FIGURE 3-2: SAMPLE CLINICAL PATHWAY FORM (8 OF 14)

Patient Assessment
Vascular Surgery

Standard (If standard not met explain in space provided or in Narrative Notes)	Date ___/___/___ Time _____	Date ___/___/___ Time _____	Date ___/___/___ Time _____
Cardiovascular	Rhythm: ☐ Regular ☐ Irregular Telemetry: ☐ Yes ☐ No Rhythm _____ Ectopy _____ Specific Pulse Checks: DP PT Radial R L Key: + Present, - Absent, Dop-Doppler	Rhythm: ☐ Regular ☐ Irregular Telemetry: ☐ Yes ☐ No Rhythm _____ Ectopy _____ Specific Pulse Checks: DP PT Radial R L Key: + Present, - Absent, Dop-Doppler	Rhythm: ☐ Regular ☐ Irregular Telemetry: ☐ Yes ☐ No Rhythm _____ Ectopy _____ Specific Pulse Checks: DP PT Radial R L Key: + Present, - Absent, Dop-Doppler
Respiratory -Regular & unlabored -No cough -Lung sounds clear bilaterally -On room air	☐ Meets Standard O_2 _____	☐ Meets Standard O_2 _____	☐ Meets Standard O_2 _____
Gastrointestinal -Soft & non-distended -Bowel sounds present	☐ Meets Standard BM within last 8h? ☐ Yes ☐ No	☐ Meets Standard BM within last 8h? ☐ Yes ☐ No	☐ Meets Standard BM within last 8h? ☐ Yes ☐ No
Neuromuscular/Safety -Alert & oriented -Speech clear & coherent -Moves all 4 extremities equally -Hand grasps strong & equal -Gait steady -Swallows without difficulty	☐ Meets Standard	☐ Meets Standard	☐ Meets Standard
Skin -Warm, dry & intact -Color normal	☐ Meets Standard	☐ Meets Standard	☐ Meets Standard
Surgical wound	☐ N/A	☐ N/A	☐ N/A
Urinary -Voiding, continent -Clear, yellow urine	☐ Meets Standard	☐ Meets Standard	☐ Meets Standard
Drainage tubes (describe)	☐ N/A	☐ N/A	☐ N/A
Peripheral Edema -Absent	☐ Meets Standard	☐ Meets Standard	☐ Meets Standard
IV Therapy -No redness -No swelling/tenderness -Site and tubing < 72h old	☐ N/A ☐ Meets Standard Site _____ Fluid _____	☐ N/A ☐ Meets Standard Site _____ Fluid _____	☐ N/A ☐ Meets Standard Site _____ Fluid _____
Special Equipment (describe)			
Discomfort (describe)			
Signature/Title			

Page 8 of 14

FIGURE 3-2: SAMPLE CLINICAL PATHWAY FORM (9 OF 14)

Inter-disciplinary ActionPlan	POD 1 Date: ___/___/___	Initials N|D|E	Time	Interdisciplinary Progress Notes
Consults	Case manager			
Tests	BCP I prn Hematology profile prn Room air pulse oximetry (DC O2 if sat ≥ 92%) DC O2			
Treatments	Discontinue arterial line INT for 24h			
Medication reminders	Resume all routine meds ASA 325 mg q day Oxycodone/Acetaminophen 1-2 tabs q 3h prn pain LOC			
Nutrition	Advance diet as tolerated Type _____ Bkfst: All ¾ ½ ¼ 0 NPO Lunch: All ¾ ½ ¼ 0 NPO Dinner: All ¾ ½ ¼ 0 NPO			
Activity/ Safety	Up in Chair then increase to up ad lib ♦ *Risk Management protocol* ☐ Yes ☐ No Implemented @ _____ Visually checked q 2 h♦ Bed in low position and locked Call light in reach Siderails up x 2♦ ID armband on patient			
Assessment	VS q 4h x 24h Neuro check q 4h DC continuous pulse oximetry Discontinue intermediate care Discontinue telemetry			
Patient/ family education				
Discharge planning	Assessment of potential discharge needs Social services referral as needed			

Expected Outcome	Outcome Met?	Initials	Reason outcome not achieved *(circle one)*	If outcome not met, record intervention(s) *Continue to address until outcome is achieved*
Transfer from Intermediate Care	☐ Yes ☐ No		a. Hypotension requiring inotropic support b. Hypertension requiring vasodilator support c. Unstable neurological state d. Unstable respiratory state e. Other	

♦ Reflects changes if Risk Management protocol implemented.

Initials/Signature   Initials/Signature   Initials/Signature

___/_____   ___/_____   ___/_____

___/_____   ___/_____   ___/_____

FIGURE 3-2: SAMPLE CLINICAL PATHWAY FORM (10 OF 14)

Patient Assessment
Vascular Surgery

Standard (If standard not met explain in space provided or in Narrative Notes)	Date ___/___/___ Time _____	Date ___/___/___ Time _____	Date ___/___/___ Time _____
Cardiovascular	Rhythm: ☐ Regular ☐ Irregular Telemetry: ☐ Yes ☐ No Rhythm _____ Ectopy _____ Specific Pulse Checks: DP PT Radial R L Key: + Present, - Absent, Dop-Doppler	Rhythm: ☐ Regular ☐ Irregular Telemetry: ☐ Yes ☐ No Rhythm _____ Ectopy _____ Specific Pulse Checks: DP PT Radial R L Key: + Present, - Absent, Dop-Doppler	Rhythm: ☐ Regular ☐ Irregular Telemetry: ☐ Yes ☐ No Rhythm _____ Ectopy _____ Specific Pulse Checks: DP PT Radial R L Key: + Present, - Absent, Dop-Doppler
Respiratory -Regular & unlabored -No cough -Lung sounds clear bilaterally -On room air	☐ Meets Standard O_2 _____	☐ Meets Standard O_2 _____	☐ Meets Standard O_2 _____
Gastrointestinal -Soft & non-distended -Bowel sounds present	☐ Meets Standard BM within last 8h? ☐ Yes ☐ No	☐ Meets Standard BM within last 8h? ☐ Yes ☐ No	☐ Meets Standard BM within last 8h? ☐ Yes ☐ No
Neuromuscular/Safety -Alert & oriented -Speech clear & coherent -Moves all 4 extremities equally -Hand grasps strong & equal -Gait steady -Swallows without difficulty	☐ Meets Standard	☐ Meets Standard	☐ Meets Standard
Skin -Warm, dry & intact -Color normal	☐ Meets Standard	☐ Meets Standard	☐ Meets Standard
Surgical wound	☐ N/A	☐ N/A	☐ N/A
Urinary -Voiding, continent -Clear, yellow urine	☐ Meets Standard	☐ Meets Standard	☐ Meets Standard
Drainage tubes (describe)	☐ N/A	☐ N/A	☐ N/A
Peripheral Edema -Absent	☐ Meets Standard	☐ Meets Standard	☐ Meets Standard
IV Therapy -No redness -No swelling/tenderness -Site and tubing < 72h old	☐ N/A ☐ Meets Standard Site _____ Fluid _____	☐ N/A ☐ Meets Standard Site _____ Fluid _____	☐ N/A ☐ Meets Standard Site _____ Fluid _____
Special Equipment (describe)			
Discomfort (describe)			
Signature/Title			

Page 10 of 14

FIGURE 3-2: SAMPLE CLINICAL PATHWAY FORM (11 OF 14)

Inter-disciplinary ActionPlan	POD 2 Date: __/__/__	Initials N|D|E	Time	Interdisciplinary Progress Notes
Consults	Case manager			
Tests				
Treatments	Discontinue INT			
Medication reminders	Resume all routine meds ASA 325 mg q day Oxycodone/Acetaminophen 1-2 tabs q 3h prn pain LOC			
Nutrition	Type _____ Bkfst: All ¾ ½ ¼ 0 NPO Lunch: All ¾ ½ ¼ 0 NPO Dinner: All ¾ ½ ¼ 0 NPO			
Activity/ Safety	**Consider discharge** Up ad lib ♦ *Risk Management protocol* ☐ Yes ☐ No Implemented @ _____ Visually checked q 2 h♦ Bed in low position and locked Call light in reach Siderails up x 2♦ ID armband on patient			
Assessment	VS q 8h Neuro check q 8h			
Patient/ family education	Risk factor modification Wound care Follow-up appointment Activity Diet Complications Medications			
Discharge planning				

Expected Outcome	Outcome Met?	Initials	Reason outcome not achieved *(circle one)*	If outcome not met, record intervention(s) *Continue to address until outcome is achieved*

♦ Reflects changes if Risk Management protocol implemented.

Initials/Signature

____/_____

____/_____

Initials/Signature

____/_____

____/_____

Initials/Signature

____/_____

____/_____

FIGURE 3-2: SAMPLE CLINICAL PATHWAY FORM (12 OF 14)

Patient Assessment
Vascular Surgery

Standard (If standard not met explain in space provided or in Narrative Notes)	Date ___/___/___ Time _____	Date ___/___/___ Time _____	Date ___/___/___ Time _____
Cardiovascular	Rhythm: ☐ Regular ☐ Irregular Telemetry: ☐ Yes ☐ No Rhythm _____ Ectopy _____ Specific Pulse Checks: DP PT Radial R L Key: + Present, - Absent, Dop-Doppler	Rhythm: ☐ Regular ☐ Irregular Telemetry: ☐ Yes ☐ No Rhythm _____ Ectopy _____ Specific Pulse Checks: DP PT Radial R L Key: + Present, - Absent, Dop-Doppler	Rhythm: ☐ Regular ☐ Irregular Telemetry: ☐ Yes ☐ No Rhythm _____ Ectopy _____ Specific Pulse Checks: DP PT Radial R L Key: + Present, - Absent, Dop-Doppler
Respiratory -Regular & unlabored -No cough -Lung sounds clear bilaterally -On room air	☐ Meets Standard O_2 _____	☐ Meets Standard O_2 _____	☐ Meets Standard O_2 _____
Gastrointestinal -Soft & non-distended -Bowel sounds present	☐ Meets Standard BM within last 8h? ☐ Yes ☐ No	☐ Meets Standard BM within last 8h? ☐ Yes ☐ No	☐ Meets Standard BM within last 8h? ☐ Yes ☐ No
Neuromuscular/Safety -Alert & oriented -Speech clear & coherent -Moves all 4 extremities equally -Hand grasps strong & equal -Gait steady -Swallows without difficulty	☐ Meets Standard	☐ Meets Standard	☐ Meets Standard
Skin -Warm, dry & intact -Color normal	☐ Meets Standard	☐ Meets Standard	☐ Meets Standard
Surgical wound	☐ N/A	☐ N/A	☐ N/A
Urinary -Voiding, continent -Clear, yellow urine	☐ Meets Standard	☐ Meets Standard	☐ Meets Standard
Drainage tubes (describe)	☐ N/A	☐ N/A	☐ N/A
Peripheral Edema -Absent	☐ Meets Standard	☐ Meets Standard	☐ Meets Standard
IV Therapy -No redness -No swelling/tenderness -Site and tubing < 72h old	☐ N/A ☐ Meets Standard Site _____ Fluid _____	☐ N/A ☐ Meets Standard Site _____ Fluid _____	☐ N/A ☐ Meets Standard Site _____ Fluid _____
Special Equipment (describe)			
Discomfort (describe)			
Signature/Title			

FIGURE 3-2: SAMPLE CLINICAL PATHWAY FORM (13 OF 14)

Inter-disciplinary ActionPlan	Date: __/__/__ POD 3	Initials N|D|E	Time	Interdisciplinary Progress Notes
Consults	Case manager			
Tests				
Treatments	Neck staples out			
Medication reminders	Resume all routine meds ASA 325 mg q day Oxycodone/Acetaminophen 1-2 tabs q 3h prn pain LOC			
Nutrition	Type _____ Bkfst: All ¾ ½ ¼ 0 NPO Lunch: All ¾ ½ ¼ 0 NPO Dinner: All ¾ ½ ¼ 0 NPO			
Activity/ Safety	**Discharge** Up ad lib ♦ *Risk Management protocol* ☐ Yes ☐ No Implemented @ _____ Visually checked q 2 h♦ Bed in low position and locked Call light in reach Siderails up x 2♦ ID armband on patient			
Assessment	VS q 8h Neuro check q 8h			
Patient/ family education	Risk factor modification Wound care Follow-up appointment Activity Diet Complications Medications			
Discharge planning				

Expected Outcome	Outcome Met?	Initials	Reason outcome not achieved *(circle one)*	If outcome not met, record intervention(s) *Continue to address until outcome is achieved*
Discharge			a. Hypotension b. Hypertension c. Unstable neurological state d. Severe wound infection e. Discharge planning needs incomplete f. Respiratory complications g. Other	

♦ Reflects changes if Risk Management protocol implemented.

Initials/Signature

____/_____

____/_____

Initials/Signature

____/_____

____/_____

Initials/Signature

____/_____

____/_____

FIGURE 3-2: SAMPLE CLINICAL PATHWAY FORM (14 OF 14)

Carotid Endarterectomy Clinical Pathway
Guidelines:

General Information:
- RN's, SN's, LPN's, MD's and related disciplines may document on this form.
- The clinical pathway serves as a guide for patient care and does not replace the physician's orders.
- All initials have one-time signature verification.

Page 1:
- Initiate the clinical pathway by stamping it with the patient's stamp plate and recording your signature in the blank at the top of the page.
- Indicate the achievement of desired patient outcomes by recording the date of achievement and your initial.
- All intermediate care discharge criteria must be addressed upon transfer out of the intermediate care area.
  All discharge criteria must be addressed prior to or upon discharge.
- If a patient fails to meet a particular outcome, place an asterisk beside it and note a rationale in the interdisciplinary notes.

Page 6:
- Record the vital signs and other information indicated on the post arteriogram assessment and the intermediate care assessment.

All Clinical Path/Assessment Pages:
- Enter the correct date at the top of each column.
- Initial the completion of each intervention in the columns of the respective shift for which the item occurred.
- If an item does not apply to the patient, strike through it using a single line.
- Individualize the interventions on the pathway by writing in items particular to that patient.
- Gray shaded areas indicate that no nursing signature is required for that particular item.
- Update the clinical pathway each shift. Document assessment each shift.

- Indicate the achievement of each daily outcome by marking the block "Yes or No" and sign your initials to the right of the "Yes or No" column.
- If there is an outcome that is not met, circle the reason/cause for the variation.
- To the right of the circled reason/cause, indicate the action taken and the date that the variance was resolved.

All Interdisciplinary Action Plan Pages:
- ♦ If Risk Management protocol implemented during shift, write in time of implementation and follow protocol. Protocol includes visual check q 1 h; bed in low and locked position; call light in reach; siderails up x 4 at all times and ID armband on patient.

Page 14 of 14

VIPS

One last method of documentation is the VIPS method. The VIPS model for documentation of nursing care in patient records was scientifically developed in 1991 with the aim of supporting systematic documentation of nursing care and promoting individualized care (Ehrenberg, Ehnfors, & Thorell-Ekstrand, 1996). The model, which is accepted and used in many parts of Sweden, is based on four key concepts: well-being, integrity, prevention, and safety (yielding the acronym VIPS in the Swedish spelling).

The VIPS documentation model consists of keywords on two levels. The first level corresponds to the nursing process model, with the keywords nursing history, nursing status, nursing diagnosis, goal, nursing intervention, nursing outcome, and nursing discharge note. The second level of keywords consists of subdivisions for nursing history, nursing status, and nursing interventions. The VIPS model seems to be useful in different care areas. However, in some areas, systematic inquiries concerning documentation are lacking or partly lacking, such as in psychiatric care, perioperative care, anesthesia care, and hospital outpatient clinics. Geographically, this system seems to be disseminated to most parts of Sweden, indicating general acceptance in Sweden's nursing practice.

SELECTING A DOCUMENTATION SYSTEM

Selecting a documentation method that ensures optimal communication, simplifies the charting process, and meets required regulations is difficult. It is important to consider the staffing mix of the hospital or unit. If unlicensed assistive personnel are part of the staff, their role in documentation must be evaluated. On an all-RN unit, documentation may be at a more sophisticated level than on a unit staffed by health care providers with a mix of educational backgrounds.

The knowledge and skills of the staff must also be considered. Nurses have varying degrees of exposure to different types of documentation, and their age, educational background, and work experiences influence their documentation skills. Nurses may resist a new documentation method if they do not have the knowledge and skills to understand the process.

Changing documentation systems can be costly; therefore, determining the financial outlay of a new documentation system is essential. Cost estimates should include planning and preparation time, printed materials, design and development of new forms, and educational time.

Another critical consideration in the process of changing documentation methods is education. A sound educational program must be developed and repeated as often as necessary. Following implementation, the process will need monitoring for compliance and troubleshooting for any problems that may develop.

CONCLUSION

Several common documentation methods have been presented. Each has advantages and disadvantages. Institutions and specialty units must select the method that works best for their specific needs. When selecting a documentation system, JCAHO standards, state and federal regulations, and legalities must be considered. Because health care reimbursement is in a state of flux and regulators and regulations continually change, new documentation systems must be designed with care. The emphasis on measuring outcomes of care may require many institutions to make changes in their documentation methods. When developing new documentation methods, feedback must be obtained from risk management and legal counsel to ensure the changes are legally sound.

EXAM QUESTIONS

CHAPTER 3
Questions 16-21

16. The oldest and probably most time-consuming method of documentation is

    a. APIE.

    b. CBE.

    c. Focus notes.

    d. narrative notes.

17. POMR charting became popular in the late 1960s and includes

    a. SOAPIER and APIE.

    b. narrative notes and process recordings.

    c. CBE and care pathways.

    d. nursing process and Kardex.

18. A major advantage of Focus charting is it

    a. is difficult to construct and lacks accuracy and logical judgment.

    b. requires nurses to change their thinking processes.

    c. promotes the nursing process and provides structure to the process.

    d. must be closely monitored to avoid becoming narrative notes.

19. A major *disadvantage* of CBE documentation is

    a. trends in the patient's status are difficult to follow.

    b. it requires repetitive charting of routine care.

    c. the system was designed for an all RN staff.

    d. it's emphasis on the chronology of problems.

20. Clinical pathways define a patient's progress through managed care and

    a. are only nursing focused and do not communicate continuity of care.

    b. patients and their families are not included in the planning process.

    c. there is no need to address the knowledge and skills of the staff mix.

    d. are based on DRGs, contain key elements, and promote coordination of care.

21. When selecting a documentation method, an institution should

    a. consider the education level of staff and the staffing mix.

    b. disregard other regulations.

    c. keep the process secret until it is ready for implementation.

    d. not worry about the costs involved with changing the method.

CHAPTER 4

COMPUTERIZED NURSING DOCUMENTATION

CHAPTER OBJECTIVE

After completing this chapter, the reader will be able to discuss the move toward computerized nursing documentation and describe at least three requirements necessary when using computerized nursing documentation.

LEARNING OBJECTIVES

After studying this chapter, the reader will be able to

1. identify the evolution of computer use for nursing documentation.

2. specify six advantages of using computerized nursing documentation.

3. indicate a major disadvantage of using computerized nursing documentation.

4. identify requirements for computerized documentation implementation and education.

5. indicate three legal concerns with the use of computerized documentation.

6. discuss future predictions for computerized nursing documentation.

INTRODUCTION

The latest trend in nursing documentation is the move toward computerized documentation. Computerized information systems are becoming the norm in most health care facilities. Getting nursing data into computerized information systems requires that they be defined and structured to fit the parameters of a computer without losing the essence of nursing. This chapter addresses the evolution of computerized documentation, its advantages and disadvantages, implementation and education requirements, legal concerns, and predictions for the future.

EVOLUTION OF COMPUTERIZED CHARTING

Most medical institutions began using computers for tracking admissions, discharges, and transfers. Demographic data was collected and usually tied to finances and billing. Computers then began appearing on nursing units and were first used to order supplies, laboratory tests, and other diagnostic tests and procedures. The unit secretary was usually the person who handled the entries for the procedures and was the most computer-literate person on the unit.

In the mid-1980s, software began to be developed that could be used for nursing documentation. The earliest uses involved care plans that could be individualized, printed out, and placed on a patient's chart. In many cases, individual departments purchased computers and software that were specific to the department. Challenges related to the incompatibility of systems resulted from the rapid development and increasing number of software companies that began developing programs for a variety of services.

The reporting of laboratory and other test results to the nursing units computer terminal occurred early in the development of hospitals becoming computerized. Systems were developed for computerizing patient supply charges, which led to more accurate hospital billing.

One of the next steps in computerizing the medical record was to add order entries. Many physicians resisted order entry because they were uncomfortable with computer technology, could not type, or felt that direct entry is too time-consuming. The most desirable method of data entry is to have physicians input their orders directly into the computer. This process reduces the chances of transcription error from being unable to read and decipher physician handwriting.

Adding pharmacy systems to electronic capabilities further reduces the chances for error. A pharmacy system that provides a printed medication administration record reduces the risk associated with transcription of orders and provides a clear, legible record. Some systems permit the nurse to chart the administration of medications directly on the computer.

Currently available electronic documentation systems use wall-mounted (touch screen), handheld, or other portable devices to record patient data, such as assessment information, routine care, medication administrations, treatments, and changes in condition. These devices provide the ability to continually update information and access to the information by multiple health care providers. The ability to have the whole hospital networked with compatible programs has greatly enhanced the use of computers.

Some newer nursing information systems suggest nursing diagnoses based on predefined assessment data that has been entered. More recent systems are interac-

tive, prompting the nurse with questions and suggestions about the entered information. These questions and diagnostic suggestions make documentation quick and thorough. All the documentation information is available in the computer program so that it may be added or changed to individualize the plan of care.

Future developments will lead to a comprehensive system that makes use of various data collection components and the broad scope of computer capabilities. Computerized documentation is flexible and expandable enough to meet the evolving needs of each clinical specialty and subspecialty. As knowledge bases and sophistication in the use of information grow, so must computer systems.

BARRIERS TO COMPUTERIZED NURSING DOCUMENTATION

Nursing is often the last department to receive adequate and updated software for documentation. Nurses must convince administrators that the computerization of nursing information will provide tangible results. Successful nurses use the power of their group size to become involved in the selection, integration, and use of information management technology. The lack of a unified nursing language, nursing's unique information requirements, lack of good software, and use of incompatible systems have caused barriers. With the advent of nurses who specialize in informatics and the involvement of nurses in the development of computer documentation programs and software, many of these barriers are being overcome.

ADVANTAGES OF COMPUTERIZED DOCUMENTATION

The age of the computer has arrived; computers have become an economic necessity. They assist health care providers to improve the quality of health care. Additional advantages of using computers and computerized documentation are listed in Table 4-1.

DISADVANTAGES OF COMPUTERIZED DOCUMENTATION

Despite the long list of advantages of computerized documentation, there are some disadvantages. Mostly related to confidentiality and security, these disadvantages are listed in Table 4-2.

IMPLEMENTATION AND EDUCATIONAL REQUIREMENTS

The transition to computerized documentation presents a unique challenge to nurses and nurse-managers. The successful implementation of a computerized documentation system requires preparation, involvement, and commitment from the entire nursing staff. It also requires thoughtful, deliberate planning.

TABLE 4-1: ADVANTAGES OF USING COMPUTERS AND COMPUTERIZED DOCUMENTATION

Computers

- play an increasing role in the education process.

- can be interactive, allowing for computer-assisted diagnosis.

- allow for computer-generated prescriptions and interaction with the pharmacy, which reduces the incidence of medication errors.

- can be programmed to generate reminders for follow-up testing and assessments.

- can assist in the decision-making process.

- are capable of assisting in the identification of allergies and drug-drug and food-drug interactions.

- provide printouts that are completely legible, therefore taking the guesswork out of interpreting handwriting.

Computerized Documentation

- makes retrieval of demographic information, consultant's reports, and laboratory and other test results is made easier.

- improves productivity and quality of care.

- saves time and reduces costs.

- supports clinical research.

- is helpful when standardizing treatment protocols.

- saves data entry time, allowing the nurse more time for patient contact.

- decreases the ability to tamper with records.

- supports the use of the nursing process and facilitates individualized patient assessments.

- reduces redundancy in documentation. Data are entered once and the information is automatically sent to all appropriate places on various forms.

- software can be designed so that documentation can be sorted and printed out in ways not possible with paper systems.

- provides analysis of data compiled from several patients' records can lead to conclusions about achieved outcomes.

- includes storage of discharge instructions, which can be individualized and printed for patients' use.

(Daniels, 1997; Holly, 2003; Iyer & Camp, 1999; White & Hemby, 1997)

TABLE 4-2: DISADVANTAGES OF COMPUTERIZED DOCUMENTATION
• Use of computerized documentation may result in loss of confidentiality and unauthorized disclosure of information.
• Sophisticated security systems must be developed.
• Equipment may not be reliable and may lack quick responsiveness.
• Some people question the accuracy and reliability of data input by computer operators.
• Downtime may disrupt the usability of the system.
• Hospital policy may require daily printouts of data, resulting in voluminous amounts of paper.
• Software limitations may force nurses to omit key information about the patient.
• Resistance to change and inadequate numbers of terminals can affect the acceptance of computers.
• Costs for purchase of hardware and software, education of all health care providers, licensing fees, and continual needs for upgrades may be prohibitive.
(Daniels, 1997; Iyer & Camp, 1999; White & Hemby, 1997)

Knowledge of change theory is helpful when trying to implement new documentation methods. The classic change theory developed by Kurt Lewin (1951) is often used. Lewin states that change occurs in three phases: unfreezing, moving, and refreezing:

- During unfreezing, a disruption in the balance or equilibrium occurs within the system. Dissatisfaction with current documentation practices provides the need for change. Data should be gathered in regard to the strengths and limitations of the current documentation method.

- During the moving phase, there is a move to a new goal. Resistance to change occurs because most people are uncomfortable with change. New ideas are developed and implemented. Committees are formed, goals are developed, systems are redesigned, and pilot studies are conducted. This phase is the longest in the change cycle.

- Finally, in the refreezing phase, consolidation and adoption of new ideas occur. Monitoring and evaluation of the changes take place. Resource people must be available for user support. As staff become more comfortable with the new documentation method, acceptance of the method increases and resistance decreases.

A plan must be developed to provide the institution with a clear understanding of the changes involved in computerized documentation. Collaboration and communication are necessary between all levels of employees. Establishing goals and time frames keeps the project on target.

Staff development is a critical part of implementing computerized documentation. Staff members must stay informed about the progress of the change and their input is necessary to make sure all questions and concerns are addressed. Specific, detailed classes must be offered, and all staff members must have the opportunity to attend in-service sessions. Self-learning modules and videotapes of class presentations are necessary to educate people who are unable to attend classes or for those who want to review the process.

Once the staff has been educated, the implementation process begins. Small-scale pilot projects may be used to implement the changes. Specific units are selected for the pilot study and, eventually, every unit in an institution can be included. Communication and follow-up are key elements in the success of implementation.

The process does not stop at this time. Continued monitoring and evaluation are necessary to determine if the overall plan for change is being met. Monitoring and evaluation are critical in determining the degree of compliance and the identification of any unforeseen problems. Ongoing education, refresher courses, and introduction to new software help maintain compliance and keep staff up-to-date.

LEGAL AND SECURITY CONCERNS

The security needs of an electronic documentation method are different from those of handwritten methods. Electronic records require additional security measures to ensure that they are reliable and authentic. Security for electronic records includes the protection of documents, files, systems, and network areas from unauthorized access and damage or loss from fire, water, theft, mutilation, or unauthorized alterations or destruction.

Computerized medical records present new challenges to nurses' ethical and legal obligations to safeguard confidential patient information. Security measures must be developed to strictly control the ability of others to access computerized records from distant sites. Even the placement of computer screens must be taken into consideration. Likewise, medical records must be protected from destruction by computer viruses introduced via floppy disks or the Internet.

There are a variety of federal laws that protect credit information; however, few laws protect the computerized medical record. Health Insurance Portability and Accountability Act (HIPAA) regulations require increased security for computers and computer users. (HIPAA is discussed in detail in Chapter 5). With the rapid growth of the Internet, an explosion of high-technology crime and related illegal activities has occurred. Increases in cybercrime have necessitated development of technologies and systems to combat these problems. Therefore, breach of security is a very serious con-

cern. Users should only have the level of access necessary to do their jobs. Most often, codes are set up so that staff working on certain units have access only to information about the patients on that unit and not every patient in the hospital. Some hospitals have fired personnel for giving their passwords to unauthorized individuals, and illegally obtaining someone's password is considered a crime.

Lastly, the proliferation of electronic records requires both records managers and archivists to redefine their roles. Plans must be made for the preservation and accessibility of records beyond the useful life of the systems that created them. Decisions must be made regarding storage of electronic records, ease of retrieval, and length of time the records are retained. Electronic data take up much less space than paper records; however, accessibility to records over time requires that the record be reproduced in a reliable and authentic format. The length of time medical records must be retained varies from state to state. Therefore, when an institution decides to use computerized documentation, all parties involved as well as legal counsel must work together to ensure that all requirements from every health care provider, department, and regulator are met.

CONCLUSION

The benefits of computerized records are many. They free up physical space in an institution, provide health care providers ready access to complete patient data, and are legible and easy to read. Computerized documentation results in better standardization of care plans and more efficient use of nurses' time. It also improves the quality of patient care. Computers are becoming easier to use, and bedside terminals are becoming more common. Bedside systems using standard keyboards, touch-sensitive screens, handheld units, palm-sized terminals, voice-activated systems, and other devices allow nurses to promptly document vital signs, routine care, and changes in status. Implementing electronic medical records as part of a complete electronic patient management program can significantly improve patient safety and ultimately save lives.

Many developments in computer programs are rapidly taking place. The Institute of Medicine has promoted the vision of having fully computerized medical records in all hospitals by the end of the decade. New systems are being developed because there are currently no systems available that can support a completely computerized medical record. Future plans include the development of a computerized system that fully integrates medical records and acts as a repository for lifelong medical information. Computer chips that contain medical information are already being implanted into human bodies. Work is still needed and software programs must be developed before nurses will see a completely computerized medical record. A sample of a computerized medical record is displayed in Figure 4-1 on pages 67-68.

FIGURE 4-1: SAMPLE COMPUTERIZED MEDICAL RECORD (1 OF 2)

Last Name
First Name
Middle Intital

Place bar code label here

Print date: 10/07/03

Last Name	First Name	Middle Initial	ID#	MRN
Maternal Birth Date	Language	Mothers Education	Admission to Hospital	Phycisian

Admission

Date and Time	Arrival	Reason for Admission	Advance Directives

Status	Allergies	Specific Problem	Att !	Detail

Health Care Providers

Obstetrician	
Nurse Midwife	
Newborn's Physician	

Pregnancy History

Gravida	Term	Preterm	SpAb	IndAb	Born Alive	EDC- LMP	Gestational Age

Obstetrical History

Date	Delivery GA	Route of Delivery	Birth Weight (g)	Sex	Labor	Anesthesia	Place of Birth	Born Alive	Preterm Labor	Comment/Complications

Test Name	Results	Comments

Maternal Problems	Current status

Home Medications

Current List	Medication	Start	Stop	Dose	Unit	Frequency	Route

Vital Signs

VE

ROM

OBSTETRIC ADMITTING RECORD

Page 1 of 2

FIGURE 4-1: SAMPLE COMPUTERIZED MEDICAL RECORD (2 OF 2)

Last Name

First Name

Middle Intital

Place bar code label here

Patient Height:		Prepregnancy Weight:		Current Weight:	
Status	Examination		Date	Finding	

Medical History				
Status	Category	Specific Problem	Att !	Detail

Status	Assessment/Screens	Item	Detail

Status	Psychosocial	Item	Explanation

Biophysical Profile												
Child	Date	GA	BPP	B	T	V	A	Test	Test Reason	Test Result	Comment	User	Location

Ultrasound Examination													
Child	Date	GA	Est Weight (g)	CRL	BPD	OFD	HC	TAD	APAD	AC	FL	Comment	User	Location

RN Electronic Signature

EXAM QUESTIONS

CHAPTER 4
Questions 22-27

22. The use of the computer for nursing documentation first evolved in the

    a. 1960s.
    b. 1970s.
    c. 1980s.
    d. 1990s.

23. An *advantage* of using computerized documentation is

    a. reliability of equipment and quick responsiveness.
    b. printouts are legible compared to handwriting.
    c. hardware and software do not require upgrades.
    d. unauthorized personnel cannot access records.

24. A *disadvantage* of using computerized documentation is that

    a. downtime may disrupt the usability of the system.
    b. nurses will have more time for patient contact.
    c. it reduces redundancy in documentation.
    d. the decision-making process can be facilitated.

25. A hospital has decided to move toward computerized documentation and hires you as a consultant. As you help the hospital implement a computerized documentation system, you keep in mind the need to

    a. implement the new system throughout the hospital at one time.
    b. do on-the-job training sessions with all of the nursing assistants first.
    c. set up small-scale pilot projects that may be used to implement the changes.
    d. terminate your services as soon as the computers are located on the units.

26. The security needs of an electronic documentation method are different from those of hand-written methods. The hospital must be aware of the need for

    a. less strict control to prevent distant site access.
    b. handling records that are more difficult to retrieve and retain.
    c. allowing staff access to information about all patients in the hospital.
    d. a backup system to prevent down time which may disrupt usability.

27. Predictions for the future indicate that nurses will document

    a. with the same systems that are presently in place.

    b. with handheld units, palm-sized terminals, and voice-activated systems.

    c. with all narrative notes methods that require hours of additional overtime.

    d. with paper and pens, necessitating the need to continue to interpret others' handwriting.

CHAPTER 5

DOCUMENTATION STRATEGIES

CHAPTER OBJECTIVE

After completing this chapter, the reader will be able to describe charting techniques and strategies to improve documentation.

LEARNING OBJECTIVES

After studying this chapter, the reader will be able to

1. specify five do's of documentation.

2. specify five don'ts of documentation.

3. identify three techniques or strategies to improve documentation.

4. indicate three rules for good charting.

5. describe four characteristics of effective written communication.

6. indicate the significance of HIPAA.

7. identify patient confidentiality issues and ways to protect patient confidentiality.

INTRODUCTION

Good charting means that findings and interventions are properly documented. All health care providers can easily follow up and ensure timely continuity of care for the patient. To make sense and be meaningful, documentation must communicate what was intended. Excellent documentation is not a substitute for providing nursing care, but excellent clinical care must be accompanied by appropriate documentation. Although the patient record is a permanent legal document that details nurse-patient interactions, it is not unusual to find critical omissions in nursing documentation as well as meaningless, repetitious, and inaccurate entries. This chapter presents characteristics of effective written communication, including documentation techniques and strategies to improve nursing documentation. Additionally, rules for ensuring good charting and patient confidentiality will be presented.

CHARACTERISTICS OF EFFECTIVE WRITTEN COMMUNICATION

Communication may be defined as the exchange of information through verbal or written means. It is a two-way process that involves sending and receiving information. It also involves the sharing of experiences, feelings, and emotions. Nurses who have effective communication skills are better able to establish successful relationships with patients, colleagues, and other health care professionals. Effective communication can also prevent many errors that can lead to legal incidents.

Basically, a communication system involves a sender, message, channel, receiver, and response or feedback. The sender transmits an original message to a receiver in verbal or written form. The receiver interprets the message and provides a response or feedback. If the message was not interpreted correctly or if additional information is needed, the process starts again. Communication is an ongoing process, and the roles of the sender and receiver are interchangeable.

Verbal communication allows the process of instant clarification and reinterpretation of the message. This process is not possible with written communication because the decoding or interpretation may occur when the writer is not present and may occur long after the information was written. Therefore, it is important that written information be clear so that it can be interpreted correctly. Written communication must contain appropriate language and terminology; correct grammar, spelling, and punctuation; logical organization; and appropriate statements without judgment. Language and terminology must be appropriate for the age, education, reading level, and cultural background of the reader. Using correct grammar, spelling, and punctuation provides clarity for the reader. If written materials are well organized, they are logical and easy to follow. When documenting information in a patient's chart, only the facts should be recorded, without any judgments or assumptions.

Effective communication and documentation of patient care increases awareness of patient needs. When documentation is complete, accurate, and clearly understood by all health care professionals, the quality of patient care improves. Clear documentation also provides adequate defense in the event of a lawsuit. Therefore, all nurses need techniques and strategies to improve documentation of patient care.

TECHNIQUES AND STRATEGIES TO IMPROVE DOCUMENTATION

Documentation begins with a complete assessment and appropriate plan of care. A patient's medical record is used to document the nursing process and fulfill the nurse's obligation to commu-

nicate vital information. Nurses must make sure their documentation meets the standards of their states' nurse practice acts and administrative codes or rules, national professional standards, applicable federal regulations, accrediting body requirements, and the standards of their institutions.

When a nurse documents, he or she should support what is being written with facts. Documentation includes observations, such as volumes, totals, amounts, and values, as well as physical assessment findings, patient comments, and information collected by other health care providers. Comparison of current findings to the initial documented physical assessment helps the nurse determine if changes in the patient's condition are occurring.

Negative as well as positive findings need to be recorded. This helps identify changes in a patient's condition. Chart so that the reader can tell that you were at the bedside and evaluated the patient (see Table 5-1). If a nurse assesses a patient and finds a difference from a previously documented assessment, he or she can readily see this is a change in the patient's status.

TABLE 5-1: CLEAR DOCUMENTATION
DON'T:
"No c/o voiced or signs of distress."
DO:
"Resting quietly. Denies pain or shortness of breath."

It is very important to write legibly and use correct grammar, spelling, and terminology. Most institutions have a list of approved abbreviations. This list is important because not everyone may know what you mean by a particular abbreviation. In addition, because many medical abbreviations have more than one meaning, it is better to spell out what you are trying to say. For example, "Voiding qs" is frequently seen documented in patients' charts. Does this mean that patient was voiding "every shift" or voiding "quantity sufficient"? Likewise, how much is considered "sufficient"? It is much better to document the exact amount, such as "Voided 250 cc clear yellow urine." The exact amount and color provides clearer information.

Use measurable terms to describe sizes and amounts. It is better to provide specific dimensions than comparisons to other objects such as fruits and vegetables. Not everyone has the same concept of fruit and vegetable sizes. This may necessitate having a small measuring device in one's pocket. This is a change from past recommendations; however, exact measurements are accurate and are not misleading (see Table 5-2). Take and remember the exact measurements of parts of your hand. For example the width of your thumbnail, length of your index finger, width of your hand, distance from the tip of your thumb across your palm to the tip of your little finger (octave span), and so forth. These measurements can be very helpful when determining sizes.

TABLE 5-2: DOCUMENTING SIZE
DON'T:
". . . size of a pea"
DO:
"1.5 cm in diameter"
(Yocum, 2002)

It is important to chart for quality. Information should be complete, concise, and thorough. Concise information is easy to understand. A long report is difficult to read, may be boring, and wastes time. Sketchy or abbreviated notes may imply the nurse was in a hurry and did not document all the details. Clear, succinct documentation provides essential information and avoids unnecessary words and irrelevant details. Some simple do's of charting that may prove helpful are listed in Table 5-3 on page 74.

PITFALLS OF DOCUMENTATION

Many of the pitfalls of documentation are just the reverse of the proper documentation tech-niques. Review the pitfalls displayed in Table 5-4 (found on page 75) and those discussed here.

Write Legibly

It is important to document so that others can read what has been written. It is very embarrassing to appear at a deposition or on a witness stand years after an event, be asked to read what you wrote, and have to admit that you cannot read your own writing. Patient injuries may occur if information cannot be read, and illegible handwriting can form the basis for a lawsuit.

Negative impressions of a nurse are portrayed if misspelled words and poor grammar are used. It may be necessary to keep standard and medical dictionaries close at hand. If a nurse has problems with long medical terms, describe the observation with clear, concise descriptions. Errors in grammar or incorrect use of words may lead to some very humorous situations. For example, review the errors in grammar and use of incorrect words presented in Table 5-5 on page 76.

It is permissible to use first-person pronouns ("I") in charting. Doing so allows a nurse to be very clear and exact when charting actions and who performed those actions. Clearly identify the subject of the sentence and read what you have written to make sure you have said what you really mean. For example, in Table 5-6 on page 76, did the physician call or did the nurse call the physician? To clarify the statement, it should say, "'I telephoned the physician and left message with answering service for physician to return call.' C. Nurse, RN." Simply turning the words around could make the documentation clearer, for example, "Called the physician" or "Telephoned the physician." By putting the verb first, it implies that the nurse called the physician. In addition, by documenting "Dr. Jones returned call, orders received. See order sheet." it is very clear who called who and what action was taken.

TABLE 5-3: SOME DO'S OF CHARTING FOR QUALITY

- Document pain accurately.
- Mean what you say and say what you mean.
- Follow professional standards for nursing care and documentation.
- Name anyone who becomes involved in the patient's care, including managers and primary care providers.
- Think before you abbreviate.
- Follow the same rules with flow sheets.
- Write neatly and legibly.
- Sign every entry with your name and title.
- Document in blue or black ink only, depending on your institution's requirements.
- Use graphic records to record vital signs.
- Make sure the patient's name is on every page (clearly identify patients with the same name).
- Take care with confidential information, (i.e., recording the status of a HIV test).
- Transcribe orders carefully.
- Question inappropriate or illegible orders.
- Document omitted care or medications.
- Document complete information about medications.
- Document allergies to medications and foods.
- Document sites of injections.
- Record all details of intravenous therapy and blood administration.
- Record the report of abnormal laboratory findings to primary health care providers.
- Chart promptly.
- Avoid block charting.
- Chart after delivery of care.
- Fill in blanks on charts and forms.
- Document exact quotes.
- Eliminate bias from written descriptions of the patient or other health care providers.
- Document changes in the patient's condition.
- Notify the primary health care provider of a patient's changes and document the information reported.
- Chart only care you give or supervise.
- Correctly identify late entries.
- Document noncompliance.
- Describe unauthorized personal items found at the patient's bedside.
- Document the patient's response to treatments.

(Daniels, 1997; Habel, 2003a; Yocum, 2002)

Acknowledge Written Comments

The nurse providing care to a patient and who documents care given, must sign at the end of each entry. Usual practice is to write the initial of the first name, full last name, and status (level of education, i.e. RN, LPN, etc.). When charting flows over to another page, the nurse should sign the first page and, at the top of the new page, note the date, time, and "continued from previous page." The nurse should also properly sign the end of the documenta-

TABLE 5-4: PITFALLS OF DOCUMENTATION

Records that do not clearly show that the nurses and institution are meeting the basic standards of care acceptable for the nursing area can cause you to lose any lawsuit brought against you or the facility. That is why you need to follow correct documentation guidelines. You also need to avoid several pitfalls that can decrease your record's viability in a court of law.

DO NOT:

- Fail to follow nursing law and regulations, and professional standards.
- Fail to follow facility policies and procedures in relationship to care and documentation.
- Fail to document clinical condition or changes in the patient's condition.
- Fail to follow-up on earlier documented events, doctor orders, changes in condition, or one-time orders.
- Fail to write legibly.
- Falsify records or make fraudulent entries.
- Under estimate the importance of flow sheet documentation.
- Fail to follow policy and procedures relating to how to use a flow sheet.
- Fail to read what you are signing when documenting on the flow sheet, do not just document where the shift before has charted.
- Use ditto marks or apothecary symbols.
- Document for someone else unless absolutely necessary. If necessary, clearly identify who did the task.
- Sign anyone else's nurses notes.
- Leave blank lines or spaces in documentation or on forms.
- Chart before the event, such as giving medications. Your initials on the medication records means the medication has been given. To sign your initial prior to giving it is seen as falsification by Boards of nursing.
- Express opinions or assumptions.
- Criticize or blame other team members or refer to staffing difficulties.
- Tamper with a record, including any official logs kept on the unit.
- Use correcting fluid, tape, or erasures to correct errors and to completely eradicate the information.
- Back-date records.
- Lie or misrepresent information.
- Try to prejudice the reader.
- Insert information between lines.
- List account numbers from credit cards when inventorying valuables.
- Document that an incident or occurrence report was filed.
- Fail to document communication with doctors and the content of that communication.
- Use unmeasurable or vague terms such as good, better, negative, appears, and seems.
- Fail to document incidents.
- If you have information that should be added talk to the facility lawyer.
- Do not add information to a chart that will be used in a law suit.
- Allow anyone to pressure you from documenting the acts by adding or withholding information. Report anyone who applies pressure to your supervisor. If your supervisor is pressuring you, go to the next person in the chain of authority, the risk management director, or the hospital lawyer.
- Discard part or all of a medical record.
- Alter anyone else's notes or documentation. Report to your supervisor any evidence that a chart or notation has been altered.
- Document in a biased or negative manner. Do not demean the patient with words such as *useless, lazy, bum, drunk,* or *disagreeable.* Chart the facts.
- Use unapproved abbreviations or shorthand notations when documenting. Write out words. For example, do not use T3 or TYL 3 for Tylenol #3.
- Use erasable ink.

Note. From *Documentation Skills for Quality Patient Care* by Fay Yocum (1999), president of Awareness Productions (http://www.awarenessproductions.com). Reprinted with permission.

TABLE 5-5: ACTUAL SENTENCES FOUND IN PATIENTS' HOSPITAL CHARTS

- She has no rigors or shaking chills, but her husband states she was very hot in bed last night.
- Patient has chest pain if she lies on her left side for over a year.
- On the second day, the knee was better, and on the third day, it disappeared.
- The patient is tearful and crying constantly. She also appears to be depressed.
- The patient has been depressed since she began seeing me in 1993.
- Discharge status: Alive but without my permission.
- Healthy appearing decrepit 69-year old male, mentally alert but forgetful.
- The patient refused autopsy.
- The patient has no previous history of suicide.
- Patient has left white blood cells at another hospital.
- Patient's medical history has been remarkably insignificant with only 40-pound weight gain in the past three days.
- Patient had waffles for breakfast and anorexia for lunch.
- She is numb from her toes down.
- Patient has two teenage children but no other abnormalities.
- Large brown stool ambulating in the hall.
- While in ER, she was examined, X-rated, and sent home.
- Occasional, constant infrequent headaches.
- Patient was alert and unresponsive.
- Both breasts are equal and reactive to light and accommodation.
- I saw your patient today, who is still under our car for physical therapy.

TABLE 5-6: WHAT WAS THE ACTION?

"Physician telephoned."

"Physician called."

tion. Some institutions allow the use of first and last initials following documentation, especially on flow sheets and the medication administration record (MAR). Normal practice is to have a specified place on these forms where the full name of the nurse appears and the initials are indicated so that the nurse may be correctly identified.

Some institutions have policies about documenting when a supervisor or other health care providers are notified. If you do not document that you notified your manager or supervisor and did not include his or her name, then there is no proof that you followed the chain of command. Include the supervisor's name and title. This makes it very clear

to whom you communicated your concerns. Likewise, document the name of any other health care provider who participated in the patient's care. Naming names is an important standard of quality care. Anyone reading your documentation at a later date should be able to tell exactly who participated in the patient's care.

The person doing the documentation should be the person providing the care. If you chart a procedure that was performed by someone else (such as unlicensed personnel, another nurse, or the physician) make sure you chart the name and title of the person performing the procedure or care and the procedure or care that was given (see Table 5-7).

It is sometimes necessary to cosign someone else's notes, such as a student nurse's. Cosigning implies that the instructor or the precepting nurse

TABLE 5-7: PROCEDURES PROPERLY DOCUMENTED
6/24/03, 9:30 AM. Patient admitted to LR #3 in active labor. C. Smith, RN, started IV of 1000 cc lactated Ringer's solution with #16 angiocath in patient's rt. forearm. N. Horn, RN, Charge Nurse, notified Dr. Jones. Dr. Reed on standby until Dr. Jones could arrive. Admission assessment completed. Patient gowned, fetal monitors attached, and patient prepped for delivery. _____ C. Rains, RN.

approved the care given and is assuming responsibility for that care. Students are rarely named in lawsuits; however, if a plaintiff initiates a suit against a student, the cosigner, instructor, school, agency, physician, and other nurses could all be included.

Use Ink to Document

Most institutions require that all charting be done in blue or black ink. Other colors do not reproduce well if a chart must be photocopied. It is wise to use only one pen during a shift to avoid looking like the documentation has been altered or additions made at a later time. Chemical tests and computerized analysis can now be conducted on written charts to determine if the ink corresponds to ink that would have been used at the time of original documentation.

Make sure you include the date on each entry to add clarification and provide logical sequencing of care provided. Many institutions use military time, or the 24-hour clock, to avoid confusion between AM and PM times, especially if the AM or PM has been omitted from the charting. Military time is easy to determine. Once you get past 12:00 noon, which is 1200, you add 12 to the time. Therefore, 1:00 PM would be 1300, 10:00 PM would be 2200, and midnight would be 2400.

Avoid Block Charting and Chart Promptly

Block charting refers to documentation is entered to cover a broad time frame, frequently a whole shift. If a nurse documents a note to cover a 12-hour shift, such as 7 AM to 7 PM, there is no clear indication that he or she was in the patient's room during that period. Specific time entries

indicate that the nurse was actually at the patient's bedside and performed care. It is especially critical to date and time a change in a patient's condition and the interventions taken when the change was noted. Attorneys are quick to point out when a patient's change in condition was not documented and when the physician was not notified of the change in a timely manner. It is also critical to document that the change of condition was reported to the primary health care provider.

The nurse should chart as soon as possible after an observation or procedure. Information that is charted immediately is more accurate and detailed. Everyone knows that, in a time of emergency, it is not always possible to document immediately. In such cases, the nurse should make notes on a scrap of paper or a paper towel to later record the exact events and their time of occurrence.

Documenting and Transcribing Orders

Verbal and phone orders may be discouraged at some institutions. When taking verbal or phone orders, the nurse must be sure she has heard the order correctly and written it correctly. With phone orders, the physician may misdiagnose the problem and give a wrong order. This is especially problematic if an on-call physician gives an order for a patient with whom he or she is not familiar. Repeating the order back to the physician, along with the patient's name, is now the standard of practice. If there are any concerns about the credibility of or familiarity with a physician, another nurse may listen to the telephone conversation and cosign the order with the nurse receiving the order. Always document in the nursing notes that an order was received; then write the order on the order sheet.

Guidelines for documenting a phone or verbal order are addressed in Table 5-8.

It is essential that orders be transcribed accurately. Many institutions have standing orders printed for specific diseases, surgeries, or conditions. The physician simply checks the items requested. This reduces errors when transcribing orders. Nursing standards and codes require that nurses assume responsibility and accountability for nursing judgments and actions. That means nurses must be able to question orders and spot errors. It is the responsibility of the nurse to call the physician to question orders that are illegible or appear inappropriate.

Numerous medication errors have been made because a decimal point was misplaced or the wrong dosage of medication was ordered. The nurse should document in the nursing notes a call for clarification of orders and what changes were made, if any. If a physician cannot be reached, the nurse should hold the medication and document in the nursing notes that attempts were made to contact the physician. It is wise to write in a memo the details of such an event, with the measures taken to resolve the problem, and send the memo to the nursing supervisor.

Handling and Documenting Other Phone Calls

Sometimes, parents of children or family members of a patient in an intensive care unit are given unit telephone numbers so that they may telephone to ask questions about their child or family member.

It is wise to establish some type of code system so that the nurse taking the call knows that the caller is truly authorized to have the information. One must be very careful about giving information out over the telephone to avoid violations of the Health Information Portability and Accountability Act (HIPAA).

On occasion, someone from an insurance company or a news reporter may try to get information by calling the unit on which a patient is staying. Once again, it is very important to not give out any information that could be considered a violation of confidentiality. It is not wise to even acknowledge that fact that the patient is on your floor or unit. Direct all calls of this nature to public relations. The legal department may also need to get involved.

Any other calls should be handled professionally. For example, a nurse may receive calls from other departments requesting clarification of orders. If the order was not clearly written and the nurse did not call the physician, he or she may need to do so in order to answer the other department's questions. Remember to always be courteous and professional with any telephone caller.

Documenting Medication Administration

Institutions have specific guidelines for documenting medication administration and omissions. The dose, date, time, and nurse's initials must be documented for each medication given. Failure to do so could lead to overmedicating a patient. For

TABLE 5-8: GUIDELINES FOR DOCUMENTING A PHONE OR VERBAL ORDER
1. Write the date and time of the order.
2. Document the order as it is being given to you.
3. Read the order back to the physician to verify accuracy.
4. Document "V.O." for a verbal order or "T.O." for a telephone order, followed by the name of the physician, your name, and your status (for example, T.O. Dr. Waitley/R. Mooney, RN).
5. Transcribe the order according to your agency's policy. This order should be confirmed on the phone as follows: "Dr. Waitley, you have ordered Halcion zero-point-five milligrams P.O. for Bertha McGuire. Is that correct?"

(Iyer & Camp, 1999)

example, if a nurse believes the medication has not been given he or she may remedicate the patient. It is wise also to document immediately after giving the medication—not before, in case the patient refuses or is not on the unit at the time the medication should be given.

If medications are not given, the nurse must indicate on the MAR that the dose was omitted and then document in the nursing notes the reason the dose was omitted. For example, if a patient is to receive digoxin and the patient's pulse is only 48, the nurse would hold the dose. If the nurse notifies the physician of these findings, this too should be included in the nursing notes. Following hospital policies regarding documentation of medications is vitally important in preventing double-doses or missed doses of medications.

When giving injections, the site of administration as well as the time and the nurse's initials should be documented. If the patient sustains an injury from an injection, it may be easily traced to the time and site of an injection. Thus, every nurse who gave an injection would not have to be questioned if a lawsuit develops from the injury. A scenario in regard to an incident that could have resulted in a lawsuit is presented in Table 5-9.

All details of intravenous (IV) therapy and blood administration must be properly documented. When an IV line is started, the date, time, size of needle, type of IV solution, rate, site, and ease of insertion should be documented. Likewise the nurse starting the IV line must be included if different from the one documenting the information. Failure to monitor IV fluids or blood administration is a common source of nursing liability. Lack of fluids as well as too-rapid administration could cause damage to neonates, infants, and elderly patients. Observations of IV sites must be clearly documented. This type of documentation is frequently noted on flow sheets. Additional documentation should be provided in the nursing notes if a problem develops with the IV site, for example, infiltration, swelling, or redness.

RULES FOR GOOD CHARTING

Many of the techniques and strategies to improve nursing documentation could be considered rules for good charting. Using common sense in documenting is also a good practice. Institutions require that no blanks be left on any nursing notes or flow sheets. A blank space raises questions, so a line should be drawn through the space. "Not applicable" (NA) can also be written in a space. However, the nurse may want to wait until close to the end of a shift to add "NA" in case a change of condition requires documentation sometime during the shift. It is wise to only document a procedure or medication after administration because the information may be inaccurate if chart-

TABLE 5-9: AVOIDING A LAWSUIT

Nurse Jane gave a patient an injection in the right gluteus muscle, and the patient immediately began complaining of pain and numbness in her right leg. A neurologist was called in to evaluate the patient. When he put pressure on a reddened pinpoint area on the patient's right gluteus, the patient reported the same complaint of pain and numbness. The patient was also experiencing footdrop and difficulty walking. A nurse expert reviewed the record and discovered that Nurse Jane did not document the location of the injection but did write a note in the nursing notes in regard to the patient's comments about the injection. The neurologist's report provided clear evidence that the injection was the probable cause of the patient's problems. The nurse expert advised the institution's legal counsel to settle the case because the injection most likely caused the injury to the patient. The patient's length of stay was extended and the institution absorbed all the cost of the hospitalization and the additional costs of treatment necessary to overcome the patient's problems with footdrop, numbness, and pain in the right leg. Quick action by legal counsel avoided a lawsuit.

ed before delivery of care. Review the rules for good charting presented in Table 5-10.

As stated before, all documentation should be based on fact, not on opinions or assumptions. Negative words may imply that the patient did not receive adequate care. Use the five senses when observing situations and document those findings. It is appropriate to document exact words that the patient, family members, or visitors say. Using quotation marks indicates that the comment is a direct quote.

CHANGES IN THE PATIENT'S CONDITION

One area on which attorneys capitalize is the lack of documented changes in patient conditions (see Table 5-11). In addition, the initial admission assessment is commonly not completed. Therefore, there is no baseline to which comparisons can be made. It is critical that nurses document changes in the patient's status, the interventions taken, what was reported to the primary health care provider, and what changes in orders, if any, were received. Recording the physician's name leaves no question about who was called, what information was given, and what

TABLE 5-10: TWENTY RULES FOR GOOD CHARTING

1. Follow hospital policy regarding notes, and supplement that policy with sound professional judgment.

2. Record only on the proper forms. Enter the date and time before each note.

3. Properly sign each entry.

4. Chart in chronological order, recording on every line so the note cannot be altered.

5. Correct errors appropriately according to your institution's policy; do not erase or use correction fluid or tape.

6. Record information as close as possible to the time you deliver care. Do not document in advance and do not leave important notations until the end of the shift. The higher the situation risk, the greater the effort you should make to record as soon as possible.

7. Write notes only for patients you are caring for; do not let others chart for you.

8. Record what you can see, hear, smell, and touch. Report factual events.

9. Eliminate bias from your notes.

10. Do not generalize. Chart facts.

11. Document the patient's history; it is part of the permanent record.

12. Include written nursing care plans.

13. Include progress notes to deal with problems identified.

14. Use flow sheets to chart routine care.

15. Use a problem-oriented approach or the approach designated by your institution.

16. Ensure continuity. Chart problems as they occur, the interventions used, and any positive or negative change in the patient's status.

17. Record the patient assessment before and after administration of medications.

18. Document all medical visits and consultations, whether in person or by phone.

19. Document discussion of questionable medical orders and the directions the physician gave confirming, canceling, or modifying the orders. Make sure to include the time, the date, and your actions.

20. Prepare a discharge plan and send instructions home with the patient.

(Philpott, 1986)

TABLE 5-11: REASONS TO NOTIFY THE PHYSICIAN
You should call the physician about any changes in the patient's condition or if any of the following situations occurs: <ul><li>Unusual occurrence</li><li>Accidents or falls</li><li>Abnormal test results</li><li>Errors in medications</li><li>Inability to carry out physician orders</li><li>Questions about an order</li><li>Patient failing to take appropriate action</li><li>Usual monitoring test not being ordered (to verify that a monitoring test was not accidentally missed)</li><li>Family concerns and questions</li><li>Information that affects discharge planning.</li></ul>(Yocum, 1993)

actions were to be taken. Good documentation depends on characteristics of effective written communication (see Table 5-12). Remember, attorneys believe that if care was provided but not documented, the care was not given.

TABLE 5-12: EFFECTIVE WRITTEN COMMUNICATION
6/27/03, 9:30 PM. Dr. Smith notified of patient's condition; BP 86/45, P 100, weak and thready; skin pale and clammy. Pt. vomited 300 cc bloody emeses. Order received. See order sheet. Dr. Smith to come in._____J. Jones, RN

PATIENT CONFIDENTIALITY

Confidentiality is the statutorily protected right and duty of health professionals to not disclose information acquired during consultation or care of a patient. Respecting and protecting the privacy and security of health information is a professional obligation, one that all nurses should take seriously. Confidentiality has always been an essential element in nursing practice. However, privacy is not always an absolute right and must be balanced with the safety of the patient and others.

The Code for Nurses defines nurses' responsibility for safeguarding patient rights by protecting information of a confidential nature. The release of confidential information and destruction of medical records are problems with written, paper charts. If someone telephones the unit or otherwise begins asking questions about a patient, the nurse should refer the caller to the public relations department or to the institution's legal counsel. As a safety precaution, it is a good idea to complete an incident form and initiate the chain of command to make everyone aware of the situation.

Faxing patient records is another privacy concern. Fax machines are a quick way to obtain medical records from a physician's office or to send orders, such as sending medication orders to the pharmacy. However, the location of the fax machine is a major privacy concern. It must be in a secure place so that only authorized personnel have access to it. The patient's privacy must be protected when using a fax machine (see Table 5-13).

The consequences of releasing private health information can be severe, including ruined careers, public ridicule, social rejection, and economic devastation of patients and families. A nurse who does not protect patient privacy is liable for civil and criminal penalties for violating patient privacy

TABLE 5-13: PROTECTING PATIENT PRIVACY WHEN USING A FAX MACHINE

- Place all fax machines in secure areas where they can be observed by staff.

- Call the recipient before sending a fax to alert him or her of the fax.

- Add the word "confidential" to the cover sheet.

- Make sure your phone number and fax number appear on the cover sheet.

- Add to the cover sheet that the information should be returned to you if it is accidentally sent to the wrong machine.

- Ask the recipient to call or send a fax message that the document has been received.

- Check the fax machine's internal log to determine where the fax was sent.

- If information went to the wrong number, send another fax to the wrong number asking them to destroy the information.

- When sending a fax, check the number before you dial; check the number on the fax machine display, and recheck it before you push the send button.

(Habel, 2003b; Iyer & Camp, 1999)

rights. The only time confidential information should be disclosed is when withholding the information could cause harm to the patient or to others.

Computerized medical records present yet another challenge with regard to protecting patient privacy and confidentiality. The ability for anyone to retrieve computerized information from a distant site requires strict security measures. The most important privacy safeguard is the appropriate use of each staff member's security code. In addition, computer screens must be placed so that other patients and visitors cannot view them.

Many computer systems are designed for limited access. For example, two levels of entry code may be required or nurses' codes may limit access only to patients on their units. In some places, passwords, keys, badge readers, and biometrics may be required to gain access. Much of this technology is expensive; however, it is becoming more widespread and necessary.

PRIVACY RULE

In 1996, Congress passed HIPAA as a means to improve health care delivery. HIPAA required the U.S. Department of Health and Human Services (DHHS) to adopt national standards to maintain the privacy of patient health information. HIPAA includes standards with compliance dates for:

- electronic transactions, privacy, security, and a unique identifier for employers, and proposed standards for enforcement with civil and criminal penalties

- unique identifiers for health care providers and health plans

- an electronic signature.

(McCartney, 2003)

In August of 2002, DHHS finalized the requirements and mandated that all health care providers implement systems by April 14, 2003, to comply with the new federal regulations. HIPAA preempts state laws controlling confidentiality unless the state law mandates a stricter regulation than HIPAA.

The DHHS Office of Civil Rights enforces the rules. If a patient complains that his or her right to privacy was violated, the health care provider may face a penalty of $100 for each breach of privacy or disclosure of patient information. Penalties of disclosure for commercial advantage, personal gains, or malicious harm may include fines up to $250,000 and 10 years in prison. Complaints should be filed with the DHHS Office for Civil Rights at (800) 368-1019 or www.hhs.gov/ocr/hipaa/ (Basler, 2003).

Health care providers who have direct treatment relationships with patients in any practice setting that conducts electronic transactions for payment or authorization of referrals are governed by these regulations. HIPAA is the first federal law to protect medical privacy. Every doctor's office, clinic, hospital, pharmacy, and health plan is now required to build privacy protections into how they do business. The new rules cover all medical records and other individually identifiable health information used or disclosed by health care providers in any form, whether electronically, on paper, or orally. The privacy rule does allow practices and providers to design their own policies and procedures for compliance, thereby adjusting the system to fit the practice. Figure 5-1 on page 86 presents an example of a well-designed HIPAA document presented to patients.

The HIPAA privacy rule protects patients' medical records and health information by:

- giving patients more control over their health information

- setting boundaries on the use and release of health records

- establishing appropriate safeguards to protect the privacy of health information

- holding violators accountable by imposing civil and criminal penalties for violating patient privacy rights

- striking a balance when public responsibility supports disclosure of some forms of data, for example, to protect public health.

HIPAA now provides for universal access by patients to review and copy their own medical records. Under HIPAA, the patient can also request that corrections or amendments be made to the record and may request restrictions on the uses and disclosures of the information. The patient can request a history of disclosures that have been made to third parties.

The right to request the records of a minor patient resides with the parent or the legal guardian. In the case of divorced parents, the custodial parent has the right to access for a minor child. For a deceased patient, the administrator of the estate may request the medical records (Gudgell, 2003). All patients have privacy rights (see Table 5-14).

TABLE 5-14: PATIENTS' RIGHTS

Under the new medical privacy rule, patients have the following rights:

- to see, copy, and request corrections to their medical record

- to know how health care providers intend to use and disclose their medical information

- to prohibit employers and marketing companies from obtaining medical records without a patient's written authorization

- to request that medical information be sent to an address other than the one officially listed

- to tell hospitals not to release any information about the patient's condition—or even reveal the fact that patient is in the hospital— to relatives and the public.

Note. From "Medical Privacy – What Are Your Rights" by American Association of Retired People (AARP), *Your Health,* (July/August 2003), Washington, DC: Author. Reprinted with permission. Retrieved from www.aarp.org

The privacy rule recognizes that communication about patient care must occur freely and quickly; however, steps to avoid disclosure to a third party must be taken. Health care providers must understand current anxieties about the ways in which health information is handled and learn the rules and apply them. They must also accept that unrestrained access to personal health information is a thing of the past and that skilled information management is among the many tools needed for modern clinical practice. The guidelines in Table 5-15 may help you better understand HIPAA regulations.

Although HIPAA has restricted the release of medical records and patient information, some types of confidential information must be disclosed.

TABLE 5-15: STEPS TO PREVENT ACCIDENTAL DISCLOSURE OF PATIENT INFORMATION

- An office should have a formal confidentiality policy in effect, and patients should receive individual confidentiality statements informing them of the policy.

- Computers must be password protected, and screens must be kept hidden from public view.

- Computers should be surveyed and tracked and kept clear of viruses. A disaster plan should be in place to preserve the confidentiality of information.

- Medical records, lab reports, and faxes should only be accessible to staff .

- Formal, documented procedures should be used to preserve patient confidentiality when transferring information, x-rays, or specimens to or from other areas.

- All faxes and e-mails should have confidentiality statements included and should be transmitted in a secure mode.

- All sign-in sheets, patient schedules, and medical conversations containing confidential information must be concealed from other patients.

- Formal privacy and security procedures should be in place to limit access to confidential information, including office computers and medical charts.

- Before new staff can access patient information, they should be trained in confidentiality and security procedures.

- Patients should sign consent forms for any information transferred.

HIPAA Exceptions:

Although the HIPAA privacy rule generally requires providers to protect the privacy of their patients' health information, restrictions do not apply in the following circumstances:

- disclosures to or requests by a health care provider for treatment purposes

- disclosures to the person who is the subject of the information

- uses or disclosures made pursuant to authorization by a patient

- uses or disclosures required for compliance with HIPAA

- disclosures to DHHS when disclosure of information is required under the privacy rule for enforcement purposes

- uses or disclosures that are required by other law.

(Ramos, 2003; Starr, 2003)

States vary in their requirements; therefore, every nurse must be aware of the requirements of the state in which he or she practices. All states require that specific contagious diseases (such as syphilis and gonorrhea) and cases of acquired immunodeficiency syndrome be reported to the health department. Other mandatory disclosures are presented in Table 5-16. Once again each nurse is advised to check institutional and state laws regarding mandatory reporting.

HIPAA regulations have become a reality. Patient records containing individual, identifiable information must be secured so that they are avail-able only to those who need the information to carry out care, operate a practice, or obtain reimbursement for services rendered to patients. Helpful web sites for obtaining more information about HIPAA are listed in Table 5-17.

CONCLUSION

Documentation must be a conscious effort by the nurse. The suggestions presented in this chapter are intended to improve nurses' documentation. Because the information in a medical chart

TABLE 5-16: MANDATORY DISCLOSURES

1. The reporting of births and deaths, certain wounds, and accidents or other violently incurred injuries

2. Fatalities due to blood transfusions and certain medical devices

3. Workers' compensation claims, seizures, and certain congenital diseases such as the inborn error of metabolism, phenylketonuria.

4. Induced termination of pregnancy

5. Occupational diseases

(Gudgell, 2003, p. 44)

TABLE 5-17: HELPFUL WEB SITES

- U.S. Department of Health and Human Services, Final Rule:

  http://www.aspe.dhhs.gov/adnmsimp/index.shtml

- Code of Federal Regulations:

  http://www.gpoaccess.gov/cfr/index.html

- Office for Civil Rights:

  http://www.hhs.gov/ocr/hipaa

- Health Privacy Project:

  www.healthprivacy.org

(Basler, 2003)

provides the only evidence that appropriate care was provided, good documentation helps defend nurses against lawsuits. By using good charting techniques and strategies, good rules for good charting, characteristics of effective written communication, and guidelines for protecting patient confidentiality, a nurse has documented that quality care was provided to the patient and also protected patient rights. The new HIPAA rules require nurses to be cognizant of protecting patient privacy, providing confidentiality of medical records and patient information, and documenting properly to protect patient confidentiality.

FIGURE 5-1: SAMPLE NOTICE OF PRIVACY PRACTICES (1 OF 7)

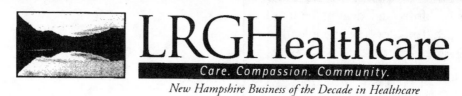

New Hampshire Business of the Decade in Healthcare

Dear Patient:

LRGHealthcare's primary concern is your health and well-being. We understand that information about your health can be very personal. We want you to be confident that we have always been, and continue to be, committed to protecting your privacy.

We want to make sure you are aware of your rights related to the privacy of your healthcare information. The attached document, distributed under the Healthcare Insurance Portability and Accountability Act (HIPAA), outlines those rights and our responsibilities for protecting your privacy.

If you have any questions about HIPAA or this document, please feel free to call our Health Privacy Officer at 524-3211, ext. 3186.

Thank you for choosing LRGHealthcare.

Sincerely,

Tom Clairmont
President and CEO, LRGHealthcare

Lakes Region General Hospital • 80 Highland Street, Laconia, NH 03246 • 603.524.3211 • www.lrgh.org

Lakes Region General Hospital | Franklin Regional Hospital
Affiliated Medical Practices | HealthLink | Occupational Health | Rehabilitation Services
Community Wellness Centers | Adult Day Health Care | Holistic Health

FIGURE 5-1: SAMPLE NOTICE OF PRIVACY PRACTICES (2 OF 7)

LRGHealthcare Notice of Privacy Practices
Effective April 14, 2003

**THIS NOTICE DESCRIBES HOW MEDICAL INFORMATION ABOUT YOU
MAY BE USED AND DISCLOSED AND HOW YOU CAN GET ACCESS TO
THIS INFORMATION.
PLEASE REVIEW IT CAREFULLY.**

Each time you visit your doctor, a hospital, or other healthcare provider, a record of your visit is made. This record usually contains your symptoms, examination or test results, diagnosis, treatment, a plan for any future care or treatment you may need, and often, it also includes payment information. This is called your health or medical record.

Although your medical record is the physical property of the healthcare provider or facility that compiled it, the information it contains belongs to you. For the purpose of this document, we will refer to that information as "Protected Health Information," or "PHI."

I.   YOUR HEALTH INFORMATION RIGHTS

You have the right to:

- Obtain a paper copy of this notice, or upon your request, any future revisions of this notice.

- Request a restriction on certain uses and disclosures of your PHI (though we are not required to agree to any such request).

- Review and get a copy of your PHI.

- Request that we correct or update your PHI if you believe that there is a mistake in your record, or an important piece of information is missing.

- Obtain a list of disclosures of your PHI made after April 14, 2003, for purposes other than treatment, payment, or healthcare operations.

- Receive confidential communications of PHI, choose how we send PHI to you if you prefer an alternate form of communications to traditional mail (ie. Email), and choose if you wish to have your PHI sent to a different address.

- Withdraw your authorization to use or disclose your PHI except to the extent that action has already been taken.

All requests for the release of PHI must be made in writing, and must be signed by the patient or responsible party. Requests may be made through Health Information Management Services of the LRGHealthcare hospital, physician, or practice where you were seen and treated.

FIGURE 5-1: SAMPLE NOTICE OF PRIVACY PRACTICES (3 OF 7)

II. OUR RESPONSIBILITIES REGARDING YOUR PHI

LRGHealthcare is required to:

- Maintain the privacy of your PHI.

- Provide you with a notice as to our legal duties and privacy practices with respect to information we collect and maintain about you, and abide by the terms of this notice.

- In the event that we deny your request to review and get a copy of your PHI, we will inform you in writing and explain whether you can appeal your denial, and if so, how that process works.

- Notify you in writing if we deny your request to change your PHI, which we may do if we find that your medical record is accurate and complete; it was not created by us; your requested change is to information to which we are not required to provide access; or if your requested change is to information that is not part of our records.

- Notify you if we are unable to agree to a requested restriction.

- Accommodate reasonable requests you may have to communicate health information by alternative means or at alternative locations.

We reserve the right to change our privacy practices and to make those changes effective for all protected health information we have collected prior to the date of the change. Should our information practices change, we will make available to you, at your request, a revised paper copy of our Notice of Privacy Practices. Our current Notice of Privacy Practices will always be posted on our website at www.lrgh.org.

III. HOW WE MAY USE AND DISCLOSE YOUR PROTECTED HEALTH INFORMATION

There are many ways in which hospitals and providers use and disclose patient PHI. For some of these uses, we are required to get your written consent; for others, we are not. Below please find a list of how we may use and disclose your PHI:

A. Uses and Disclosures Relating to Treatment, Payment, or Health Care Operations.

We may use and disclose your PHI without your prior consent for the following reasons:

1. **For treatment**. We use your health information to provide you with healthcare treatment and services. For example, information collected by a nurse, physician, or other member of your healthcare team will be recorded in your record and used to determine the course of treatment that should work best for you. Your physician will note in your record his or her expectations of

FIGURE 5-1: SAMPLE NOTICE OF PRIVACY PRACTICES (4 OF 7)

the members of your healthcare team. Members of your healthcare team will then record the actions they took and their observations. In that way, your physician will know how you are responding to treatment.

2. **For payment**. We may use or disclose your health information so that we may bill and receive payment from you, an insurance company, or another third party for the healthcare services you receive from us. For example, a bill may be sent to you or your insurance company. The information sent with the bill may include information that identifies you, as well as your diagnosis, procedures, and supplies used.

3. **For health care operations.** We may use or disclose your health information in order to perform the necessary administrative, educational, quality assurance, and business functions of our facilities. For example, members of the medical staff, the risk management director, or members of the quality improvement team may use information in your health record to assess the care and outcomes in your case and others like it. This information will then be used in an effort to improve the quality and effectiveness of the healthcare and services we provide. While we may also provide your PHI to our accountants, attorneys, consultants, business associates, and others in order to make sure we are complying with the laws and business practices that affect us and to conduct hospital business, we will make every effort to protect the privacy of your PHI.

B. **Uses and Disclosures for Patient Directories and to Persons Assisting in Your Care.**

Generally, we will get your verbal consent before using or disclosing PHI in the following ways. However, in certain situations, such as an emergency, we may use and disclose your PHI for these purposes without your consent.

1. **Patient directories.** We may include your name, location, general condition, and religious affiliation in a patient directory for use by clergy and visitors who ask for you by name.

2. **Disclosures to family, friends or others.** We may provide your PHI, including your condition and status, to a family member, friend, or other person that you indicate is involved in your care or the payment for your health care. In addition, we may disclose health information about you to an entity assisting in a disaster relief effort so that a family member or other person responsible for your care can be notified about your condition, status and location.

FIGURE 5-1: SAMPLE NOTICE OF PRIVACY PRACTICES (5 OF 7)

C. Other Uses and Disclosures that Do Not Require Your Authorization

We may use and disclose your PHI without your consent or authorization for the following reasons:

1. Appointment Reminders: We may use and disclose PHI to contact you as a reminder that you have an appointment for tests or treatment.

2. Treatment Alternatives: We may use and disclose PHI to tell you about or recommend possible treatment options or alternatives that may be of interest to you.

3. Health-Related Benefits and Services: We may use and disclose PHI to tell you about health-related benefits or services that may be of interest to you.

4. Research: We may disclose information to researchers when their research has been approved by an institutional review board that has reviewed the research proposal and established protocols to ensure the privacy of your health information.

5. To Avert a Serious Threat to Health or Safety: We may use and disclose your PHI when necessary to prevent a serious threat to your health and safety or the health and safety of the public or another person. Any such disclosure, however, would be to someone able to help prevent the threat.

6. Organ and Tissue Donation: If you are an organ donor, we may release PHI about you to organizations that handle organ procurement or organ, eye or tissue transplantation or to an organ donation bank, as necessary to facilitate organ or tissue donation and transplantation.

7. Military and Veterans: If you are a member of the armed forces, we may release PHI about you as required by military command authorities.

8. Workers' Compensation: We may release your PHI for workers' compensation or similar programs. These programs provide benefits for work-related injuries or illness. The exception to this occurs when the information is particularly sensitive (such as drug and alcohol testing results and AIDS results): in those cases, a written release is required.

9. Public Health Risks: We may disclose PHI about you for public health activities. These activities generally include the following:

    a. Preventing or controlling disease, injury or disability;
    b. Reporting births and deaths;
    c. Reporting child abuse or neglect;
    d. Reporting reactions to medications or problems with products;
    e. Notifying people of recalls of products they may be using;
    f. Notifying a person who may have been exposed to a disease or may be at risk for contracting or spreading a disease or condition.

FIGURE 5-1: SAMPLE NOTICE OF PRIVACY PRACTICES (6 OF 7)

10. Victims of Abuse, Neglect or Domestic Violence: We may notify the appropriate agencies if we believe a patient has been the victim of abuse, neglect or domestic violence. We will only make such disclosures if you agree or when required or authorized by law.

11. Health Oversight Activities: We may disclose your PHI to a health oversight agency for activities authorized by law. These oversight activities include, for example, audits, investigations, inspections, and licensure.

12. As Required By Law: We will disclose your PHI when required to do so by federal, state or local law. We may also disclose PHI about you in response to a court or administrative order, in response to a subpoena, discovery request, or other lawful process.

13. Law Enforcement: We may release your PHI for law enforcement purposes as required by law or in response to valid legal process. We are also required to report to law enforcement all information regarding the treatment of injuries believed to be caused by a criminal act. The exception to this is in the case of sexual assault victims over the age of 18, unless that patient is also being treated for a life-threatening injury.

14. Coroners, Medical Examiners and Funeral Directors: We may release PHI to a coroner or medical examiner. We may also release PHI to funeral directors as necessary to carry out their duties.

15. National Security and Intelligence Activities: We may release your PHI to authorized federal officials for intelligence, counterintelligence, and other national security activities authorized by law.

16. Protective Services for the President and Others: We may disclose your PHI to authorized federal officials so they may provide protection to the President, other authorized persons or foreign heads of state or conduct special investigations.

17. Inmates: If you are an inmate of a correctional institution or under the custody of a law enforcement official, we may disclose to the institution and its agents health information necessary for your health and the safety of other individuals.

18. Fundraising: We may contact you as part of a LRGHealthcare fundraising effort.

D. All Other Uses and Disclosures
In any situation not described in sections III. A, B, and C above, we will ask for your written consent before using or disclosing any of your PHI.

FIGURE 5-1: SAMPLE NOTICE OF PRIVACY PRACTICES (7 OF 7)

IV. For More Information or to Report a Problem
If you would like more information, or you believe your privacy rights have been violated, please call the LRGHealthcare Privacy Officer at 524-3211, ext. 3186. or write to her attention at LRGHealthcare, 80 Highland Street, Laconia, NH 03246.

You may also file a complaint with the Secretary to the Department of Health and Human Services at:

Office of Civil Rights, U.S.
Department of Health and Human Services
Government Center
J.F. Kennedy Federal Building - Room 1875
Boston, Massachusetts 02203
Phone: (617) 565-1340   Fax: (617) 565-3809
TDD: (617) 565-1343

Government regulations require that healthcare organizations must state in their privacy notices that no retaliation will be taken against any person for filing a complaint. Consistent with this regulation, LRGHealthcare will not take any action that would penalize you for exercising your rights as outlined in this privacy notice. Your choice to file a complaint will not affect your current or future care at LRGHealthcare or any of our providers.

We welcome your feedback.

V2003-1

EXAM QUESTIONS

CHAPTER 5
Questions 28-40

28. Nurse Molly is documenting her patient Sue's response to an intervention to reduce pain. Nurse Molly should

    a. sign someone else's name to the note.

    b. express opinions and assumptions.

    c. follow professional standards for nursing care and documentation.

    d. leave blank lines so the supervisor can come back and add a comment.

29. An appropriate method of documentation would include

    a. documenting that the patient is stupid and does not follow orders.

    b. charting that the primary nurse took an extended lunch break.

    c. not documenting the patient's response to treatments.

    d. recording the patient's statements, identified with quotation marks.

30. From a legal standpoint, if you provide care and do not document it, then the care was

    a. done.

    b. not done.

    c. done by yourself and a coworker.

    d. only half-done.

31. Documentation pitfalls that could lead to legal problems include

    a. documenting what you mean and meaning what you document.

    b. documenting in blue or black ink only, depending on your facility's requirements.

    c. using unapproved abbreviations or shorthand notations when documenting.

    d. naming anyone who becomes involved in the patient's care, including managers and primary care providers.

32. To improve her documentation, Nurse Rose

    a. uses her own set of abbreviations so she can chart more quickly.

    b. describes sizes using fruits as indicators.

    c. signs her name so that no one can read it so she will not get called for deposition.

    d. writes neatly and legibly, using ink to document, date, and time all entries.

33. To document contact with a physician, Nurse Carol should write

    a. "physician telephoned."

    b. "physician called."

    c. "called physician; left message with answering service."

    d. "physician never returned call, so called again."

34. Rules for good charting include

    a. leave no blanks, eliminate bias, and do not generalize.

    b. chart as thoughts come to you, leave flow charts with blank areas, and use white out.

    c. leave charting until tomorrow, record on every other line, and document in advance.

    d. ensure continuity, send the patient home without instructions, and do not question physician orders.

35. The physician should be notified if

    a. the patient responds appropriately to the treatment given.

    b. there was no inability to carry out the order and it was done on time.

    c. family members left several telephone numbers where they could be reached.

    d. the lab report indicates abnormal findings.

36. Communication, the giving or exchanging of information through verbal or written means

    a. is a one-way process.

    b. is vague and ambiguous so it may be interpreted correctly.

    c. should contain appropriate language and terminology.

    d. relays no facts and is given with judgments and assumptions.

37. Rose, RN, needs to fax a patient's medical record to another department. To protect the patient's privacy, she should

    a. ask the recipient to call or send a fax message that the document has been received.

    b. send the fax without a confidential cover sheet.

    c. use the fax machine in the lobby of the patient waiting room.

    d. place the information on the unit secretary's desk and ask her to fax it when she has time.

38. Patient confidentiality includes

    a. the right and duty of health professionals to respect and protect patient privacy.

    b. relaying information over the telephone to an inquiring caller.

    c. sending information via fax to an unsecured receiver.

    d. talking in the elevator to another nurse about the HIV status of a patient.

39. HIPAA was enacted to

    a. allow physician office staff to sell lists of patients' names with cardiac problems to drug companies.

    b. allow staff to list all patients' names with room numbers on an easily accessible display board.

    c. provide individuals with no legal access to their own records.

    d. safeguard individual privacy and discourage misuse of patient records.

40. If a patient believes his or her right to privacy was violated, the health care provider may

    a. reassure the patient it will not happen again.

    b. release information about the patient to a drug company for research.

    c. be fined for each breach of privacy or disclosure of patient information.

    d. call out the patient's full name and address when bringing the patient back to an examination room.

CHAPTER 6

WHAT SHOULD BE DOCUMENTED

CHAPTER OBJECTIVE

After completing this chapter, the reader will be able to use the nursing process to improve sound documentation.

LEARNING OBJECTIVES

After studying this chapter, the reader will be able to

1. use assessment to make accurate nursing diagnoses and set priorities.

2. indicate a plan for interventions.

3. identify three suggestions for developing care plans.

4. indicate two essential features of documenting patient education and discharge planning.

5. specify three ways that interventions promote health care.

6. select the appropriate documentation for evaluation of nursing care provided.

INTRODUCTION

Nursing documentation must be both comprehensive and flexible enough to retrieve critical data. In order to maintain quality and continuity of care, it must also reflect current clinical practice guidelines and track patient outcomes. A well-documented patient record is hard evidence with which nurses can successfully defend themselves against legal action. In contrast, a poorly documented patient record can serve as powerful evidence in support of a suit, even when the accusations are trivial. When in doubt, it is safe to document everything as long as you are documenting facts and not charting any inferences, opinions, or hearsay. This chapter provides information about using the nursing process to improve nursing documentation, with hard evidence for sound defense.

ASSESSMENT

The initial assessment helps establish a baseline for all future assessments and should be considered the first step in patient care. Facilities may use a variety of databases to identify each patient's physical, psychological, and social needs. Many institutions use assessment forms designed as standardized flow sheets or checklists that include data pertinent to patients in specific settings. The database should focus on common problems seen in the specific setting, such as skin care for elderly or paraplegic patients, prenatal concerns for obstetric patients, and developmental milestones for pediatric patients.

Assessment charting should specifically document, in either checklist or narrative form, what has been observed, inspected, palpated, auscultated, or percussed, plus whatever the patient has disclosed about his or her personal history and current condition. The time frame for completing the initial database is defined by institutional policy and may vary by clinical area. Joint Commission on Accreditation of Healthcare Organizations (JCAHO) policies indicate that a patient's history, physical examination, nursing assessment conducted by a registered nurse (RN), and any other screening assessments must be completed within 24 hours of admission. This standard applies to all days of the week and includes holidays.

Data collected during the initial assessment is important for establishing the patient's priority needs and for identifying nursing diagnoses or problems. Short- and long-term plans can be established and patient educational needs identified. The charting tips in Table 6-1 can be used to assist in completing the initial assessment.

During the initial assessment, the nurse should discuss and document factors that may contribute to patient injury, such as falls, pressure ulcers, suicidal or violent tendencies, physical or emotional abuse, substance abuse, and ability to provide self-care following discharge. Previous hospital admissions and medical problems must also be documented. The documentation of self-care abilities provides information about the patient's and significant others' involvement in discharge planning.

Most institutions now require that patients have advance directives — living wills and power of attorney documents. The 1990 federal Patient Self-Determination Act requires hospitals, long-term care facilities, home health providers, hospice, and other health care providers to present, at admission, information about patient rights. Questioning

TABLE 6-1: CHARTING INITIAL ASSESSMENT

- Describe physical assessment findings in detail.
- Write another note if necessary to fully describe findings if the information is too much for the form.
- Describe what is seen, heard, felt, and smelled or comments the patient makes.
- Use the PQRST mnemonic to gather data about patient problems or pain.

  P = Provocative/palliative. What does the patient do to cause, bring on, or relieve the problem pain?

  Q = Quality/quantity. What does the problem feel, look, or sound like? How much is present?

  R = Region/radiation. Take one finger and point to the pain. Does the pain spread (radiate) to other parts of the body?

  S = Severity. Use a 10-point scale (1 = little or none to 10 = worst) to describe the pain. How does it affect the patient's activities? Is it sharp or dull?

  T = Timing. When does the pain/problem begin? Is it worse during a specific time of day? How often does it occur? Is it gradual or sudden?

- Use the patient's own words to describe the reason for hospitalization.
- Indicate symptoms the patient denies as well as negative physical findings.
- Indicate the reason the patient cannot respond or indicate who provided the information.
- Include information on developmental levels on pediatric forms.
- Document disposition of valuables and personal items. Encourage a family member to take the patient's personal belongings home.
- Identify and record drug and food allergies and the patient's reactions.
- Keep in mind that although other health care providers may document some of the assessment, such as vital signs, the RN is responsible for completing the initial physical assessment.
- Document whether the patient has an advance directive.

(Eggland, 1995; Iyer & Camp, 1999; Lewis, 2002)

patients on admission about advance directives is common practice. The information should be provided, kept on file, and updated. Documentation of advance directives and where they can be found should be made.

In many cases, patients do not have advance directives. In such a case, the nurse should encourage the patient to talk with family members about his or her desires. A statement can be handwritten by the patient and placed in the patient's chart. An advance directive becomes effective when an institution has a copy and the attending health care provider determines that the patient lacks decision-making ability.

Patient and family education is an area that infrequently appears in nursing notes. Nursing care plans or checklists that include educational needs have increased nursing documentation of patient education. The initial assessment of educational needs and subsequent encounters help keep educational needs up-to-date, and the teaching that has occurred can then be documented.

Documentation of the initial assessment is only the beginning. Frequent reassessments provide continual updates that allow nurses and other healthcare providers to evaluate the patient's progress. The frequency of nursing reassessment depends on patient needs and institutional and reimbursement requirements. Many institutions require nurses to document reassessment every 8 hours; in some extended-care facilities, this documentation is required every 24 hours. Reassessment occurs more frequently if the patient's condition requires it. Reassessment should include observations and physical findings as well as statements made by the patient or family members. Learning needs may also change and require reassessment. Reassessment of key information at appropriate intervals demonstrates proper use of the nursing process.

NURSING DIAGNOSIS AND PLANNING

Documentation of planned care becomes the next part of the patient's record. The planning phase of the nursing process involves formulating nursing diagnoses, establishing desired patient outcomes, selecting appropriate interventions, and documenting the plan of care. After gathering and analyzing the assessment data, the nurse formulates nursing diagnoses based on problems defined by the North American Nursing Diagnosis Association or the institution's adopted problem list.

During the planning phase, identification and documentation of expected patient outcomes is necessary. This provides information for evaluating the patient's progress. Outcomes should be patient-oriented, realistic, measurable, observable, clear, and concise. They should be established collaboratively with the patient and designated with a time frame for meeting the goal. Planning should be deliberate and thoughtful to be effective. It should include discharge and educational needs to allow the patient to manage after discharge. Planning patient care helps nurses provide quality care.

DOCUMENTING INTERVENTIONS

The next step is to determine and document interventions. Nursing interventions are those actions taken to assist the patient moving from the present level of health to that planned in the expected outcomes. They include any direct care, treatment, or procedure that a nurse performs to or on behalf of a patient. Documenting interventions and outcomes is a vital link between planning and evaluating care. The documentation should be timely, chronological, consistent, and complete.

Interventions should be documented specifically enough to clearly describe what was done. Interventions should describe the type of care given, the frequency with which the intervention was carried out, and who provided the care. The tips presented in Table 6-2 for documenting interventions may be helpful.

TABLE 6-2: DOCUMENTING INTERVENTIONS
• Interventions should be generated from nursing diagnoses.
• Interventions should be specific and clearly describe facts.
• Interventions should be individualized and mutually developed with the patient.
• Interventions should be realistic and based on the patient's length of stay, resources available, and expected outcomes.
• All interventions must be dated and signed or initialed to establish professional accountability.
(Eggland, 1995; Iyer & Camp, 1999)

Discharge planning should be started on admission. If discharge needs are not addressed, the patient may remain in the hospital and receive care longer than necessary. The patient could also be discharged too early and not receive adequate education or preparation if discharge planning has not been done. A form may be developed or some area designated on the nursing care plan to help remind health care providers to document discharge planning.

Once educational needs have been identified, the nurse prioritizes these needs. Documentation of the teaching provided is critical but is often omitted in nurses' notes. JCAHO emphasizes patient teaching; however, it does not require formal teaching plans. JCAHO does require documentation of teaching, and teaching plans can be helpful with this requirement.

A written teaching plan defines outcomes and identifies who should provide the teaching. Standardized teaching forms may be used for patients with complex educational needs, such as those with diabetes or heart disease. The teaching plan should provide in-depth information that can

be used for teaching. A patient education record provides the nurse with a standard form on which to document the outcomes of teaching.

Some institutions document teaching outcomes as met, partially met, or not met, whereas others may use such comments as content presented or demonstrated, content reviewed, return demonstration, and outcome achieved. The achieved status should be dated. When possible, teaching should be supplemented with written materials to which the patient may refer at a later date. Document all educational material and instructions given to a patient.

When interventions are documented, this indicates that some action by the nurse has been implemented, thus providing evidence of the care given. This documentation facilitates reimbursement and promotes continuity of care. Flow sheets or any of the documentation methods discussed in Chapter 3 can be used to chart nursing interventions.

Documenting implementation of the nursing process provides a clear, chronological description of patient care. Specific documentation of interventions and the patient's response to those interventions provides the best defense if malpractice litigation should occur.

DOCUMENTING EVALUATION

Follow-up, or evaluation, is a final step in the nursing process that should be clearly documented. Evaluation flows from the outcomes defined in the plan of care. It is an expectation of nursing care that the interventions carried out will be evaluated to see if they have met the patient's needs. Both the American Nurses Association and JCAHO require nurses to document a patient's response to an intervention and any revisions to the nursing diagnosis, outcomes, or plan of care that are needed. Reasons for documenting the evaluation of interventions are to determine the results of specific care and treatment of patients and their families, to improve the effectiveness of care, and to help institutions better understand and improve their own systems.

Evaluation can be formative (occurring on a periodic basis) or summative (occurring at the end of a specified time). Periodic evaluation depends on institutional policies, regulatory standards, the health care setting, the charting system, standards of care, nursing diagnoses, outcome time frames, and nursing interventions.

Summative evaluations usually occur at the time of patient transfer or discharge. Patient needs should be evaluated so that another agency, the patient, or family members will be able to continue care. Discharge summaries document the care provided and indicate that patient education has been completed.

The evaluation of outcomes is documented on flow sheets, progress notes, and discharge summaries. Typical evaluation documentation would address the items listed in Table 6-3.

TABLE 6-3: EVALUATION DOCUMENTATION
• Progress toward achieving outcomes
• Response to pain or other as-needed medications
• Response to change of activity
• Tolerance of treatments or position changes
• Ability to perform activities of daily living
• Responses to diet and changes in diet
(Iyer & Camp, 1999)

Nurses must evaluate their teaching to make sure patients will be able to continue with proper care at home. Specific documentation of teaching should also include evaluation of the teaching. Several methods can be used to evaluate teaching: return demonstration, written tests, diaries, discussions, observations, questionnaires, and simulations.

The scope of patient education documentation has expanded to include documenting that the patient, family, or both understand the teaching that was given to them. Giving a patient an instruction sheet may reinforce what was taught. Written information provides reminders to facilitate follow-up and continuity of care.

CONCLUSION

Using the nursing process to improve documentation is no guarantee against legal action. It can, however, provide evidence to safeguard against patients who threaten legal action, function as a safety net when allegations are made, and decrease liability losses when suits are successful. Conscientious and thorough documentation improves and supports outstanding quality of care. In this chapter, information was presented to improve nursing documentation during assessment, establishment of nursing diagnoses and planning, implementation of interventions, and evaluation. Emphasis on education, in all phases of the nursing process, was included.

Note: Effective January 2006, the Joint Commission on Accreditation of Healthcare Organizations (JCAHO) requires hospitals and other health care organizations to document each patient's language and communication needs, as applicable, in the patient's medical record, along with other key patient information.

EXAM QUESTIONS

CHAPTER 6
Questions 41-46

41. An RN must complete the initial patient assessment within

    a. the first hour after admission.

    b. 24 hours of admission.

    c. the time of the patient's stay.

    d. the moments prior to discharge from the institution.

42. The planning phase of the nursing process involves

    a. asking the nursing assistant to complete the assessment.

    b. asking the patient's family to hire evening sitters.

    c. leaving the plan of care for another nurse to document.

    d. establishing outcomes and interventions.

43. Care plans are developed for a patient based on

    a. initial assessment, patient needs, and expected patient outcomes.

    b. type of surgery, age of patient, and time of year.

    c. history of disease process, physicians' schedules, and nurses' workloads.

    d. staff mix, patient's knowledge, and patient's needs.

44. Discharge planning and patient education begin

    a. at discharge.

    b. 1 hour before discharge.

    c. at the time of admission.

    d. whenever the nurse has time.

45. Interventions promote good health care by being

    a. generated from nurses' needs.

    b. guided by the nurses' time schedule.

    c. undated and unsigned.

    d. realistic and based on length of stay.

46. The *best* example of appropriate documentation for evaluation of the patient's response to nursing care provided is

    a. "Pt reports that pain is a '2'- out of '10'(10 being worst) on the pain scale."

    b. "Pt. received Demerol 50mg Q4hrs for post op abdominal pain."

    c. "Pt. is lazy and uncooperative and refused his respiratory treatment today."

    d. "Patient's pressure ulcer on his bottom is now the size of a pea."

CHAPTER 7

LEGAL ASPECTS OF CHARTING

CHAPTER OBJECTIVE

After completing this chapter, the reader will be able to discuss charting practices that decrease liability risk.

LEARNING OBJECTIVES

After reading this chapter, the reader will be able to

1. indicate how good documentation is one of the best ways to keep a nurse out of court.

2. specify two recommendations to create a comprehensive and defensive medical record.

3. distinguish why it is legally important for nurses to be familiar with the documentation standards in their area.

4. identify the proper techniques of documentation to meet patients' clinical and safety needs and all legal requirements, while avoiding pitfalls of documentation.

INTRODUCTION

There are no stereotypical characteristics about a patient who may file a lawsuit. Unfortunately, in the environment in which nurses practice today, they must assume that any patient may file a lawsuit.

Because lawsuits are filed months to years after an incident, an accurate record of each patient encounter may help the nurse recall a situation. It is impossible to recall every patient encounter; however, a well-documented patient medical record may help a nurse remember the patient and the situation in question. Therefore, it is important to document everything, no matter how trivial the situation may appear at the time. This chapter addresses charting practices to decrease liability risk, the best ways to keep a nurse out of court, recommendations for creating a comprehensive and defensive medical record, and the nurse's role in understanding documentation standards. Legal cases will be used to help demonstrate documentation concerns.

CHARTING PRACTICES TO DECREASE LIABILITY

A legible, accurate medical record is an important document that communicates significant patient information to numerous health care providers. If a lawsuit occurs, the medical record may become the basis for the plaintiff's case or the defense of the nurse, other health care provider, or institution. The medical record is an important piece of evidence in the evaluation of a nursing or medical malpractice claim. It is necessary that health care institutions maintain complete, accurate, and timely medical records. The importance of medical records as evidence in legal proceedings cannot be overemphasized. The medical record is used to reconstruct events involved with any alleged negligence in the care of the patient. Nurses and other health care providers are permitted to review a patient's chart prior to giving a deposition or going to trial.

Medical records are admitted as evidence in court. The court assumes that the information is accurate, that it was recorded at the time the event took place, and that it was not recorded in anticipation of specific legal proceedings. Whatever the situation, the medical record must be complete, accurate, and timely. If the plaintiff can show the record is inaccurate, incomplete, or made long after an event, its credibility as evidence is diminished.

Some basic measures can be taken to improve accuracy and decrease liability. As stated before, documentation should be based on fact, not opinions or assumptions. When charting, avoid words that present a negative attitude or connotation. A jury could interpret the negative words as substandard care or as indicators of a nurse's dislike for a patient. Instead of using negative words, clearly describe the patient and the situation. Words to avoid in documentation are presented in Table 7-1.

TABLE 7-1: WORDS TO AVOID IN DOCUMENTATION	
Complainer	Aggressive
Abusive	Crazy
Drunk	Obnoxious
Lazy	Nasty
Spoiled	Disagreeable
Problem patient	Bad
Difficult	Failed
Hostile	Excessive
Rude	Sufficient
Demanding	Prolonged
(Iyer & Camp, 1999; Tiller, 1999)	

One of the goals when documenting is to provide an accurate report of a patient's care, health status, and stay in an institution. Therefore, information must be complete, unbiased, legible, and understandable today and in the unspecified future. The chart should contain descriptive, objective information. Chart what you see, hear, feel, and smell, not what you suppose, infer, conclude, or assume. Documentation may contain subjective information, but that information must be supported by documented facts. It is always better to document clear facts (see Table 7-2).

TABLE 7-2: DOCUMENTING CLEAR FACTS
Subjective:
"Patient appears restless."
Objective:
"Patient tossing and turning in bed."
(Tiller, 1994)

For example, in Table 7-2, what does "patient appears restless" mean? This is not a description; it is a vague and ambiguous conclusion. An entry like this is not very helpful and may even be dangerous. At a trial, which usually takes place years after an incident, such an entry could create a damaging exchange between a nurse and the plaintiff's attorney, such as in Table 7-3.

TABLE 7-3: QUESTIONING AT TRIAL	
Attorney:	"What made you think she was restless?"
Nurse:	"I cannot remember."
Attorney:	"You cannot remember? This is important. We are trying to reconstruct the events surrounding the incident. What did you actually observe?"
Nurse:	"I cannot recall."
(Tiller, 1999)	

"I cannot remember" is an acceptable answer; however, it does not provide the jury much of a choice because the plaintiff always says he or she can remember minute details. Even if you do remember, the plaintiff's attorney can discredit your testimony. If you had written, "patient is tossing and turning in bed," the attorney could not attack your entry or your credibility.

Likewise, using the word "appears" does not clarify the facts. The jury may think you are hedging. If you chart what you see, feel, hear, or smell, you protect yourself and provide an accurate, complete description of the incident. Review Table 7-4 for common charting errors.

TABLE 7-4: FIVE ERRORS THAT COMMONLY APPEAR IN CHARTS THAT COME TO LITIGATION
1. Incomplete initial history and physical
2. Failure to observe and take appropriate action
3. Failure to communicate changes in a patient's condition
4. Incomplete or inadequate documentation
5. Failure to use or interpret monitoring appropriately
(Tiller, 1999)

When reviewing medical records, one would be amazed at the number of times initial history and physical forms are not completed. Without the initial assessment, there is no baseline data from which comparisons can be made. If the initial history and physical are incomplete, the basic plan of care will prove useless and unanticipated problems may arise. Therefore, changes in the patient's status have no basis for comparison. Nurses must be aware that a key legal expectation of a professional nurse is the ability to foresee harm. A thorough admission assessment is a solid source of information that proves the nurse covered all bases.

Nursing knowledge and judgment are crucial. Although the physician is responsible for medical management, it is the nurse who must assess the patient's immediate status and recognize situations that require interventions. All interventions, whether simple or complex, are viewed as legally significant.

A nurse may make observations and take appropriate actions; however, if they were not document-ed, there is no way to determine what observation was made or what care was provided. It is important to document all observations and interventions. If documentation is complete, the plaintiff's attorney cannot question what was done.

As a registered nurse, you are legally accountable for your practice. Competence is judged against a standard of usual practice in a similar situation using the knowledge and skills of the profession. The best defense against becoming involved in a malpractice suit is to maintain clinical skills and practice according to the standard of care.

One area that plaintiffs' attorneys capitalize on is failure to notify physicians or other health care providers in a timely manner. Nurses are legally responsible for keeping physicians and other health care providers informed of changes in patients' conditions. A nurse may indeed have telephoned the physician; however, without charting the telephone call and what the physician was told, there is no evidence that the call was made.

After recognizing that a physician's intervention is necessary, the nurse must provide the physician with enough specific information to make a reasonable medical judgment. The nurse must communicate expectations; if the nurse believes the physician is needed on the unit, he or she must say so. Do not expect a physician to be able to read your mind.

In addition to being timely, the call to the physician must be effective. "Timely" means calling when appropriate, and "effective" means that all necessary information has been gathered and clearly relayed to the physician. The example in Table 7-5 is timely; however, it is an ineffective telephone conversation between a nurse and a physician. The situation in Table 7-5 makes the nurse look ridiculous, lowering her credibility in future interactions with the physician. Anything less than timely, clear, and complete information increases the liability of the nurse. If reconstructed properly, the telephone conversation in Table 7-5 might proceed as in Table 7-6.

TABLE 7-5: TIMELY BUT INEFFECTIVE TELEPHONE CONVERSATION

Nurse: Dr. Jones, this is nurse Sue Smith at General Hospital in labor and delivery. Your patient Mrs. Jarvis is 5 cms dilated and her blood pressure suddenly shot up to 150/102.

Doctor: What are her reflexes?

Nurse: They were 2+ on admission...

Doctor: Well, what are they now?

Nurse: Well, I was so concerned about the blood pressure I have not taken them yet. Do you want to hold on while I do?

Doctor: No, never mind. What is the urine protein running?

Nurse: It was trace on admission and she has not voided since. Do you want me to get her to try?

(Tiller, 1994)

TABLE 7-6: RECONSTRUCTED TELEPHONE CONVERSATION

Nurse: Dr. Jones, this is nurse Sue Smith at General Hospital's labor and delivery. Your patient, Mrs. Jarvis is 5 cms dilated and her blood pressure suddenly shot up to 150/102. The blood pressure has previously been 100/76 to 118/84. I checked her reflexes and they are 4+ with 2 beats of clonus. Her urine was trace for protein on admission but is now 2+. She said her vision is blurred. The fetal heart rate is basing at 140 bpm with adequate variability and no decelerations.

Doctor: Start magnesium sulfate per protocol, and I'll be over to evaluate her.

Nurse: Dr. Jones, please let me read Mrs. Jarvis' order back to you. "Start Magnesium sulfate per protocol and you are coming in." Thanks.

(Tiller, 1994)

In this example, the physician received the information needed to develop a plan of medical management. There was no need to "fish" for information. Likewise, the nurse saved time by having all the information necessary and knowing what was needed.

Inadequate and incomplete documentation is another area that plaintiffs' attorneys emphasize. Years later, if a case comes to litigation, the medical record is the only valid record of events. Careful, defensive charting is the only evidence that a nurse provided quality care, acted appropriately, and notified the physician as soon and as clearly as possible.

A bad chart can make a good nurse look bad. The medical record must show that standards of care were met and that the nurse followed the policies and procedures of the institution. A complete and adequate chart defends itself and those who wrote it. The nurse must document not only an awareness of a problem but also appropriate actions and the resolution. Remember, if it was not documented, it was not done.

Lastly, failure to use and interpret monitoring appropriately is a major concern, especially fetal monitoring in obstetric cases. Nurses can and should document observations using the appropriate terminology for deviations in fetal heart tones (early, late, and variable decelerations). Misinterpretation of fetal monitor strips is a common problem. The nurse should document completely the interventions taken and the telephone call made to the physician. The fetal monitoring mode (external or internal) should also be charted. Another serious omission is neglecting to continue fetal monitoring in the delivery room. If monitoring is not continued as indicated, the nurse is practicing below the standard of care, and thereby increasing liability. Awareness of the risks is an important beginning, but developing and using strategies to deal with risks is a dynamic process that should become part of every nurse's practice.

DOCUMENTING TO AVOID COURT

Malpractice is defined as "professional misconduct, improper discharge of professional duties, or failure to meet the standard of care of a professional that results in harm to another" (Pozgar, 2002, p. 459). Negligence is described as the "omission or commission of an act that a reasonably prudent person would or would not do under given circumstances. It is a form of heedlessness or carelessness that constitutes a departure from the standard of care generally imposed on members of society" (Pozgar, 2002, p. 459). In order for a nurse to avoid charges of malpractice or negligence, documentation must be timely, complete, and accurate.

By applying the principles addressed here and in previous chapters, nurses can improve documentation and reduce their chances of ending up in court. Malpractice may be avoided if proactive actions are taken (see Table 7-7).

TABLE 7-7: PROACTIVE NURSING ACTIONS
Respond to the patient
Educate the patient
Comply with the standards of care
• Supervise care
• Adhere to the nursing process
• Document
• Follow-up
(Hall & Hall, 2001, p. 148)

The best defense against being included in a lawsuit is to practice non-negligently. One vital defense against allegations of any negligent conduct is the inability of the plaintiff to prove the elements of the cause of action: duty, breach of duty, proximate cause, and injuries or damages. These elements do not prohibit a case from being filed; however, they can prohibit a verdict against the defendant.

The plaintiff's attorney has to prove that there was a duty owed to the client; that the nurse, doctor, or institution breached that duty; that an injury or damage in fact occurred; and that the breach caused the alleged injury or damage. If the plaintiff cannot prove that all four elements occurred, the plaintiff is unlikely to have a favorable verdict returned. To prove negligent behavior requires proving that the defendant placed the injured party in danger of a recognized risk and then pursued unreasonable conduct.

In the past, plaintiffs' attorneys have sued for negligent acts by nurses using one of four legal theories: *respondeat superior*, "captain of the ship," borrowed servant, and ordinary negligence. In the first three theories, someone other than the nurse is held responsible for the nurse's actions, such as the physician, nursing supervisor, or hospital.

Under *respondeat superior*, or "let the superior answer," the employer is held responsible for the legal consequences of the acts of a nurse or other employee acting within the scope of employment. The basic idea behind this theory comes from the concept that the employer possesses the right to control the acts of the employee. In other words, the hospital is held responsible for the actions of the nurse. Likewise, the nursing supervisor can be held responsible for staff nurses' actions. Usually, a plaintiff files suit against both the nurse and the institution. One reason for doing this is because the institution usually has more money to cover a judgment.

In the past the physician was held responsible for all actions of nurses. This is no longer the case today, however, the "captain of the ship" rule still applies in some situations. It holds a chief surgeon to be the one who controls, and is therefore responsible for, all individuals in the operating room. Basically, the employees in the operating suite become the surgeon's temporary employees, and any injury during the course of a surgery becomes the vicarious responsibility of the chief surgeon.

The *borrowed servant* approach is a special application of the *respondeat superior* theory. This theory applies when an employer, such as a hospital, sends one or more of its employees to work for a separate, unaffiliated organization. The sending or loaning employer is often referred to as the general employer and the receiving or borrowing employer is the special employer. The employee, even though he or she remains the servant of the general employer, is directly under the supervision of the special employer. Therefore, the general employer is usually not liable for injury or negligence caused by the servant while in the services of the special employer. Liability is imposed upon the employer who is in the best position to prevent the injury. This is very similar to the captain of the ship doctrine.

According to borrowed servant, a nurse or other employee who is working for a hospital, can also be working for a staff physician for a particular purpose. The nurse is responsible for his or her own actions, however, the hospital would also be held responsible. Under certain circumstances, the physician who borrows the servant may also be responsible for the nurse's negligence.

With ordinary negligence, nurses are sued personally, and the allegedly negligent conduct is compared with the conduct of a reasonably prudent person, not a reasonably prudent nurse. Ordinary negligence is conduct that involves undue risk of harm to someone. For example, if an orderly sees water on the floor but fails to wipe it up resulting in a patient fall, the orderly would be held responsible for damages suffered by the patient. Professional negligence is different from ordinary negligence because professionals are held to professional standards of care.

Today, the captain of the ship and borrowed servant theories still apply in the operating room. Nurses are held liable for malpractice or professional negligence in all other settings. Nurses' increased responsibilities and the fact that many nurses carry personal malpractice insurance makes them financially attractive to plaintiffs. However, a plaintiff does not inquire if a nurse has his or her own private policy, and just because a nurse carries a personal policy does not mean that he or she is more likely to be sued. Further discussion about malpractice insurance is found in chapter 8.

The best way for a nurse to secure self-protection is to make sure that documentation covers all aspects of the nursing process and any changes in the patient condition. Timely and complete reporting to the physician and responses from the physician must be documented as well. Good nursing practice is both moral and legal. Malpractice law enforces the moral value to do no harm to the patient. The law represents the minimum standard of nursing practice. The standards of good nursing practice include assessment, planning, implementation, and evaluation.

RECOMMENDATIONS FOR CREATING A COMPREHENSIVE AND DEFENSIVE MEDICAL RECORD

It has been rumored that a national standardized medical record or chart format may be developed in the future. Until that happens, it is important for each nurse to create a comprehensive and defensive medical record.

Inherent in a nurse's documentation responsibility — to ensure objective, timely, comprehensive, relevant, and legible documentation of patient care — is the need to ensure that the ethical values of professional practice are understood and fulfilled. Such values include protecting confidentiality, ensuring informed consent, and respecting the values and rights of individual patients.

Complete and proper medical record documentation is important because it permanently reflects the nursing care given and provides proof of meeting professional standards. Likewise, appropriate documentation provides information about the progress of services, care, and monitoring provided to the patient. The patient's medical record serves as a primary communication format to direct and coordinate services between the many health care providers involved with the patient's care. An institution's ability to adequately defend itself in the event of a lawsuit largely rests on the extent of the documentation regarding an incident in question. Steps that can be taken to monitor and help improve documentation are listed in Table 7-8.

Nurses who provide comprehensive and defensive medical records use the nursing process and the required institutional documentation method to record care provided, patient education, discharge planning, interventions, reactions, and evaluation of patient outcomes. To re-emphasize: always document, no matter how trivial it may seem; If it was not documented, it was not done! The more completely and accurately the nurse documents in the

medical record, the more helpful the medical record will be if litigation should occur. As a reminder, review Table 7-9 for recommendations about creating a comprehensive and defensive medical record.

NURSES' ROLE IN UNDERSTANDING DOCUMENTATION STANDARDS

Health care institutions are required to maintain medical records for their patients in accordance with accepted professional standards and practice. The requirements for these records are commonly set forth within each state's public health laws. Medical records are to be complete and must contain all relevant information about the daily care and treatment of a patient. As stated before, medical records must be complete, accurate, current, readily accessible, and organized systematically so as to defend themselves.

TABLE 7-8: DOCUMENTATION CHECKLIST

- During orientation and as needed, provide nurses with in-service training about the importance of the medical record and maintain documentation standards.

- Routinely complete random record reviews and audits to assure compliance.

- Address documentation deficiencies through individual counseling or further staff training.

- Track documentation of incidents involving patients for consistent clinical observations, nursing interventions, patient response to nursing care, and appropriate periodic re-evaluation following an incident.

- Never reference incident reports in a patient's medical record to limit discoverability by a plaintiff's attorney and to retain its privileged internal status (depending on jurisdiction).

- Document in a timely manner all family and physician notification of any incident, change in condition, alteration of treatments, or room change regarding the patient.

- Document and keep all patient appointments and referrals in the patient's record.

- Send a physician consultation form with each patient to appointments in order to obtain recommended care and treatment information based on the physician's assessment. When this form is returned with the patient, immediately transfer the information in it to the patient's record and care plan, if indicated, and place the consultation form in the patient's chart.

- Immediately notify the patient's physician of any abnormal test results and the date, the time, and to whom the results were given. Document the name and title of the staff member relaying the results in the record.

- To protect the facility against liability, formally document the exchange of all information with a signature obtained from the patient or the individual with health care decision-making power.

(GuideOne Insurance, 2004)

TABLE 7-9: GENERAL DOCUMENTATION GUIDELINES

- Contents of a medical record must meet all regulatory, accrediting, and professional organization standards. Common requirements specific to nursing documentation include but are not limited to nursing assessment and care provided, informed consent for any and all procedures, teaching provided either to the patient directly or to the family, and response and reactions to teaching recorded.

- Use black or blue permanent ink for entries.

- Date, time, and sign all entries. Use first initial, last name, and title. Full signature and title must be on file in the institution.

- Entries are to be legible, with no blank spaces left on a line or in any area of the documentation. If space is left on a line, draw a line through the space to the end of the line. For large areas not used on a form or page, use diagonal lines to mark through the area.

- If an error is made, draw a line through the error, write "error," and then initial and date the line. Do not attempt to erase, obliterate, or "white out" the error.

- Entries are to be factual, complete, and accurate and should contain observations, clinical signs and symptoms, patient quotes when applicable, nursing interventions, and patient reactions. Do not give opinions, make assumptions, or enter vague, meaningless statements (for example, "is a good parent"). Be specific.

- Use correct grammar, spelling, and punctuation.

- Place the patient's name and other identifying information on each medical record page.

- Be sure to use only those abbreviations approved by your institution.

- Always record a patient's noncooperative or noncompliant behavior.

- Never document for someone else or sign another nurse's name in any portion of the medical record.

- Documentation should occur as soon after the care is given as possible. Note problems as they occur, resolutions used, and changes in the patient's status.

- When leaving messages, document the time, name, and title of the person taking the message as well as the telephone number you called.

- Record patient assessment before and after you administer medications or other treatments.

- Document any discussion of questionable medical orders and the specific directions the doctor gave. Include the time and date of the discussion, your actions, and any subsequent directions given.

- Chart an omission as a new entry. Do not backdate or add to previously written entries.

- When an unusual incident occurs, document the incident on a special incident or occurrence report form. Do not write "incident report filed" in the medical record. Document what happened to the patient and the actions taken to assure the patient's safety in the medical record.

- Record only your own observations and actions. If you receive information from another caregiver, state the source of the information.

- Record the date, time, and content of all patient-related telephone communications.

- Remember, if you did not document it, it did not occur.

The medical record is an essential and necessary part of patient care. Its contents are regulated by many sources, including licensing, accrediting, and professional organizational standards; case law; and state practice acts. The regulating bodies were discussed in Chapter 2. All nurses must be familiar with the regulating bodies and must follow the guidelines and documentation methods established at the institution where they work. If nurses are familiar with regulatory documentation requirements, they may be able to avoid lawsuits.

The defense of a professional negligence suit requires time, effort, and strategy. Probably the best defense is to avoid being included in a suit. Although this may be easier said than done, and even though there is no absolute way a nurse can avoid being named in a suit, many nurses avoid inclusion by following the rules and regulations of professional practice and all the other documentation regulators' guidelines. Knowing the regulations and following the elements in Table 7-10 may assist a nurse in avoiding inclusion in a lawsuit.

USING DOCUMENTATION TECHNIQUES TO AVOID PITFALLS

Three cases that have gone to litigation are presented for review of completeness of documentation. Read the cases; then, using all the documentation techniques you have learned, decide what you would have documented to prevent litigation. All cases are reprinted with permission from Andrew Lopez, RN.

Case One

Clinical Nursing Malpractice Case Studies
January 29, 2002

Coleman v. East Jefferson General Hospital,
747 So.2d 1044-LA (1999)

Summary: Starting intravenous (IV) lines and performing venipunctures are basic nursing skills in acute care or hospital settings. In this case, a female patient accused a male nurse of negligence that resulted in injury when he needed three attempts to successfully start an IV catheter.

The female patient came to the hospital with vague complaints of abdominal pain and was evaluated in the emergency department. The physician's

TABLE 7-10: STEPS TO PREVENT INCLUSION IN A LAWSUIT

- Practice nursing in accordance with licensing standards, professional standards, well-developed policies and procedures of the health care institution, and accreditation standards.

- Ask for orientation to a new position.

- Review the job description of the position.

- Document care in accordance with accreditation and licensing standards, agency policy, and applicable national standards of documentation for nursing care.

- Maintain open lines of communication with fellow health care workers and patients and their families.

- Maintain and update credentials and certifications for areas of nursing practice, including specialty areas of practice.

- Keep current on nursing practices, procedures, and other developments in the delivery of nursing care.

- Carefully evaluate professional liability insurance coverage, including whether to purchase a personal policy, the type of policy, and policy obligations.

- Practice within the scope of nursing practice, including any specialty areas of nursing.

(Brent, 2001, pp. 88-89)

orders for treatment included IV medications, for which a line would need to be started.

A male nurse was assigned to the patient when the IV catheter was to be placed. The nurse was having difficulty finding veins in the woman's arms. He then attempted twice to start a line in her hand and was successful on the third attempt.

It was the policy of the hospital at that time that a nurse may attempt an IV catheter insertion no more than two times before calling for assistance. For the remainder of the patient's treatment at the hospital, it would be documented that the patient complained of discomfort at the IV site and tolerated it poorly. Pain or discomfort at the site of an IV insertion should present a "red flag" to an experienced nurse.

There was no indication in the hospital record that other signs and symptoms of a complication existed, other than the discomfort. This may have been positional, due to the location of the IV site in the patient's hand. There was no indication that placement of another line was either offered to or refused by the patient.

"When an IV lawsuit is argued in court, top-notch IV skills do not mean much unless they are backed up by appropriate, accurate, and concise documentation. Unfortunately, documentation is where many nurses fall short." (Satarawala, 2000) Following her discharge, the patient filed a suit alleging negligence in the skill of the nurse and hospital. Specifically, she claimed a poorly performed catheter insertion caused her to develop reflex sympathetic dystrophy in her right hand.

Summary judgment was entered for the hospital finding that no negligence was evident. The patient appealed.

1. Was the nurse negligent in his catheter insertion technique? Were certifications and hospital policies and procedures followed?

2. Were standards of care specific to IV catheter insertions adhered to?

3. Was it plausible that the IV caused the patient's reflex sympathetic dystrophy?

On review of the chart and following expert testimony, no deficiencies in technique could be found in the placement of the catheter. By his employment record and training, the nurse was fully qualified to place IV catheters as a part of his scope of practice as a licensed nurse. It was noted that the hospital's standards allowed for a maximum of two attempts before calling for assistance. The nurse questioned attempted three times. On further review, the community standards, which were the measures used for this case, allowed four insertion attempts. By this standard of care, the nurse was within reasonable limits by trying three times.

Expert testimony addressed the issue of causation of the patient's reflex sympathetic dystrophy. In statements made, no direct causative link could be established between the starting of the IV catheter, and a diagnosis of reflex sympathetic dystrophy. At best, the plaintiff's expert stated that it was a slim possibility that a link could be made. The physician offered no support to the claim that the plaintiff's alleged injuries were caused by the catheter insertion.

The appeals court affirmed the judgment of the lower court. It should be noted that IV therapy, although a basic part of nursing practice, is extremely prone to complications and resulting malpractice and negligence actions. (Lopez, 2002)

Case Two

Cytomegalovirus Test Result Misinterpreted by Nurse. Did Negligence Lead to Child with Birth Defects?

Duplan v. Harper, 188 F.3d 1195 OK (1999)

Summary: Nurses access and report confidential and sensitive test results to case managers, insurance companies, physicians, and other nurses as a matter of course each day. It is commonly accepted that only a physician can interpret what a test result implies for a specific patient. By training, nurses have a general knowledge of basic lab values and what they may represent. In this case, a nurse reporting a result misinformed a pregnant woman with an active cytomegalovirus (CMV) infection. Had an accurate explanation been given, a therapeutic abortion might have been performed.

The pregnant woman was in her first trimester. She took ill and discovered that CMV was involved. The patient was aware that CMV was associated with birth defects when contracted during a pregnancy. Fearing harm to her child, an obstetrician was consulted. The physician had her worked up to determine the nature and extent of the infection. The results showed that the woman had an active infection, with CMV noted as the primary infecting organism.

It would have been prudent at this point for the physician to discuss the possibility of a child with birth defects being born. With this knowledge, the woman and her husband could have made an informed decision on whether to continue with the pregnancy. Instead, the physician instructed a nurse to inform the patient of the test result. Apparently, there was no further follow up with the patient by the physician to discuss the results. Specifically, the physician did not ask the woman if she wished to continue the pregnancy in light of the high risk of birth defects.

When the nurse spoke to the patient, she initially only told her the test was "positive." The patient, not understanding what that meant, called the nurse to question her again about it. At this point, the nurse should have either asked the physician or told the patient she needed to talk to the doctor about what the test result meant and how it might affect her pregnancy. Instead, the nurse explained what she thought was correct to the patient.

The pregnant woman left the conversation believing that there was little or no risk of birth defects to her child. The nurse had stated that positive results of the test meant that "she was immune" to CMV. The nurse disclosed no mention of the high

risk of birth defects due to the active CMV infection during the conversation. No further discussion of the issue was documented between the patient and the obstetrician. The pregnancy continued to term. When born, the child had severe birth defects characteristic of a CMV infection during pregnancy. The parents brought suit for wrongful birth against the clinic physician, nurse, and agency contracting for the U.S. Air Force at the time.

The suit alleged that the birth of a severely deformed child could have been prevented or at least anticipated. The plaintiffs argued that had an accurate interpretation of the test result been presented, the high-risk pregnancy would have been terminated. The pregnant woman was prepared to request a therapeutic abortion when the initial possibility of CMV infection and birth defects was made known to her. Based on the misinformation presented by the nurse, the decision was made to continue the pregnancy.

The child would require significant supervision and medical care throughout his life. The court award was in excess of $3,000,000.

1. Was the nurse acting within her scope of practice when she interpreted the test result as it applied to that patient's condition?

2. Was an accurate description provided to the pregnant woman of what the test result meant and potential risks it could pose for her unborn child?

3. Was the physician ultimately responsible for informing the patient of the potential consequences of continuing the pregnancy?

The argument can be made that a practicing licensed nurse in an obstetrician's office can reasonably be expected to know about CMV. This was not the case. It seems the doctor assumed that the nurse was familiar with the disease process and the implications of a CMV infection in a pregnant woman. The nurse went beyond telling the patient that the test was "positive" by adding it meant that the patient was immune to CMV. This amounts to negligence, in that the information given was incorrect and, even worse, misleading. It did not inform the pregnant woman of the possible risks and consequences of continuing her pregnancy despite the CMV infection.

The plaintiff justifiably focused the case on the nurse who gave the results and interpretation and the physician who had ordered the test. The physician, aware of the pregnant woman's active CMV infection, left the situation entirely in the hands of the nurse. The mother never had the option to consider the likelihood of her child being born with deformities. Because neither the physician nor the nurse properly informed the mother, she could not discuss the issue with her husband. Had they been aware that the pregnancy carried a high risk of birth defects, it is likely they would have chosen to end the pregnancy. Through negligence, this option was denied to them. (Lopez, 2000a)

Case Three

Trauma Patient in Shock and in Decline;
ED Physician Does Not Transfer

Gladney v. Snneed, 724 So.2d 642-LA (1999)

Summary: When a patient from a trauma scene arrives at a hospital, initial assessments and evaluations are critical. In this case, a patient involved in a motor vehicle collision (MVC) was brought in with symptoms indicating shock. On evaluation, the decision was made to treat the patient on site. The patient died soon after admission. Should the emergency department (ED) physician have transferred the patient?

The female patient was transported to the hospital via ambulance following a MVC. The facility she was brought to was a rural hospital and not well equipped to deal with trauma emergencies. The attending ED physician was a second-year pediatric resident. The patient's initial physical symptoms — cool, clammy skin and falling blood pressure (95/55

mm Hg on arrival) — were later opined to be highly indicative of shock.

The physician ordered X-rays and IV fluids at a rate of 200 cc per hour. Attempts to stabilize the patient were initiated. Despite the efforts of the physician and nursing staff, the patient coded 3 hours following her admission. Attempts to resuscitate the patient were not successful.

An autopsy on the patient's body identified "treatable shock" as the most likely cause of death. The family brought suit against the driver of the other vehicle involved, the physician, and the hospital and nursing staff. The court found for the plaintiff and ruled that the attending physician was not qualified to treat a trauma patient. A ruling was handed down and responsibility assigned at 10% to the physician and 90% to the hospital and nursing staff. An award of $900,000 was reduced to $500,000 pursuant to a statutory cap. The hospital appealed.

1. Was the initial assessment of the patient accurate, and was adequate testing performed to identify the patient's condition? Based on the presentation of the patient, were adequate measures initiated by the ED physician?

2. Was the ED physician, a second-year pediatric resident, medically qualified to assess and treat a patient in the condition of the young woman who presented that day?

3. Was the facility adequately staffed and equipped to handle a trauma emergency on site, or should arrangements have been made to transfer her to a more suitable facility for that purpose?

4. Was another facility within reasonable distance to which the patient could have been transferred?

5. Was the patient stable enough to be transferred, had another facility been within reasonable distance?

6. Was the treatment the patient received delivered in a timely and responsible fashion? Were there delays or negligence on the part of the hospital and nursing staff?

Expert witnesses testifying at the trial examined the documentation, including initial assessments by both the medical and nursing staff and the test results from the X-rays and labs performed. They stated that the initial presentation of the woman was strongly indicative of shock and required treatment that the rural facility simply was not equipped to offer. Upon completion of the initial assessments, immediate arrangements for transfer to a trauma center would have been justified and prudent.

The evidence to justify the patient's transfer was overwhelming when examined by an emergency medicine physician expert witness. It was then revealed that the hospital had no policies or procedures in place for transfer to larger facilities. Trauma patients such as the young woman in question were not frequent, common, or expected at this facility. The decision to transfer the patient should have been based on the patient's presentation, which was strongly indicative of a trauma case that the physician and facility could not safely handle. The decision to transfer the patient was laid squarely in the lap of the emergency physician, who did not give the order.

Testimony and documentation from the chart revealed that the nursing staff discussed transferring the patient with the physician at the time. The nursing staff, in addition to the symptomatology indicating shock, told the physician the patient had active vaginal bleeding of unknown origin. The expert testimony of both nurses and physicians indicated that the decision to transfer was for the physician to make. If the physician in this situation would not arrange for transfer of the patient, it was the responsibility of the hospital and nursing staff to inform the on-duty supervisors and administrators of the situation. Had this been done, and had the record shown that the administrative, nursing, and hospital staff were aware and recommended that the patient be transferred, the assignment of responsibility would have shifted from the hospital to the individual physician.

Based on the evidence (nursing staff testimony and documentation of the need for transfer and their discussion with the physician about transfer), the appeals court shifted the hospital's responsibility from 90% to 75% and increased the physician's liability from 10% to 25% (Lopez, 2000b).

CONCLUSION

Many guidelines affect the legal aspects of documentation. As nurses learn and incorporate these guidelines into their practice, the guidelines will become second nature. Nurses should become aware of situations and practices that could create problems when trying to defend nursing care in a lawsuit. The documentation in a plaintiff's medical record should reflect that appropriate care was provided. With most cases, the medical record becomes the only source of information years after the incident. Remember, the medical record is the only witness that never dies and never lies. Keep yourself out of court by documenting completely and appropriately every time.

EXAM QUESTIONS

CHAPTER 7
Questions 47-55

47. One of the *best* ways nurses can keep themselves out of the courtroom is through proper documentation. A good documentation guideline is to

    a. write facts, be specific, and avoid giving opinions.

    b. always reference incident reports in a patient's medical record.

    c. assist other staff members by charting or signing for them.

    d. fully obliterate any errors written on the chart using white-out.

48. To create a comprehensive and defensive medical record, the documentation should be

    a. subjective, long-winded, and timely.

    b. incomplete, timely, and detailed.

    c. timely, concise, and complete.

    d. timely, concise, and subjective.

49. Malpractice may be avoided if the nurse uses proactive actions, such as

    a. not documenting accurately, timely, and completely.

    b. not responding to or educating the patient in a timely manner.

    c. documenting by using old block-style narrative notes.

    d. adhering to the nursing process and complying with the standards of care.

50. A hospital may be held liable for the negligent acts of its employees under which theory of liability?

    a. Strict liability

    b. Respondeat superior

    c. Contributory negligence

    d. Ostensible agency

51. Nurse Jones, RN, followed the procedure suggested in the nursing literature for irrigating a patient's IV line. If the IV became infected as a result of the policy and Jones is sued for malpractice, the best defense is

    a. hospital policy was followed.

    b. hospital policy was flawed.

    c. the standard of care had changed.

    d. Jones tried to convince management to change the procedure.

52. Nurse Jones opens a home health agency corporation. A practical nurse helping a patient to the bathroom falls with the patient. Nurse Jones, as the employer of the practical nurse,

    a. worries, knowing that, as the employer, she has personal liability for everything that happens in the business and could lose everything.

    b. does not worry, knowing that the practical nurse was instructed to call for help when transferring the patient and therefore the supervision was not negligent.

    c. worries, knowing that the business is liable under respondeat superior.

    d. does not worry, because malpractice insurance will protect against a lawsuit.

53. In order for the theory of respondeat superior to apply, there must be

    a. the absence of any other theory of liability.

    b. at least 50 employees employed at the institution.

    c. an employer-employee relationship.

    d. injury to a patient.

54. One method to help prevent inclusion in a lawsuit is to

    a. limit communication with coworkers and patients.

    b. practice beyond your scope of practice.

    c. practice nursing according to licensing standards.

    d. avoid professional liability insurance coverage.

55. Nursing documentation standards are regulated by all of the following sources *except*

    a. the ANA and JCAHO.

    b. federal laws and JCAHO.

    c. nursing journals and ANA.

    d. federal laws and state laws.

CHAPTER 8

PREPARATION FOR DEFENSE

CHAPTER OBJECTIVE

After completing this chapter, the reader will be able to discuss personal professional liability insurance and the steps to take when preparing for the defense of a malpractice lawsuit.

LEARNING OBJECTIVES

After studying this chapter, the reader will be able to

1. indicate the two types of nursing malpractice insurance.

2. identify three steps in preparation for a lawsuit.

3. describe the four elements of negligence that must be proven by the patient.

4. indicate how an attorney prepares a nurse for a deposition or trial.

5. describe the process of a deposition and trial.

INTRODUCTION

The aspects of patient care called "nursing" should be limited to the activities that are specifically covered by the state nurse practice act and included in the scope of nursing practice. Nursing practice involves all tangible and intangible activities that nurses do whenever they interact with a patient. If nurses practice ethically, then that practice is almost always legal nursing practice.

On occasion, nurses become named in lawsuits against their institutions. When that happens, the nurse may want to seek legal counsel. The institution will commonly provide this; however, a nurse may want additional representation. Normally, institutions carry liability insurance that covers the institution and its employees. Nurses who are comfortable with the type of insurance and coverage at their institution may not need to purchase additional personal liability insurance. There is a belief that when a nurse has a personal liability insurance policy, he or she may become a source of an additional payout to the plaintiff, thereby making the nurse more likely to be involved in a lawsuit. However, that is generally not true because patients do not ask if nurses carry individual policies. Nurses may purchase individual policies to help cover their best interests in case a lawsuit does occur.

Because of the increased fears that many nurses have about legal liability and legal actions against them, it is important for nurses to know how they can protect themselves and, if they are named in a suit, how they can prepare for their defense. This chapter discusses professional liability insurance, how to prepare for a lawsuit, the essentials of a successful malpractice case, preparing with the attorney, and how to conduct oneself at a deposition or trial.

PROFESSIONAL LIABILITY INSURANCE

From a historical viewpoint, litigation against health care providers is a relatively recent development. Since the 1940s and World War II, the development and sophistication of health care has lead to prolonging life through use of medical and nursing interventions. With advanced medical technology, nurses' skills and standards of practice enhance the life-saving efforts of medicine.

Unfortunately, with increased emphasis on technology, some patient treatment has become less personalized. Possibly because patients no longer have close, personal relationships with health care providers, some patients have become more inclined to use litigation as a means of retribution.

In the 1970s, the malpractice crisis exploded and all health care providers began recognizing the devastation of lawsuits that could potentially be filed. During this period, a medical malpractice suit could basically be filed by any patient at almost any time. Physicians were early targets for litigation and began increasing their liability coverage. Nurses, however, were much slower to obtain malpractice coverage, probably because lawsuits against nurses were less common and few insurance companies provided nurses with malpractice coverage. Even today, with numerous companies and policies available, nurses vacillate between obtaining and not obtaining individual malpractice coverage. Most nurses are covered to some degree by their employers' insurance policies; however, the primary goal of an institution's policy is to protect the institution, not the nurse.

As nurses deal with increasingly complicated technology, as well as with patients who are older and more critically ill, things may go wrong, and the patient, the patient's family, or the patient's estate may file a lawsuit and name the nurse. Because the ethical principal of accountability is one of the key elements in the nursing profession, nurses must be responsible for their actions as professionals. By accepting responsibility for their right and wrong actions, nurses acknowledge the fact that they do sometimes make mistakes. In the litigious atmosphere of today's society, it is logical for nurses to carry malpractice insurance. Individual policies can be used to cover the cost of a defense attorney should the nurse require legal counsel.

A liability policy is a written agreement between the nurse and an insurance company stating that, in exchange for a premium (payment by the nurse), the insurance company will pay compensation (money) to a patient for injuries caused either by an act of omission or commission by the nurse. Nurses are encouraged to get and keep current professional liability insurance for the entire life of their nursing practice. It is one of the least expensive and best tools a nurse can have because nursing practice exposes nurses to potential risks for liability issues every day that the nurse engages in the practice of nursing. Even nurses who are found completely innocent of charges may have to pay attorney fees and other court costs. A personal liability policy covers those fees.

Types of Liability Insurance

There are basically two types of liability insurance policies: occurrence-based policies and claims-made policies.

An occurrence-based policy covers injuries that occur during the period in which the policy is in effect, which is known as the policy period. Occurrence policies are recommended because once the coverage is in place, the nurse is insured regardless of when a lawsuit occurs, even if the policy has not been renewed or the nurse no longer works at the institution in which the incident occurred.

A claims-made policy applies only if the injury occurred during the policy period and the claim was reported to the insurance company during the policy period or during an uninterrupted extension of the policy period with the addition of a tail. A tail provides coverage for periods when the nurse is exposed to professional liability but no longer has the claims-made policy. To further explain, if a nurse left nursing practice in 1998 and had a claims-made policy, he or she could purchase a tail to cover potential lawsuits for acts of negligence that occurred in 1998 or earlier. The tail assures the nurse of protection if a claim is made in the future.

Tails must be maintained for long periods of time, as much as 21 years, and can be very expensive. The length of time a tail should be maintained depends on the statute of limitations in the state where the nurse practices. Statute of limitations is a procedural law that specifies the time during which a plaintiff may file a lawsuit. Every state has different time limits and different guidelines for determining the time frame during which a lawsuit may be filed. Nurses should be aware of their states' statutes.

Employing agencies typically carry claims-made policies. If a nurse is sued and the institution's insurance covers the nurse, the insurer has a duty to provide a complete defense, including assigning an attorney to handle the entire case. The insurer pays the attorney fees as well as any investigation costs involved. Therefore, nurses are covered under their institutions' policies. However, if a nurse is named, a personal policy assists with paying individual attorney fees if the nurse elects to obtain personal counsel. If for some reason the institution cancelled their policy and did not buy a tail and the nurse did not have personal insurance, the nurse being sued may have to pay for the defense and the money judgment awarded to the plaintiff. If the nurse had a personal policy, the insurer of that policy would be expected to pay the claims.

An occurrence-based policy is usually the safest type of policy. Many specialty organizations offer information about personal professional policies the nurse may purchase. The purchase of an individual nursing liability policy acknowledges the nurse's responsibility for individual actions as a professional. An informed decision about whether to rely solely on an employer-sponsored policy should weigh the cost of an individual policy against the benefits that a separate liability policy offers to the nurse. Nurses who do volunteer work or otherwise work outside of their primary place of employment should consider purchasing private policies. Having professional liability insurance does not mean a nurse is protected from being named in a lawsuit. If a nurse is named in a suit, there are steps to take in order to be prepared for the suit.

PREPARING FOR A LAWSUIT

The combination of increased technology in health care systems, increased public awareness, and an aggressive legal system have led to changes in the delivery of care, exposure to potential sources of liability, and changing legal trends. Many patients subject individual health care providers and institutions to intense legal scrutiny.

Nurses are becoming the target of a growing number of malpractice charges. The current shortage of nurses leads to the speculation that negligent actions may be a direct result of increased workplace stress, decreased morale, and distraction from focusing clearly on patient care. Mistakes do happen, and nurses may be open to being sued at any time for numerous valid and invalid reasons. Although it is impossible to completely eliminate the risk of litigation, a nurse can use good documentation techniques and other critical factors to reduce the threat of a lawsuit. Critical factors include maintaining open communication with patients and family members, practicing conscientiously, and maintaining autonomy. Steps for doing this are found in Table 8-1.

Even while practicing these critical factors, a nurse may be named in a lawsuit. When that happens, the nurse should work closely with the institution's attorney or a personally retained attorney. Malpractice cases are usually civil procedures, and

TABLE 8-1: REDUCING THE RISK OF MALPRACTICE LITIGATION

A. Maintain good communication.

- Be courteous, show respect, and take time to listen attentively.
- Do not belittle patients or make value judgments.
- Involve patients in decision-making.
- Explain in terminology and language that patients can understand; get an interpreter if necessary.
- Clarify and verify telephone orders; whenever possible, avoid accepting telephone orders or giving advice over the phone.

B. Maintain expertise in practice.

- Keep up-to-date in both knowledge and skills.
- Do not attempt any task or give any medication that is unfamiliar.
- Practice within the professional and statutory scope of practice.
- Be familiar with and follow institutional and professional standards of care.
- Be attentive to patients' changing health statuses.
- Communicate changes completely and in a timely manner to primary health care providers and document conversations and medical orders if any.
- Pay close attention to details and avoid distractions.
- Document objectively, thoroughly, and in a timely fashion.

C. Maintain autonomy and empowerment.

- Challenge questionable primary health care provider orders.
- Seek assistance and attention for patients with changing health statuses.
- Challenge bureaucratic structures that threaten patient welfare and safety.
- Avoid institutional settings that produce systematic and persistent threats to patient safety.

(Burkhardt & Nathaniel, 2002)

the trial practices are governed by each state's statutory requirements. Cases on a federal level are governed by federal statutory requirements.

Before any trial begins, discovery occurs. Discovery is a process in which the attorneys try to obtain evidence that might not be obtainable at the time of trial to isolate and narrow the issues for the trial, to gather knowledge of any additional evidence that may be included at trial, and to obtain leads to other evidence. Most malpractice cases take about 3 to 5 years before they go to trial or are settled out of court.

Many steps have already been completed by the time a nurse is notified of a suit (see Table 8-2). Once the plaintiff's attorney files the case in court, a sheriff serves the complaint to the defendants named in the suit. The complaint outlines the names of the plaintiff(s) and defendant(s), the allegations of the breaches of the standards of care, the damages or injuries, and the demand for an award.

When notification of a lawsuit is received, the nurse should not panic. The nurse should notify the hospital administrator and contact the insurance company that carries her or his private policy. The institution's insurance company will contact the attorney or law firm that represent the institution and the nurse. Most insurance carriers have attorneys or law firms that handle the lawsuit and all legal proceedings. Lawsuits filed against nurses are usually based on nursing negligence found in medical records. Frequently, plaintiffs' attorneys sue

TABLE 8-2: THE LEGAL PROCESS: STAGES OF A MALPRACTICE CLAIM

1. Pretrial preparation (review of medical records by attorney and expert witness; retrieval of all medical and office records as well as all patient bills)

2. Procedural process that may be required by state law:
    Prelitigation panels:

    a. Medical review panel

    b. Medical tribunal

    c. Arbitration panel

3. Petition for damages or complaint filed in court

4. Complaint or summons sent to health care provider by certified mail or served by a sheriff or process service company

5. Insurance company notified of claim by health care provider

6. Attorney or law firm assigned to health care provider

7. Answers to complaint or counterclaim filed by defendant; defenses alleged

8. Discovery stage (subpoenas may be used)

    a. Depositions

    b. Interrogatories

    c. Requests for production of documents and things

    d. Admissions of facts

    e. Physical or mental examination of plaintiff

9. Pretrial hearing

10. Settlement negotiations

11. Trial of lawsuit (may be trial by judge or jury)

12. Jury selection

13. Opening statements by plaintiff and defendant

14. Case presentation by plaintiff

15. Case presentation by defendant

16. Motion by defendant for directed verdict against plaintiff

17. Closing statements by plaintiff and defendant

18. Judge instruction to jury, if trial by jury

19. Judge or jury deliberations

20. Verdict

21. Appeal (optional)

(Aiken & Catalano, 1994; Burkhardt & Nathaniel, 2002; Tiller, 1994, 1999)

everyone who was involved in treatment or care rather than limiting the number of defendants.

Once the nurse has made the initial contacts, the defense attorney handles the rest of the proceedings. Even though being named in a lawsuit seems like a disaster, the nurse must remember that any patient can sue any health care provider for any reason at any time. Filing a case does not mean the case will go to court or that the case has merit.

ESSENTIALS FOR A SUCCESSFUL CASE

It is the responsibility of the plaintiff to prove the merit of a lawsuit by establishing the presence of four essential elements of a personal liability or medical malpractice claim. The judge or jury in a medical malpractice lawsuit must consider both the plaintiff's allegations and the defendant's answers to the allegations based on these four elements: duty, negligence, damages or injuries, and causation (see Table 8-3).

Following notification of the institution's administration and the insurance company, the nurse must refrain from consulting or talking with anyone about the case except the attorney, the risk manager, or the nursing supervisor. The nurse should have no communication about the circumstances of the case with other nurses on the staff, the plaintiff's attorney, or the plaintiff.

After the petition is received, the defense attorney files an answer on behalf of the defendant. The answer admits to, denies, or declines to answer the allegations in the petition. The attorney lists defenses to the allegations of negligence. The defenses that can be used are listed in Table 8-4.

The defense attorney tries to respond in ways that shift the responsibility from the nurse or institution back to the plaintiff. If the plaintiff did something that contributed to the injuries, then there may not be a case. Also, the lawsuit must be filed within the state's statute of limitations. Likewise, the assumption-of-risk defense argues that the plaintiff, by agreeing to have a procedure performed by a health care provider, has assumed some risk. The Good Samaritan laws usually apply in an emergency situation and cover nurses who are reasonable and who practice using the nursing standards of care as guidelines.

Sometimes the unavoidable accident is used when nothing other than an accident could have caused the plaintiff's injury. Defense of the facts contend that the health care provider's treatment was not below the standard of care, and even if the standard of care was breached, it did not cause the damage to the plaintiff. Lastly, sovereign immunity prevents suits from being filed against federal and state governments based on negligence. Many state and federal institutions are no longer protected against tort liability actions. The best defense to any malpractice lawsuit is accurate, complete, and timely documentation of facts pertaining to a patient's stay and care provided.

PREPARING WITH THE ATTORNEY

The discovery stage is a long stage, sometimes taking years to complete. During this time, the plaintiff's and defendant's attorneys try to gather and study all information and facts about the incident,

---

TABLE 8-3: ESSENTIAL ELEMENTS OF A MALPRACTICE CLAIM

DUTY presumes a relationship between the provider (defendant) and the patient (plaintiff). It says the provider has accepted a duty to care for the patient.

NEGLIGENCE is a breach of duty, a departure from the recognized standard of care. The term *standard of care* is defined as what is reasonable and prudent (ordinary) for someone with the same or similar knowledge and skills to do in the same or similar circumstances.

DAMAGES or INJURIES to the patient of a physical, emotional, psychological, or economic nature are shown to have occurred.

CAUSATION shows that the damage suffered by the patient was caused by the negligence of the provider. It includes *feasibility*; that is, but for the negligence, the injury would not have happened.

(Matthews, 2001, p. 47)

TABLE 8-4: DEFENSES TO A MALPRACTICE CLAIM

1. Contributory versus comparative negligence
2. Statute of limitations
3. Assumption of the risk
4. Good Samaritan statute
5. Unavoidable accident
6. Defense of fact
7. Sovereign immunity

(Aiken & Catalano, 1994, p. 80)

including medical records and other documents. During this period, depositions are taken.

Many malpractice suits are settled before they go to trial. However this commonly occurs after depositions are taken. A deposition is a structured interview in which the person being interviewed is placed under oath and asked questions about issues of the lawsuit. The way a person handles the questioning can be an important factor in the case. It helps establish credibility and knowledge, helps discover new information, and can be used to impeach a witness at trial.

Prior to giving a deposition, the nurse has a chance to review the medical records and discuss the case with the attorney. During the deposition, questions are presented to the nurse by the plaintiff's attorney. The defense attorney attends the deposition with the nurse, takes notes, and can object to some of the plaintiff's questions, but generally says very little during the process.

Anyone whose name appears on the medical record can be deposed. The plaintiff's attorney commonly asks questions of everyone who might have some knowledge about the circumstances surrounding the events of the alleged malpractice. Depending on the nurse's involvement with the plaintiff, the deposition may last from a few minutes to several hours. A deposition can be very stressful for a nurse being questioned. However, if the nurse has documented accurately and completely, the

chart provides the information needed for the nurse's defense.

When working with an attorney, a nurse must be open and honest. A thorough review of the situation that led to the suit and all documentation concerning the incident must be conducted. The nurse should talk with the attorney about what can be expected at the deposition or trial and who will attend both.

The nurse must be careful not to personalize anything about the suit. Although the nurse's conduct is in question when named as a defendant, the tendency to see oneself as a bad nurse or as having done something wrong is a common but unhelpful reaction. The defense attorney helps prove the nurse has done no wrong.

The nurse must rely on the advice of the attorney. The defense of any lawsuit is complicated, diverse, and foreign to most nurses. Sometimes the advice an attorney provides may not seem correct; however, the attorney is the one with the most knowledge concerning the law and its application. Nurses who cannot follow their attorneys' advice and direction should discuss their concerns with their attorneys. Both must be clear that the attorney is working as the nurse's advocate and is working toward a relationship that includes mutual trust, honesty, and open lines of communication.

The attorney works with each deponent and may even create a setting to represent a deposition for practice. Rules of discovery require that attorneys do not coach witnesses or obstruct information; however, the attorney spends time to prepare the nurse for understanding the procedure and presents some idea of the questions that might be asked. The nurse should rely on the medical record, is permitted to refer to it, and may often be asked to read from it during the deposition. The plaintiff's attorney asks all the questions at the deposition. If the defense attorney has carefully prepared the nurse and the medical record is accurately, completely, and timely documented, the nurse is able to make a strong defense.

Depending on the case and the location of the deposition, the plaintiff's attorney, the defense attorney, the nurse (deponent), and the court reporter may be the only persons present. At other times, all the defendants and, sometimes, the plaintiff are present. Frequently, the hospital attorney, if different from the one representing the nurse, the physician's attorney, and any other defense attorneys may be present. Nurses must try to concentrate on the questions the plaintiff's attorney is asking and try to shut out all others who may be present.

THE PROCESS OF A DEPOSITION OR TRIAL

After the nurse has been sworn in by a court reporter, who is present at the deposition to transcribe the information, the plaintiff's attorney begins the examination. Once the plaintiff's attorney has finished with questioning, other attorneys, including the nurse's attorney, may ask questions. When the other attorneys have finished, the plaintiff's attorney may ask more questions, as may the other attorneys. This process continues until all questions have been asked and answered.

During the process, attorneys may make objections either to a question posed or to an answer given. It is wise to take time before answering a question to allow time for the attorney to make an objection, if necessary. When a transcript of the deposition is prepared, the deponent has a chance to review it and make changes and consult with the attorney about the changes needed.

Remember that a deposition carries the same weight as testimony made in court. However, with a deposition, the defendant is entitled to a copy of the transcript and should be provided time to read and edit his or her responses. Be very careful when doing so, as changed responses in critical areas appear untruthful or evasive.

During a deposition, an attorney may ask the nurse about any subject as long as the question appears reasonably calculated to lead to the discovery of evidence. The attorney commonly spends time reviewing the nurse's background, education, training, and experience. The plaintiff's counsel wants to learn the nurse's version of the chronology of events surrounding the incident. Depositions may become extremely detailed and, at times, repetitive because attorneys are trying to find facts as well as attempting to pin a nurse down to a specific version of events. The nurse is likely to be asked about all conversations with doctors, other nurses, the patient, and family members during the time in question.

The attorney commonly questions at length the nurse's assessment of the patient, the nursing diagnosis, the plan of care, and the basis for his or her decisions. The nurse is asked to explain how certain interventions were instituted and the basis for doing so. One of the most important areas touched on in a deposition is the nurse's knowledge of the policies, procedures, and protocols of the institution where he or she was practicing. Likewise, the nurse may be asked questions about the state's nurse practice act. Therefore, it is wise to review all these documents prior to giving a deposition.

Depositions are used in several ways. As already discussed, they help the parties develop evidence needed to prosecute or defend the case. At time of trial, if the nurse testifies differently than done during the deposition, the attorney may impeach the nurse's credibility by pointing out the inconsistency. Therefore, a nurse should carefully study the deposition prior to going to trial. Nurses who cannot remember what they said in the deposition should ask for a copy of the deposition and read the comment to the judge or jury.

After discovery, if no settlement is reached, the case proceeds to trial. The trial may take place months to years after the deposition was given. Once the jury has been selected and the plaintiff has presented a case, the defense presents its evidence.

Throughout the plaintiff's presentation of witnesses, the defense has a chance to cross-examine the witnesses. The plaintiff may likewise cross-examine defense witnesses. At this time, attorneys commonly ask leading questions that require only a yes-or-no answer, without opportunity to explain or qualify.

As a defendant in a medical malpractice case, nurses must be prepared for intense scrutiny. A good defense attorney spends sufficient time to ensure that the nurse knows what to expect from the plaintiff and defense attorneys. In many cases, the defense attorney takes the nurse to a courtroom and lets the nurse sit in the witness stand to get more comfortable with the situation.

Deposition questions are similar to the questions that will be asked at trial. The same type of behavior from the plaintiff's attorney can also be expected. No matter how uncomfortable the trial may be, the nurse defendant is required to be present throughout the entire case. As one of the principals of the case, the nurse may at all times expect to be under scrutiny of jurors, spectators, and even the press. The appearance and presence of the nurse makes an impression, so attention must be paid to how the nurse dresses and acts while in the courtroom. All of this should be discussed in advance with the defense attorney, so that the nurse is viewed as a professional, competent, and caring person.

Each nurse should be well prepared before testifying at a deposition or trial. All medical records and other pertinent information must be reviewed. The nurse should notify the defense attorney if there is a diary or written account of the event. If this information is reviewed to prepare for the deposition, the plaintiff's attorney can request that a copy be attached to the deposition. Do not bring anything to the deposition because such materials may be discoverable. The tips presented in Table 8-5 on page 128 for deposition or trial may provide guidance to the process and help the nurse be aware of what to expect.

CONCLUSION

Nurses are constantly challenged by the rapid changes in medical technology and the impact of evolving health care delivery demands. As nurses function in more independent roles, use advancing technology, and assume more responsibilities, they become more at risk for potential lawsuits. Although many lawsuits are frivolous and never proceed to trial, they are stressful for the defendant. The purchasing of individual professional liability insurance may help the nurse if a suit comes to trial and there is a need to pay attorney fees and court costs. Otherwise, the institution in which the nurse works should provide coverage for any lawsuit against the nurse.

If a nurse is named in a lawsuit, it is the responsibility of the plaintiff to prove the nurse had a duty toward the plaintiff, breached that duty, and caused injury or harm to the plaintiff. Once a case is filed, the nurse must work closely with both the institution's attorney and any personal attorney to prepare for deposition and eventually trial. By appearing professional, competent, caring, and prepared, a nurse will be viewed positively at a deposition or trial. As professionals, nurses have a legal responsibility to be competent in their area of practice. Lack of knowledge is never an acceptable defense for substandard or negligent nursing care.

TABLE 8-5: GENERAL TIPS FOR DEPOSITION AND TRIAL

1. Review the records regarding anything about which you might be questioned.
2. Do not volunteer additional information if the attorney remains silent for a period after you answer.
3. Answer only the questions asked.
4. Be organized in your thinking and recollection of the facts regarding the incident.
5. Before answering, make sure you understand the question.
6. Ask to have questions that you did not hear or that you did not understand rephrased or repeated.
7. Wait until the entire question is asked before answering.
8. Take your time; before answering, wait 5 seconds to allow your attorney to make any necessary objections.
9. Listen to your attorney when he or she objects to questions. Follow the attorney's lead to determine whether you should answer a question.
10. Answer all questions verbally because the court reporter is recording answers verbatim and cannot record shaking or nodding of the head to represent "no" or "yes."
11. Explain your testimony in simple, succinct terminology.
12. Do not be intimidated or allow yourself to become overpowered by the cross-examiner.
13. Be polite, sincere, and courteous at all times. Speak slowly and clearly.
14. Be honest and truthful.
15. Do not speculate. Base your answers on the facts of the case.
16. Do not make assumptions, exaggerate, or lie.
17. Do not make excuses for other people's actions.
18. Avoid using absolutes, such as " I always take vital signs on a postop patient every 30 minutes."
19. Pay close attention to the use of pronouns when discussing events. Most people tend to speak in first person except when being evasive or deferring blame.
20. Do not be antagonistic in answering questions. Maintain your composure.
21. Do not argue, get angry, or be sarcastic with the opposing attorney.
22. Do not show any visible signs of displeasure regarding any testimony with which you are in disagreement.
23. If you do not know or cannot remember, simply state, "I do not know" or "I do not remember."
24. Do not drink caffeinated drinks; they tend to make people nervous and increase the need to go to the bathroom.
25. At deposition, if you are tired, confused, or need a break, ask for one.
26. Dress conservatively and professionally, especially at trial. A navy blue or dark-colored tailored suit is recommended.
27. If testifying in a deposition or at trial, arrive early so you can find the place and become comfortable with the surroundings.
28. Make and maintain eye contact with the questioning attorney.
29. If the question can be answered by "yes" or "no," then do so.
30. Be cautious of the "yes" or "no" trap on cross-examination. Try to add an explanation.
31. Be cautious of leading questions.
32. If the same question is asked more than once, have the court reporter read back your previous answer or hold firm to the same response no matter how many times it is asked.
33. You are not required to respond to hypothetical questions.
34. Be sure you read your deposition prior to testifying at trial.
35. Provide a resume or curriculum vitae, if requested.

(Aiken & Catalano, 1994; Brent, 2001; Pozgar, 2002; Sheeler, 2003; Tiller, 1994)

EXAM QUESTIONS

CHAPTER 8
Questions 56-65

56. An occurrence-based liability insurance policy applies so long as it is

    a. in effect at the time the incident occurs.

    b. paid in full 6 months before the claim is filed.

    c. paid in full 1 year before the claim is filed.

    d. in effect at the time the claim is made.

57. The tail added to a liability insurance policy

    a. can convert a claims-made policy to an occurrence-based policy.

    b. is free from the insurance carrier.

    c. does not have to be maintained beyond a five-year term.

    d. can convert an occurrence-based policy to a claims-made policy.

58. A structured pretrial interview, where the person is under oath to answer questions about issues pertaining to the lawsuit is known as a

    a. sovereign immunity.

    b. deposition.

    c. delegation.

    d. cross-examination.

59. If a lawsuit occurs, the nurse is notified that he or she is being sued by a

    a. pretrial preparation.

    b. petition for damages or complaint filed in court.

    c. complaint or summons sent by certified mail or delivered by a sheriff.

    d. motion by defendant for directed verdict against the plaintiff.

60. A nurse fails to keep a patient's bedrails in the upright position as ordered by the attending physician. The patient is discharged having never fallen from bed. The elements of negligence present in this scenario are

    a. duty to care and breach of duty.

    b. injury and causation.

    c. breach of duty and causation.

    d. duty and injury.

61. The elements that a plaintiff must prove in order to establish liability for malpractice include

    a. misrepresentation and worker comprehension.

    b. patient abuse and abandonment.

    c. duty, negligence, injury, and causation.

    d. disrespect, injury, and abuse.

129

62. The best defense to any malpractice lawsuit is

   a. using accurate, complete, and timely documentation of all facts.

   b. blaming another nurse in the incident report for giving the wrong medication.

   c. creating your own abbreviations used for charting on your unit.

   d. sending the plaintiff's attorney the only set of hospital records.

63. The purpose of a deposition is to

   a. discredit and impeach witnesses.

   b. assess weaknesses of opposing counsel's paralegal.

   c. prove that a nurse is lying.

   d. discover new information about the case.

64. When a nurse works with an attorney in preparation for deposition or trial, the nurse must

   a. personalize all aspects about the suit.

   b. admit to being a bad nurse.

   c. be honest and open with the attorney.

   d. admit guilt immediately.

65. While at trial and giving testimony, the nurse should

   a. answer only the questions asked.

   b. volunteer additional information to every question.

   c. never ask to have a question repeated.

   d. avoid eye contact with the questioning attorney.

CHAPTER 9

DOCUMENTATION DISASTERS

CHAPTER OBJECTIVE

After completing this chapter, the reader will be able to describe specific nursing practices that could lead to documentation disasters and potential lawsuits.

LEARNING OBJECTIVES

After studying this chapter, the reader will be able to

1. specify six areas that place a nurse at risk for potential lawsuits.

2. indicate good documentation techniques to decrease the risk of potential lawsuits.

3. identify measures the nurse may take to protect himself or herself against disasters.

INTRODUCTION

The last two decades of the 20th century brought rapid and numerous changes to the health care system that redefined concepts about health care providers: how many, what kinds, where they should practice, and how much they should be paid. As health care technology becomes more sophisticated and directed toward acute care, numerous different types of health care providers have arisen to meet medical needs. There are about 200 different allied health occupations as well as traditional professional health care providers. Some of these providers have very narrow focuses, whereas others have broad, overlapping roles. The latest redesign of health care systems and redefinitions of health care provider roles may place nurses in situations that could become disastrous. This chapter focuses on areas that require accurate, complete, and timely documentation to prevent bad outcomes and potential lawsuits. Areas addressed include use of unlicensed patient care assistants, delegation, downsizing, short staffing, floating, missing records, correcting charting errors, last entries, and other concerns. Techniques to decrease risks and ways nurses can avoid bad outcomes are integrated into each section.

SUPERVISING UNLICENSED PATIENT CARE ASSISTANTS

As nurses work toward autonomy and freedom from medical and physician control, they have taken on a greater role as primary health care givers. In the late 1980s, the American Medical Association proposed the creation of registered care technologists who would provide direct patient care and report to physicians. Nurses defending their traditional practice were able to keep this from happening (Burkhardt & Nathaniel, 2002).

Efforts at cost control have led to other new types of health care providers who are not licensed but who would provide patient care. The American Nurses Association (ANA) (1995) defines these people as unlicensed assistive personnel (UAP) or unlicensed patient care assistants. A UAP is an unlicensed individual who is trained to function as an assistant to the licensed nurse in providing patient care. The National Council of State Boards of Nursing has taken the position that UAPs should assist registered nurses (RNs) but not replace them.

The increased use of UAPs has concerned nurses for several reasons, including patient safety and nurses' accountability for UAPs' actions. Nurses have no control over the education of UAPs, and many nurses do not have the education or skills for supervising UAPs. UAPs are frequently used for delivery of care in patient care settings where only RNs or licensed practical nurses (LPNs) would be considered appropriate providers. Of special concern is medication administration by UAPs. UAPs are not licensed to administer medications, unless they have a specific pharmacology and medication administration course. Even then, a UAP still needs close supervision, especially when administering medications. Nurses are morally concerned about patient safety and any lack of professionalism of the UAP.

Normally, unlicensed personnel who work within the confines of a health care institution are covered under the license of the facility, not of a specific nurse. The nursing supervisor has the responsibility for assuring that UAPs do not perform tasks that require a license and for making sure that UAPs safely carry out appropriate tasks. Even if the task assigned is appropriate to the training of the UAP, it is the nurse's and the supervisor's obligation to monitor the correct performance of the task. The ratio of UAPs to RNs must be carefully established in order to maintain quality care for patients.

Most UAPs are allowed to collect, report, and document data including, but not limited to, vital signs, height, weight, intake and output, Clinitest and Hematest results, changes from baseline data established by the RN, environmental conditions, patient or family comments related to the patient's

care, and behaviors related to the plan of care. Other tasks the UAP may perform are listed in Table 9-1.

TABLE 9-1: TASKS A UAP MAY PERFORM
• Ambulation, positioning, and turning
• Personal hygiene and elimination care
• Feeding duties, such as cutting up food
• Assistance with activities of daily living, limited to bathing, dressing, grooming, skin care, and exercising
• Reinforcement of health teaching planned or provided by the RN
(Cutrona, 2001)

The nurse is responsible for making sure the UAP has recorded information correctly. Likewise, the nurse is responsible for all other documentation and must assess the patient and follow the nursing process for the patient's care. Any information reported to the nurse by the UAP must be validated and addressed as well as documented. All the previously discussed documentation techniques and strategies should be used.

The nurse can protect the staff and the patient by working with and observing the UAP. Knowing the job description for the UAP and the nurse's job description can help the nurse plan the UAP's activities. Each state's nurse practice act addresses UAPs and the nurse's responsibilities. Each nurse should become familiar with the act in his or her state. Once trust has been established and all are aware of the UAP's skills and job description as well as the state's delegation rules and regulations, the nurse will know the abilities and limitations of the UAP and will then be able to know how to delegate duties and appropriately assign the UAP.

WHAT CAN AND CANNOT BE DELEGATED

The ANA (1995) states that delegation is an act of transferring responsibility for the performance of an activity from one person to another, with the first individual retaining accountability for the outcome. Delegation increases a nurse's responsibility while decreasing the nurse's control over the outcome; many nurses find this an uncomfortable situation. In order to provide quality care for less money to a growing and aging population, nurses are often asked to delegate many of their responsibilities to UAPs. Delegation is believed to be a way to provide care at reduced cost, with no serious challenge to quality or safe patient care. However, nurses may resist delegation because of fears for patient safety and liability in a negative situation. The ethical concerns involved in this dilemma include patient autonomy and justice as well as nonmalfeasance and beneficence.

To meet the public's increasing need for accessible, affordable, quality health care, hospitals have been turning to the use of UAPs. Nurses, who are uniquely qualified to promote health and provide care for patients must be involved in coordinating and supervising the delivery of care by delegating nursing tasks to the UAP. The shortage of nurses working in residential care may influence the numbers of UAPs hired to meet needs of patients. About 82.5% of the 2.5 million registered nurses in the U.S. are employed in nursing (Peterson, 2001). In 2010 the projected supply of registered nurses will not adequately meet the requirements for full-time nurses. Today there are 120,000 open positions for registered nurses nationwide (CBS News, 2003) and the shortage will get bigger as many nurses reach retirement age. The Bureau of Labor Statistics indicated that the number of nurses working in residential care was 14,000 in 1992 and more than 35,000 are needed today (Solomon, 1995). Likewise, with increasing numbers of elderly patients needing assisted living or personal care homes, the use of UAPs will increase. Thus, the need for delegation decisions continues to increase.

Depending on individual state laws, RNs can delegate nursing tasks to unlicensed personnel, within certain restrictions. Because nurses are responsible for the nature and quality of all nursing care that their patients receive, under their direction, failure to properly supervise a UAP may result in loss of the nurse's license. UAPs may be used to complement nursing services, but they may not be used as a substitute for the nurse. If a UAP commits an act resulting in possible liability because of failing to properly perform a delegated task, or if the nurse failed to properly supervise the UAP, the nurse is liable. Therefore, the nurse must practice in compliance with basic requirements to avoid liability for improperly delegating nursing tasks or failure to properly supervise.

Delegation is not based on which patient requires care but rather what tasks can be performed by the UAP. Appropriate delegation requires critical thinking on the part of the nurse in deciding the needs of each patient and making sure appropriate supervision is available as needed. Remembering the five rights of delegation may help the nurse with the delegation process (see Table 9-2).

TABLE 9-2: THE FIVE RIGHTS OF DELEGATION

RIGHT TASK: Tasks that are repetitively performed, require minimal problem-solving or innovation, and are delegable for a specific patient

RIGHT CIRCUMSTANCES: Appropriate patient setting with available resources and right timing

RIGHT DIRECTION: Clear concise description of the task, including its purpose, limits, and expectations

RIGHT INFORMATION: Clear information about a patient must be communicated if any change is needed for the performance of the task

RIGHT SUPERVISION: Appropriate monitoring, evaluation, intervention, and feedback

(*Delegation Guidelines*, 2003; Perry, 1997)

The nurse must supervise the UAP and any tasks assigned to the UAP to perform. The degree of supervision required should be determined after the nurse has evaluated the patient's needs, the stability of the patient's condition, the training and capabilities of the UAP, the nature of the tasks being delegated, and the availability of the nurse to assist the UAP.

Some tasks that may not be delegated are listed in Table 9-3. Because specific tasks cannot be delegated, it is the nurse's responsibility to properly document all nursing tasks performed. The nurse would be wise to review any charting the UAP has done. Refer to the previous section regarding what activities a UAP may chart. Nurses must know and understand the delegation regulations for the states in which they practice. For example, the Georgia Board of Nursing has an excellent decision tree for delegation to UAPs (see Figure 9-1).

TABLE 9-3: TASKS THAT CANNOT BE DELEGATED
Registered nurses may not delegate the following to LPNs, LVNs, or UAPs:
• The authority for nursing care decisions
• Assessment
• Nursing Diagnosis
• Development of the plan of care
• Evaluation of patient care outcomes
UAPs may not perform patient care activities that require a license in nursing or another health care discipline. State boards of nursing define these activities.
(Cutrona, 2001; Delegation Guidelines, 2003)

Following the decision tree, making supervisory visits to the patient, and evaluating the relationship between the UAP and the patient fall under the role of the nurse. The nurse should observe and evaluate the care provided by the UAP, continually assess and evaluate the patient's status, and properly document the areas that cannot be delegated.

DOWNSIZING, SHORT STAFFING, AND FLOATING

The health care work force does not have a well-defined set of rules because rules fluctuate and change over time in response to many factors. Governments, social concerns, and definitions of health, social values, costs, consumer's expectations, and the political power of various players influence it. Managed care and capitation-based insurance have led hospitals to reduce nursing staff. This downsizing has impacted nurses by increasing their patient care workload, increasing the use of float nurses between departments, cutting support services, and increasing the use of mandatory overtime to cover staffing needs.

Downsizing

Downsizing is a set of organizational activities designed to improve organizational efficiency, productivity, and competitiveness. When defined in this positive manner, downsizing falls under the category of a management tool for achieving desired change, much like right-sizing and re-engineering. In reality, downsizing is an effort to reduce the size of a workforce; the elimination of jobs constitutes downsizing. This has led to short staffing, floating, and mandatory overtime for nurses.

Short Staffing

A major concern for institutions providing health care is the liability that could be caused by short staffing. The staffing numbers at most institutions have been decreased to the smallest complement of staff to meet patients' needs. To avoid potential liability situations caused by short staffing, nursing supervisors must be knowledgeable as well as reasonable and nursing staff must be flexible. Nurses must practice and document all the safety measures they have been taught in order to provide safe patient care.

Most health care institutions have not stated precise numbers required for adequate staffing. The

FIGURE 9-1: GEORGIA BOARD OF NURSING DECISION TREE

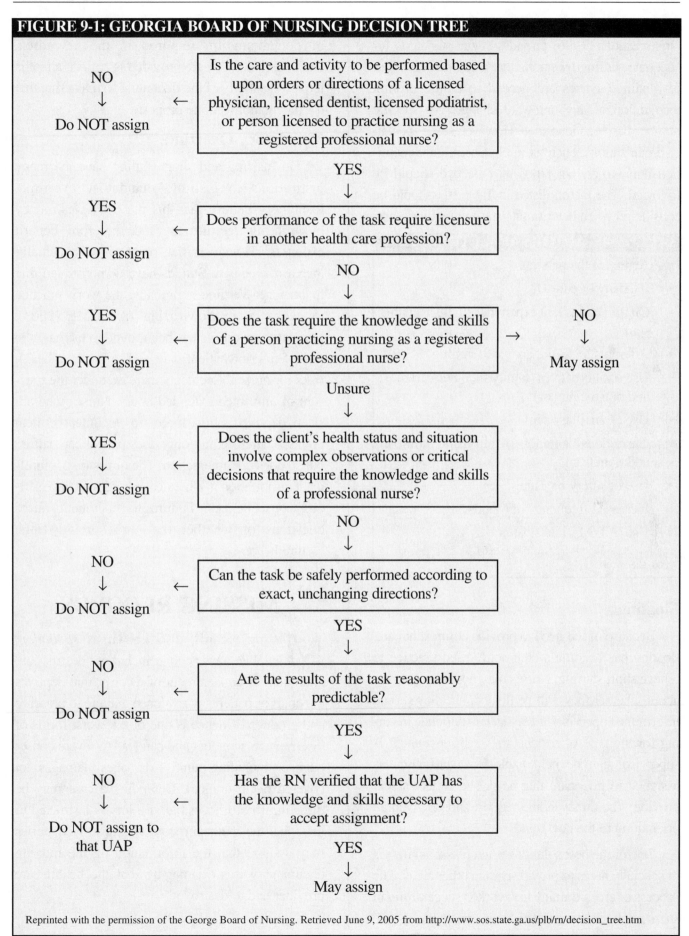

NO
↓
Do NOT assign
←
Is the care and activity to be performed based upon orders or directions of a licensed physician, licensed dentist, licensed podiatrist, or person licensed to practice nursing as a registered professional nurse?

YES
↓

YES
↓
Do NOT assign
←
Does performance of the task require licensure in another health care profession?

NO
↓

YES
↓
Do NOT assign
←
Does the task require the knowledge and skills of a person practicing nursing as a registered professional nurse?
→
NO
↓
May assign

Unsure
↓

YES
↓
Do NOT assign
←
Does the client's health status and situation involve complex observations or critical decisions that require the knowledge and skills of a professional nurse?

NO
↓

NO
↓
Do NOT assign
←
Can the task be safely performed according to exact, unchanging directions?

YES
↓

NO
↓
Do NOT assign
←
Are the results of the task reasonably predictable?

YES
↓

NO
↓
Do NOT assign to that UAP
←
Has the RN verified that the UAP has the knowledge and skills necessary to accept assignment?

YES
↓
May assign

Reprinted with the permission of the George Board of Nursing. Retrieved June 9, 2005 from http://www.sos.state.ga.us/plb/rn/decision_tree.htm

Joint Commission for Accreditation of Healthcare Organizations (1996) provides vague standards for adequate staffing by stating that a sufficient number of qualified nurses are needed to assure prompt recognition of any untoward change. No specific number has been identified. However, some specialty organizations, such as in obstetrics, have identified nurse-to-patient ratios they believe should be followed. The factors listed in Table 9-4 should be considered when determining staffing requirements.

TABLE 9-4: FACTORS AFFECTING STAFF

- Acuity of the patients
- Intensity of care
- Qualifications and experience of the available staff
- Attempts to secure adequate staffing
- Use of alternatives (family members, friends, and outside nurses)
- Use of ancillary staff
- Clear documentation of efforts to bring in additional staff
- Use of safety measures
- Increased frequency of rounds
- Use of UAPs and float nurses

(Aiken & Catalano, 1994; ANA, 1998b; Catalano, 2001; Demoro, 2000; Hickok, n.d.)

Floating

Because of the need to provide competent care, floating has become a commonly used practice to relieve short staffing. Nurses may not have a choice about whether they will be floated, but they should inform the supervisor if they lack experience in caring for the type of patients they will encounter. A supervisor can be held liable if a staff nurse is assigned to give care that he or she cannot safely provide. The nurse should request and be given an orientation to the new unit.

One of the best solutions is to cross-train nurses in specialty areas to provide care in other areas. The process of cross-training has worked successfully in such areas as labor and delivery, postpartum, and

the nursery. The nurse must inquire about the type of documentation required in the new area. Documentation of care provided is critical, and it is the responsibility of the float nurse to make sure that documentation is done properly.

Mandatory Overtime

Downsizing and short staffing have led many institutions to institute mandatory overtime. Institutions believe that this practice saves money by limiting recruitment and therefore benefit expenses. However, the practice may actually increase expenses. Studies have demonstrated that mandatory overtime is probably the worst practice to evolve from downsizing (AFSCME, 2003). Mandatory overtime has been found to increase the risk of inferior patient care and to increase health risks for nurses. Accidents increase under the pressure of unwanted extended hours. Nurses who are sleep deprived often forget to document critical points. Therefore, not only does patient care suffer, but so does documentation. The omission of significant information in a medical record may have serious consequences. Failure to document raises questions of whether the nurse provided the required care.

MISSING RECORDS

Missing records, also known as *spoliation*, involve any action, including destruction, alteration, or concealment of records, that deprives the court or patients of evidence. Failure to preserve and produce evidence is one of the worst forms of discovery misconduct and can lead to severe consequences, including punitive damages (damages not covered by insurance). Defending a case may be difficult, if not impossible, if a jury is instructed to infer that the medical record was destroyed. Juries may assume that the information on the missing document was so damaging that the health care provider had to destroy it.

Today, legal standards for maintaining records make it more difficult for medical records to be lost. A nurse should never participate in the deliberate destruction of medical records, even if the information could be damaging. The nurse should seek the assistance of the supervisor or others in the chain of command to protect the interests of all parties involved, including the institution, if someone suggests destroying all or part of the medical record.

In the past, fetal heart monitor strips were tossed in a box in a storage closet. Many physicians and nurses would help themselves to a set of strips to use for review or teaching and never return the strips to the box. Likewise, the boxes were never secured or clearly labeled. When a case was reviewed, it was not uncommon for the relevant strip to be missing. Today, fetal heart monitor strips are a legal part of the labor and delivery medical record and can now be digitalized and stored on disk.

CORRECTING CHARTING ERRORS

Errors in charting do occur, and the nurse who made the entry should correct all errors. When a charting error occurs, the nurse should follow the institution's prescribed procedure for correcting the error. If coffee or another liquid is spilled on a page, the nurse may be tempted to rewrite the page and destroy the original page. This should not be done! The damaged page should be retained along with the rewritten page. Destruction of the original gives the appearance that the record was tampered with.

Attorneys have ways of determining if a record has been tampered with or rewritten. If a page is recopied, the nurse, at the top of the new page, should write that the page was recopied, add the date, and initial it. Make sure any spaces not used on the original page are crossed out or have lines drawn through the unused spaces. Refer to Table 9-5 for ways to tell whether a record has been tampered with.

TABLE 9-5: IDENTIFYING RECORD TAMPERING AND REWRITTEN RECORDS

- The writing may appear in an unnatural order.
- Handwriting will be very uniform in style, ink used, margins, and spacing.
- The pages may be different in type, folds, style, and type of paper.
- The page may not be the form that was in use at the time of the incident.
- If several corrections or changes have been made, the date may not be correct.

(Iyer & Camp, 1999)

When an error is made in charting, the nurse should know the institution's procedure for correcting it. To begin with, all entries in a medical record should be made in nonerasable ink. Any practice used to make a jury believe the nurse altered, erased, obliterated, or otherwise tampered with an entry raises questions about the chart's accuracy and the nurse's honesty.

Nurses should never erase, use white out, or obliterate an error. Simple steps can be used to correct errors. These are displayed in Table 9-6.

TABLE 9-6: CORRECTING MEDICAL RECORD ENTRIES

1. Draw a line through the entry, making sure the original entry is still legible.
2. Write "mistaken entry" or "ME" above or beside the original words.
3. Write the date and initial next to "ME."
4. Enter the correct information next to the lined-out words.
5. If there is a question about why the entry is being altered, add a brief explanation (for example, wrong patient chart).

LATE ENTRIES

Failure to document everything diminishes a nurse's ability to confidently and persuasively testify about the details of an event. If you forget to document something and have to add it later, there are ways to do this. Late entries often raise suspicion in the plaintiff's mind, so late entries must be made in such a way as to decrease suspicion. There are times when important information needs to be added, such as when the medical record was not available at the time the nurse needed to chart or when the nurse forgot to document information. Late entries should not be squeezed into an existing note, written in the margin, or written between existing lines. Documentation standards do not support asking other nurses to leave blank lines so that other notes can be inserted.

When writing a late entry, add the entry to the first available line, label the entry "Later Entry," and date and time the entry with the current time and date. Likewise, the nurse should indicate the time and date the entry should have been made. It is helpful to cross-reference the late entry with the page where it should have appeared (see Table 9-7).

A good rule of thumb is to add a late entry as soon as possible. The longer after the fact it is added, the more the late entry may appear to be a fabrication and a response to fear of litigation. All nurses should be careful about what is added to a medical record after the fact. Trying to remember and document assessment data, times, and other details can be problematic. Any information that is added may be construed as inaccurate or as tampering.

COUNTERSIGNING NOTATIONS OF OTHERS

In no situation should the nurse chart for others or alter another nurse's documentation. If someone else performs a procedure, clearly document what was done and by whom. The person charting should clearly identify who made the entry and who actually performed the procedure.

A similar practice, discussed earlier in terms of documenting UAPs' work, is countersigning. Although countersigning does not imply that you performed the procedure, it does represent that you reviewed the entry, approved the care given, and assumed the entry was correct. If institutional policy requires the nurse to countersign a subordinate's entry, be careful. Make sure to review each entry and make sure it is clear who performed the procedure. If you signoff without reviewing the entry, or if you negligently overlook a problem the entry might raise, you could share the liability for any patient injury that results.

CONTRIBUTORY NEGLIGENCE

Contributory negligence refers to an act the patient does or does not do to contribute to her or his injury. Contributory negligence indicates that the patient failed to take reasonable care or to follow

TABLE 9-7: LATE ENTRY DOCUMENTATION		
08-31-03	1400	Late Entry: Chart in X-ray with patient on 8-30-03. See previous nursing notes, page 2. Patient stated she went to the bathroom earlier, felt faint, and fell and struck her head on sink. Patient denied any dizziness, blurred vision, or further problems. Patient stated she did not hurt herself and did not tell anyone at the time. Patient's mother encouraged her to report the incident. No bruises or lacerations. Pupils PEARL. Gait strong and steady. Patient denied pain. Dr. Douglass notified of patient's report and he examined her at 10:45. NO change in orders and new orders received. ———————— C. Dodge, RN

physician or discharge orders to prevent injury. A finding of contributory negligence may prevent the injured party from any recovery in a lawsuit. An example of contributory negligence is the patient's right to refuse care.

Right to Refuse Care

Patients do decline medical care, elect alternative procedures and sometimes act against medical advice. In so doing, they can bring about a medical condition or exacerbate an existing one. If a patient refuses care, documentation of the situation must be detailed. The nursing notes as well as the progress notes should clearly describe any behavior that specifically contradicts the instructions or care given to the patient. Accurate and complete documentation of the patient's statements, behaviors, or actions should be made. When the patient, family, or both are unable or unwilling to follow instructions, they should be advised of the consequences and the information documented in the patient's medical record. If a question arises as to the care the patient received, the documentation provides the information needed for the defense.

DISCHARGE NOTES AND OTHER DISCHARGE CONCERNS

Against Medical Advice

As previously discussed, discharge notes are the part of a medical record that summarizes a patient's initial complaints, course of treatment, final diagnosis, and directions for follow-up care. Sometimes patients decide they do not want to remain in an institution and leave against medical advice (AMA). When this happens, the nurse should clearly document all events leading to the AMA discharge, document the mental status of the patient, and quote the patient's reason for leaving.

When a patient states a plan to leave the institution and the nurse has determined the patient's reason for leaving, the nursing supervisor and the patient's physician must be notified. It is the responsibility of the physician to explain to the patient the risk of leaving without proper care. If the physician is not available to discuss the risk, the nurse should discuss the dangers with the patient. The nurse may want to take along a witness to verify what the patient was told and how the patient responded. Documentation of the conversation, including the witness's name, should be included in the nursing notes.

Many institutions have forms that should be completed and signed by the patient before he or she leaves AMA (see Figure 9-2). These forms typically require a witness or witnesses to verify the patient's signature. The form may include the procedures recommended, the potential benefits of such procedures, the risks of the refusal, and alternative treatments recommended and refused.

Most institutions include a waiver of the right to sue the institution or the health care providers in the event the patient experiences injury or death due to the refusal of treatment. Such a statement may not hold up in court, but it may make a patient aware of the situation. When the patient does sign a form, it should include that the patient was informed of the risks and consequences of leaving without continued treatment; who, if anyone, the patient left with; and the fact that the patient can return for treatment without giving a reason. If a patient refuses to sign the AMA record, the nurse should clearly document this refusal.

Refusal to Leave Facility

On the other hand, a patient may not want to leave the institution. Legally, an institution is responsible for a patient until the patient is off the property. There may be reasons a patient does not want to leave, which could include lacking transportation, having no support system after discharge, not feeling ready to leave, or having no home. A precise description of the situation and the problem-solving used must be clearly documented. If a

FIGURE 9-2: SAMPLE AMA FORM

```
                        RELEASE FROM RESPONSIBILITY
                              FOR DISCHARGE


                                    Date:  _____ , _____
                                    Time:  _____  a.m./p.m.

This is to certify that I, _____ ,
a patient in _____ , am being discharged against
the advice of the attending physician and of the hospital
administration.  I acknowledge that I have been informed of the risk
involved and hereby release the attending physician and the hospital
from all responsibility for any ill effects which may result from
such discharge.




_____        _____
Witness                              Signed By:
                                     (Patient or Nearest Relative)


_____        Relationship:  _____
Witness

NOTE:  Authorization must be signed by the patient, or by the nearest
       relative in the case of a minor; or when patient is physically
       or mentally incompetent.
```

patient is disruptive, a patient representative, security personnel, or legal counsel should be called in to assist. A formal written request from legal counsel might be presented to the patient.

If a patient is sent home by taxi, document the name of the taxicab company, time of pickup, and name and badge number of the taxi driver. Instruct the taxi driver to take the patient to the address listed as the home address and not to allow the patient to persuade the driver to go to another address. Ask the driver to contact the institution when the patient is safely home.

False Imprisonment

False imprisonment is the unlawful, intentional confinement of a person within an area so that the confined person is aware of the confinement or harmed by it. Restraints fall into the category of false imprisonment. Institutions should use restraints only as a last resort and only with a doctor's order. Most institutions have policies that require a patient to agree to remain in the institution until discharged. Retaining patients against their will has been ruled false imprisonment. Nurses must be familiar with state laws because they can be very specific regarding health care providers' and institutions' responsibilities in regard to detention, especially of vulnerable patients. Failure to understand and comply with the applicable laws can lead to liability for false imprisonment.

DO-NOT-RESUSCITATE ORDERS

The National Conference of Commissioners on Uniform State Laws proposed the Uniform Right of the Terminally Ill Act, which establishes uniform provisions in regard to powers of attorney for health care, living wills, and other directives. Most states have adopted parts of the Act (AHA, 1992). This section discusses only the do-not-resuscitate (DNR) directive.

Most statutes regulating the use of DNR orders specifically apply to medical emergencies that occur in health care institutions or in a patient's home. Most states allow DNR orders for competent and incompetent patients, but some require that DNR orders be used only with a competent patient's consent.

The majority of the statutes provide immunity for health care providers acting in good faith in reliance upon a DNR order. Professionals upholding the DNR order are protected from civil, criminal, and professional liability. This means that disciplinary action may not be taken by a licensing board and that the health care providers may not be sued by the patient or family. Additionally, the state may not criminally prosecute.

Most institutions suspend DNR orders during surgery. Although this may not be a legal practice, many surgeons and anesthesiologists are adamant about needing to be free to attempt to reverse any adverse responses to the surgery or anesthesia. They contend that it is unacceptable to expect anesthesiologists, anesthetists, and surgeons to bear the moral burdens of being able to alter or suspend normal life processes through anesthesia or surgery while being constrained from reversing the effects of their own work. Patients sometimes do not know and are not told that their DNR directives will not be honored during surgery.

A DNR order must be written for health care providers to be protected. Each institution should have policies regarding DNR orders. Such orders should have a time limit, so that they are periodically reviewed. Any discussions in regard to DNR orders with the patient or the family must be documented. If an institution has a formal DNR form (see Figure 9-3), it should explain what happens if the patient is not resuscitated. The form should be signed, dated, and witnessed by the patient or family member who consents to such an order. The patient or family members should receive a copy of the form, and a copy should remain on file or in the patient's medical record.

BLAME CHARTING

Nothing but the truth should be documented in the medical record. It is not professional practice to point fingers, make a fuss in the chart, or use sloppy documentation. For example, document each time you call a physician rather than documenting that you called again because the physician never returned the call. Opinions, use of unapproved abbreviations, speculative remarks, and ambiguous or improper words should not be used. By always charting only facts that the nurse sees, hears, smells, feels, or even tastes, the nurse's documentation will be appropriate and accurate. Review previous chapters for information about proper documentation and ways to prevent lawsuits.

PHYSICIAN'S ORDERS

Physician's orders have been discussed in previous chapters; however, they can lead to documentation problems. Make sure the order is legible and properly transcribed. Follow the institution's policy for clarifying any order that is vague or possibly in error. Misunderstandings or documentation of incorrect orders are more likely to occur when receiving verbal or telephone orders. It is also possible that the physician may misdiagnose a problem and give inappropriate orders or wrong medication orders over the telephone. Most institutions discourage verbal and telephone orders in circumstances other than emergencies because the physician may deny having given the order.

It is not wise to obtain DNR orders verbally or by telephone. If any controversy results in the death of a patient and how the DNR order was obtained, the nurse may become liable, especially if the physician disavows giving the order and refuses to sign the order. If a DNR order must be obtained over the telephone, the nurse should have a witness listen in on the call to verify the order and then document in the chart the name of the witness.

FIGURE 9-3: SAMPLE DNR FORM (1 OF 2)

PATIENT IMPRINT AREA

WellStar   Place bar code label here
Health System
☐ **Cobb**   ☐ **Douglas**   ☐ **Kennestone**
☐ **Paulding**   ☐ **Windy Hill**

PHYSICIAN ORDERS FOR LIFE-SUSTAINING TREATMENT

THIS IS A PHYSICIAN ORDER SHEET and is based on patient wishes and/or medical condition. Patient wishes may be determined through a written directive or through a personal conversation with the patient/resident or surrogate.

A.   **Resuscitation:** Patient, resident and/or surrogate decision-maker desires:

☐ **Full resuscitation.**

☐ **Desires resuscitation with the following exceptions:** Check any treatments that <u>are not to be implemented</u> for arrest/near-arrest situations based on patient or surrogate expressed wishes. If option is <u>not checked</u>, it is assumed that patient/resident/surrogate decision-maker <u>desires that treatment</u>:

     ☐   **Do not do** chest compressions
     ☐   **Do not** manually ventilate with mask/bag/valve device
     ☐   **Do not** intubate
     ☐   **Do not** place on mechanical ventilation
     ☐   **Do not** perform electrical shock/defibrillation
     ☐   **Do not** give medications to stimulate heart or to treat heart rhythm disturbances

☐ **Do Not Resuscitate (DNR):** No treatment in the event of cardiopulmonary arrest. All measures to promote patient comfort and dignity will be provided.

B.   **Care/Treatments:** Patient/resident or surrogate decision-maker desires:

☐ **Full supportive care**

☐ **Desires supportive care with the following exceptions:** Check only interventions that <u>are not to be implemented</u> based on patient or surrogate expressed wishes. If option is <u>not checked</u>, it is assumed that patient/resident or surrogate decision-maker <u>desires that treatment</u>.

     ☐   **Do not** give antibiotics
     ☐   **Do not** administer artificial nutrition (tube feedings)
     ☐   **Do not** administer artificial hydration (IV fluids)
     ☐   **Do not** give medications to support blood pressure
     ☐   **Do not** give blood/blood products
     ☐   **Do not** perform kidney dialysis
     ☐   **Do not** perform major surgery
     ☐   **Do not** insert invasive lines (arterial line, pulmonary artery line, central vein line)
     ☐   **Other**_____

☐ **Comfort care only**

C.   **Check all that apply:** The above orders are based on discussion with:
     ☐   patient
     ☐   advance directive; specify agent _____Phone #_____
     ☐   surrogate decision-maker, specify_____Phone #_____

D.   **Other:** These orders are to remain in effect during any surgical or invasive procedure. ☐ **Yes**   ☐ **No**

_____   _____
Physician Signature   *Date/Time*

PHYSICIAN ORDERS FOR LIFE-SUSTAINING TREATMENT   7/00

FIGURE 9-3: SAMPLE DNR FORM (2 OF 2)

1.   This form is to be completed for any patient requiring DNR or limited *Life-Sustaining treatment orders.*

2.   *Telephone orders are appropriate when the physician is sufficiently aware of the patient's medical condition and patient/surrogate wishes.* Two RN's (or 1 RN and 1 LPN) must hear the order and co-sign the order to this effect. The physician must then sign the order within 24 hours.

3.   The order form will be maintained as the **first document in the medical record** (in front of advance directive for final healthcare).

4.   Physician can make changes to order form only by writing "void" across the current order form and filling out a new "Life-Sustaining Treatment" order form. In order to alert staff to changes, a note must be entered in physician orders to indicate "New DNR/Life-Sustaining Treatment Orders".

5.   If orders are revoked, physician must write "cancel" or "revoke" the DNR / Life-Sustaining Treatment Orders in physician orders. RN will then write "Void" or "Revoked" across order form and note name, title, date and time. Order form should be moved to back of chart and any notations in treatment plan regarding limited treatment should be deleted.

6.   Special/surgical procedures and DNR / Life-Sustaining Treatment:: If orders are to be suspended for a special / surgical procedure, the physician must discuss this suspension with patient / surrogate and write orders to suspend the "DNR / Life-Sustaining Treatment orders" during the surgical period on specific date in the standard order sheet and check the block on the *Physician Orders for Life-Sustaining Treatment* (under "other ") and initial and date this clarification. Nurse will be responsible for amending treatment plan and communicating orders to suspend to OR and PACU staff.

The following guidelines are intended to assist the physician in writing of DNR/Life-Sustaining Treatment Orders:

A.   *Adults with decision-making capacity may express their wishes regarding withholding resuscitation and expect that these wishes be honored. Wishes may be expressed in advance through an advance directive/directive for final health care.*

B.   *An advance directive/ directive for final healthcare becomes effective when the patient/resident no longer has decision-making capacity. The assessment of decision-making capacity is a clinical judgement to be made by a physician.*

C.   *When an adult patient no longer has decision-making capacity or an advance directive/ directive for final healthcare, the patient must be determined to be a candidate for non-resuscitation prior to writing of DNR orders. The following guidelines are followed in determining that patient is a candidate for non-resuscitation*:*

   1.   *Has a medical condition which can reasonably be expected to result in imminent death of the patient <u>or</u>*

   2.   *Is in a non-cognitive state with no reasonable possibility of regaining cognitive function <u>or</u>*

   3.   *Is a person for whom cardiopulmonary resuscitation would be medically futile in that such resuscitation will likely be unsuccessful in restoring cardiac and respiratory function or will only restore cardiac and respiratory function for a brief time with expectation that repeated need for resuscitation will occur within a short time.*

   *This determination is made by attending physician with the concurrence of another physician.

D.   *In the event the patient has lost decision-making capacity, has no advance directive, and there are no surrogates for decision making, a DNR can be ordered after written concurrence by a second independent physician and review and concurrence by the Ethics Committee that the patient is a candidate for non-resuscitation.*

It is not uncommon for an office nurse to call orders, especially admission orders, to a nurse on a unit. If you receive such orders, make sure you clearly understand the orders given, the physician and the patient's name, and the name of the person calling in the orders. Make sure all this information is clearly documented in the patient's medical record.

TELEPHONE TRIAGE

The last documenting area that will be discussed covers telephone triage. Telephone triage is becoming more popular as a cost-cutting mechanism by managed care organizations. Any nurse working triage should precisely and carefully document any incoming call. Any advice given should be documented in the patient's medical record or in a logbook. Triage is important for providing an immediate response to patient needs, relieving medical staff of minor incidents, and controlling patient flow. However, telephone triage may result in potential liability for a nurse making treatment choices.

Both nurses and physicians should use caution when giving advice or prescribing treatment or medications over the telephone without seeing the patient. Nurses working telephone triage should have standard orders for reference. Telephone triage nurses should refrain from offering medical advice over the telephone and should be sure to practice within the protocol of the state nurse practice act. When in doubt, the nurse should advise the patient to come to the physician's office or go to an emergency room.

When possible, try to talk to the patient rather than another person. Determine when the symptoms began, what the patient was doing, what the patient has done or taken, and whether the symptoms are getting better or worse. If concerned, the nurse should call the patient back to find out if the recommendations made a difference. If the patient reports a worsened condition or has called more than once in 8 hours, the nurse should encourage the patient to come in for an examination or encourage the patient to go to the closest emergency room. The nurse must document the substance of the call, what the patient was told, and any needed follow-up in the patient's chart, if it is available.

CONCLUSION

Documentation is a vital component of nursing practice. Nurses are accountable for their actions; therefore, information in the record must be clear, logical, and describe exactly what happened along with all care provided. The health care environment creates many challenges for accurately documenting and reporting care provided to patients. Accurate information ensures continuity and quality of care by providing safeguards against documentation problems. By documenting facts accurately, completely, and in a timely manner, nurses may avoid disasters and provide sound defense in any lawsuits that evolve from a particular situation.

EXAM QUESTIONS

CHAPTER 9
Questions 66-71

66. Areas that may place nurses at risk for potential lawsuits include

    a. supervising their own work, delegating routine normal hygiene to a UAP, and increasing frequency of rounds.

    b. attempting to secure adequate staffing and using approved methods for correcting charting errors.

    c. having a UAP administer medications, throwing away a chart page covered with coffee, and making erasures in the chart.

    d. reviewing all entries prior to countersigning, charting facts and direct quotes, and following up on telephone triage calls.

67. Before assigning a UAP to care for a patient, the nurse must

    a. determine that the UAP is qualified to perform the necessary task.

    b. certify the UAP.

    c. determine that no other nurse is available to care for the patient.

    d. check the hospital's policies to determine if aides may receive patient assignments.

68. A staff nurse being floated to another floor should accept a patient care assignment only if

    a. the patient would otherwise be left without any nurse.

    b. he or she feels comfortable with most aspects of the needed care.

    c. he or she has been adequately oriented to the treatments and care required by patients on that unit.

    d. the union contract governing nurse employment allows it.

69. When writing your last nursing note for the day, you realize that you neglected to document the patient's 11:00 a.m. serum glucose level and the amount of insulin you administered. You correct this situation by

    a. adding no further notation, because the patient's care was not compromised.

    b. inserting the missing information where it is chronologically correct.

    c. completing an incident report and adding it to the medical record.

    d. writing the information on the next available line in the notes, clearly indicating that it is a late entry.

70. DNR orders

    a. must be oral.

    b. must be written.

    c. must have no time limits for renewal.

    d. protect the patient's family.

71. Dr. Jones knows that a patient is terminal and calls the unit with a verbal telephone order for DNR. You as the nurse

    a. refuse to take the order.

    b. write the order without any questions.

    c. let the unit secretary write the order.

    d. have a witness listen in on the call to verify the order.

CHAPTER 10

DOCUMENTATION IN SPECIFIC HEALTH CARE SETTINGS

CHAPTER OBJECTIVE

After completing this chapter, the reader will be able to describe documentation methods used in specific settings.

LEARNING OBJECTIVES

After studying this chapter, the reader will be able to

1. identify differences in documentation practices used in specific settings.

2. indicate four specific documentation forms used in various settings.

3. compare standard documentation requirements to specific setting requirements.

INTRODUCTION

Most hospitals still use the medical model and arrange departments by the services rendered. Nurses use a variety of documentation methods, and some specific departments require additional or particular kinds of documentation. Regardless of the method used for documentation, the chart is always a formal, legal document that details a patient's needs, interventions, evaluations, and progress. Additionally, nurses should use good documentation practices to provide complete and accurate descriptions of the patient's care.

The patient's medical record may be composed of a variety of forms, some of which were discussed in Chapter 1. Likewise, the institution may require nurses to document using a specific method. These methods were discussed in Chapter 3. Forms and documentation methods are used to make documentation easy, quick, and comprehensive. Most forms eliminate the need to duplicate repeated data in the nursing notes. Forms provide specific information in a format that is more accessible than long, detailed progress notes.

In all settings, nurses should use the documentation strategies discussed in Chapters 5, 6, and 7, adapting those strategies to meet their specific requirements. This chapter presents information about special documentation requirements in several specific settings. Examples of forms are displayed throughout the chapter. Each form is a representation only from the institution providing the form and is not presented as absolute truth. There are numerous other forms that many hospitals use that are not addressed.

MEDICAL-SURGICAL UNIT DOCUMENTATION

Medical-surgical, or adult health care, units may be further subdivided into specific areas of care based on illnesses or conditions or other criteria, such as gynecology, general surgery, orthopedics, and cardiology. Each unit uses the institution's approved documentation method. However, each unit may have additional forms required to better document care provided to patients. For instance, orthopedic units commonly use care pathways for different orthopedic surgical procedures; cardiology may have telemetry records. An example of an adult-health care form is found in Figure 10-1.

Various methods are used to document patient care. Each health care institution selects the method that best meets its needs. Specific medical-surgical units' documentation requirements are commonly based on standards developed by specific specialty organizations. The types of methods that can be used were presented in Chapter 3. In addition, many health care institutions have adopted computerized documentation systems. Chapter 4 addressed computerized documentation and its ability to save time, improve the monitoring of quality issues, and make it easier to gain access to patient information.

LABOR AND DELIVERY DOCUMENTATION

Labor and delivery (L&D) units in hospitals are regulated by the Emergency Medical Treatment and Active Labor Act (EMTALA) (American Hospital Association [AHA], 1992). The act requires hospitals that participate in the Medicare program to provide medical screening to determine if an emergency medical condition exists or if a woman is in labor. The patient, regardless of ability to pay, must have a medical screening examination conducted in a timely manner. Nursing assessment must be conducted and documented. If an emergency situation exists or if the woman is in labor, treatment and stabilization are required under the law before the patient may be discharged or transferred. Hospitals that violate EMTALA are subject to fines of up to $50,000 per violation. Practitioners found guilty of serious or repeated EMTALA violations can be terminated from Medicare participation and from practice in

Medicare-approved facilities as well as being fined up to $50,000 per violation.

The Association of Women's Health, Obstetric, and Neonatal Nurses (AWHONN) and the Emergency Nurses Association (ENA) jointly published a position statement in 1991 regarding the evaluation of obstetric patients in emergency departments (ENA & AWHONN, 1991). AWHONN and ENA support the development of hospital policies and procedures that specifically outline triage, care, and disposition of obstetric patients. The statement indicates that the care of a woman should take place in the area best prepared to handle her needs. AWHONN and ENA recommend that if fetal heart monitoring is used in the emergency unit, the nurse responsible for the monitoring must be educated, be properly credentialed, and meet the hospital's standards for fetal monitoring. These organizations recommend that a woman be immediately referred to the labor unit if fetal gestational age is 20 weeks or greater and the presenting complaint is labor, ruptured membranes, or vaginal bleeding.

Once a patient arrives in L&D, the unit has its own specific forms for documentation. AWHONN, the American College of Obstetricians and Gynecologists (ACOG), and the American Academy of Pediatrics (AAP) have guidelines and publications to assist nurses in identifying areas that need to be documented. AWHONN's (1998) standards and guidelines recommend that documentation follow the nursing process and that data be documented in a retrievable format.

Most perinatal units have developed assessment forms that address prenatal care, prenatal problems, a review of systems, medications, and intake of food and fluid. Maternal vital statistics, including the woman's age, number of pregnancies, parity, estimated due date, fetal gestational age, and maternal height and weight, are also documented. Numerous forms have been developed for use in L&D for a variety of procedures. Some of these forms are listed in Table 10-1 on pages 151.

FIGURE 10-1: SAMPLE ADULT HEALTH CARE FORM (1 OF 2)

| Time: | Date: | Nurse's Progress Notes |

Cognitive - Behavioral Perceptual

Loc.
- ☐ Alert ☐ Orient. Time ☐ Forgetful
- ☐ Orient. Pers. ☐ Orient. Situa. ☐ Lethargic
- ☐ Orient. Place ☐ Asleep ☐ No resp. to stimuli

Emot. Status
- ☐ Calm ☐ Fearful ☐ Withdrawn
- ☐ Cheerful ☐ Irritable ☐ Labile
- ☐ Anxious ☐ Apathetic

Pain
- ☐ Denies ☐ Present ☐ Scale (1-10) _____
- ☐ Location: _____
- ☐ Description: _____

Oxygenation - Ventilation Tissue Perfusion

Resp.
- ☐ No distress ☐ Irregular ☐ O₂ _____
- ☐ Dyspnea/rest ☐ Dyspnea/Exertion

Lung Sounds
- ☐ N/A ☐ Fine Crackles: _____
- ☐ Clear/Equal: _____ ☐ Coarse Crackles: _____
- ☐ Diminished: _____ ☐ Wheezes: _____

Cough
- ☐ Absent ☐ Productive:
- ☐ Non-Productive — A: Color: _____
- B: Amount: _____
- C: Consistency: _____

Pulses
- ☐ N/A

	R	B	F	PT	DP
R:					
L:					

- ☐ Telemetry: _____

Edema
- ☐ None   Pitting ☐ +1 ☐ +2 ☐ +3 ☐ +4
- ☐ Nonpitting   Location: _____

Nutrition - Elimination

Food Intake
- ☐ 100% ☐ 75% ☐ 50% ☐ 25% ☐ 0% ☐ NPO
- ☐ Tube Feeding: _____
- ☐ Nausea ☐ Aggravating Factors: _____

Abd.
- ☐ N/A ☐ Soft ☐ Firm ☐ Distended
- ☐ Tender ☐ N/G Suction Drainage: _____

Bowel Sounds
- ☐ N/A ☐ Absent ☐ Hyperactive
- ☐ Active ☐ Passing Flatus ☐ Hypoactive

Stools
- ☐ Not observed ☐ Loose ☐ Colostomy
- ☐ No Stool ☐ Hard ☐ Ileostomy
- ☐ Formed ☐ Incontinent ☐ Other

Urine
- ☐ Not observed ☐ Hematuria ☐ Dysuria
- ☐ Clear/yellow ☐ Foul ☐ Foley
- ☐ Cloudy ☐ Incontinent ☐ Suprapubic

Integumentary

Mucous Membranes
- ☐ Moist ☐ Dry ☐ Tender
- ☐ Intact ☐ Cracked ☐ Sores

Skin
- Skin: ☐ Warm ☐ Dry ☐ Hot ☐ Cool ☐ Diaphoretic
- Turgor: ☐ WNL ☐ Tight ☐ Loose
- Color: ☐ WNL ☐ Pale ☐ Flushed ☐ Other: _____
- Integrity: ☐ Intact ☐ Broken: _____

Incision
- Incision: ☐ N/A ☐ Not Observed
- Location: _____
- ☐ Steri Strips
- ☐ Sutures/Staples ☐ Intact ☐ Removed
- ☐ Collodian
- Edges: ☐ Well Approx ☐ Open ☐ Inflamed
- ☐ Drainage   Amt: _____ Color: _____

Wound
- Wound: ☐ N/A ☐ Not Obsv. Location: _____
- Descrip: ☐ Red ☐ Blister ☐ Yellow
- ☐ Necrotic ☐ Edema ☐ Granulating
- ☐ Drainage: _____

Dsg.
- ☐ N/A ☐ Dry ☐ Intact ☐ Changed
- Location: _____

Mobility
- Gait: ☐ Not Observed ☐ Steady ☐ Unsteady
- Extremity Movement: ☐ All ☐ RA ☐ LA
- ☐ RL ☐ LL

Signature _____

FIGURE 10-1: SAMPLE ADULT HEALTH CARE FORM (2 OF 2)

```
                          PIEDMONT HOSPITAL                Page 1
            09/24/04 Shift 1 thru 09/24/04 Shift 2              Cont'd
```

ADL'S / MISC.
 ACCU-CHEK   Q 4 HRS
 ACCU-CHEK   AC & HS
 VITAL SIGN   ROUTINE
 FEEDING   SELF
 I&O   Q SHIFT
 TOILET   B/ROOM W ASSIST
 BATH   PARTIAL/ASSIST
 TRANSPORT   *STRETCHER
 BEDREST   *W FEET ELEVATED

Diet: DIABETIC-1500 CAL

ACTIVE ORDERS
 EKG   09/23 1038
 LOWER EXT ARTERIAL EV 09/22 1212
  bilateral arterial dopplers
 VENOUS DOPPLER LOWER   09/22 1116

PRN ORDERS

TREATMENTS
 1:ACCUCHECK Q 4HR OVERNITE UNTIL POST
   FASTING LIPID PROFILE
 2:NPO after 2000 (8 pm) for fasting
   lipid profile in AM at 0800 am.
   thanks
 3:IV THERAPY (PLACE ON I&O):
   D 5 W AT 75 ML/HR
 4: IV SITE: SWELLING YES/NO
   REDNESS YES/NO   PAIN YES/NO
 5:PHARMACY NOTIFIED OF IV D/C, RATE OR
   SOLUTION CHANGE: Y/N:_____
 6:CONSULT IMS -DIABITES CONTROL
   CALLED 09/22/04 10:22
 7:__COPY OF ADVANCE DIRECTIVE ON CHART
   __FURTHER FOLLOW UP REQUIRED
   __PT'S ADVANCE DIRECTIVE NOT
     AVAILABLE
   __PT DOES NOT HAVE OR WANT ADV.DIR.
 8:PRESSURE SORE PREVENTION
   SKIN ASSESSMENT Q 72 HOURS
   INITIAL SCORE _____   DATE: _____
   CURRENT SCORE _____   DATE: _____
   REASSESSMENT DATE: _____
 9:PATIENT TEACHING: REFER TO INTER-
   DISCIPLINARY EDUCATION RECORD.

PLAN OF CARE
 * = Completed elements

PC:INFECTION, ACTUAL
DO:PT/SO VERBALIZES UNDERSTANDING OF
   INFECTION PRECAUTIONS TO TAKE AFTER
   DISCHARGE.
 1:TEACH INFECTION PRECAUTIONS FOR
   PT/SO TO TAKE HOME-SPECIFIC TO
   PATIENT'S CONDITION (DRESSING
   CHANGE, AVOID CROWDS, MONITOR
   TEMPERATURE, HAND WASHING, ETC.).
 2:TEACH PT/SO SIGNS AND SYMPTOMS OF
   INFECTION TO REPORT TO M.D.
   (INCREASED TEMPERATURE, INCREASED
   WOUND DRAINAGE, PAIN, ETC.).
EO:PATIENT WILL HAVE APPROPRIATE
   ISOLATION/INFECTION PRECAUTIONS
   TAKEN BASED ON INFECTIVE MATERIAL.
 1:FOLLOW ISOLATION PRECAUTIONS
   APPROPRIATE FOR THE PATIENT'S
   INFECTIVE MATERIAL (SIGN ON DOOR,
   ISOLATION CART, GOWN/GLOVES, MASK,
   ETC.).
 2:NOTIFY INFECTION CONTROL NURSE OF
   ANY CHANGES IN PATIENT'S CONDITION
   OR STATUS.
 3:INSTRUCT PT/SO REGARDING HOW TO
   MAINTAIN ISOLATION PRECAUTIONS IN
   HOSPITAL.

PC:AGE SPEC/ADULT AGES 18-65
DO:PATIENT WILL RECEIVE APPROPRIATE
   CARE RELATED TO SPECIFIC AGE GROUP
   AND DEVELOPMENTAL STAGE.
 1:ACTIVELY INVOLVE ADULT IN PLANNING
   AND IN DECISION MAKING.
 2:ASSESSE CULTURAL AND RELIGIOUS
   BELIEFS AND ADAPT PLAN OF CARE,
   DIET, AND PATIENT EDUCATION TO NEEDS
 3:ASSESS AND EVALUATE RISK FACTORS
   RELATED TO THE DEVELOPMENT OF HEALTH
   PROBLEMS. INCLUDE RISK FACTORS IN
   HEALTH TEACHING.
 4:INCLUDE EVALUATION OF FUNCTIONAL
   NEEDS AND HOME ENVIRONMENT IN
   DISCHARGE PLANNING.

Dx : 682.9-CELLULITIS NOS
Alg: nka+
Iso: Smk: UNK
Sgy:
                        Type: IP
                        0326500068

Phys: Level: 2

INT | SIGNATURE
_____|_____
_____|_____
_____|_____
_____|_____

Wed Sep 24,2004 0919

PATIENT CARE PROFILE   # 7

TABLE 10-1: LABOR AND DELIVERY FORMS

- Antenatal testing
- Short stay assessment forms
- Labor and delivery admission and assessment forms
- Labor progress records
- Delivery records for both vaginal and caesarean section
- Postdelivery record
- Newborn assessment forms

Some hospitals have adopted all or parts of the Hollister Labor Progress Chart® to use during the labor process. Documentation on any form has strict guidelines. AWHONN, ACOG, and AAP recommended frequencies for nursing assessment and documentation. The normal frequency of assessment and documentation ranges from every 4 hours or more frequently for maternal temperature to every 5 minutes for fetal heart tones and other maternal vital signs during active second stage labor. There are even times when maternal blood pressure is taken every minute, such as with the initial dose of epidural medications. All nurses working in L&D should be well versed in the additional parameters needed for assessment and the standards guiding documentation.

Many cases of L&D nursing negligence have been reported in the literature. The most common types of nursing negligence that appear in records that come to litigation are highlighted in Table 10-2 and were discussed earlier.

TABLE 10-2: LABOR AND DELIVERY NURSING NEGLIGENCE

- Incomplete initial history and physical examination
- Failure to assess and take appropriate action
- Incomplete or inadequate documentation
- Failure to use or interpret fetal monitoring appropriately

Avoiding liability encompasses documenting a thorough initial history and physical assessment; appropriately practicing the nursing process through ongoing assessments, interventions, and evaluations; timely notification of the health care practitioner of changes in status; and proficiency in electronic fetal monitoring interpretation. See Figures 10-2 and 10-3 on pages 152-154 for sample L & D forms.

Postanesthesia and postdelivery documentation needs to reflect recommendations by the American Society of Postanesthesia Nurses as well as AWHONN guidelines. Documentation in the record should follow the policies adopted by the institution. In addition, documentation in the postpartum period includes assessment, nursing diagnoses, interventions, and evaluations (see Figure 10-4 on pages 155-156). AWHONN recommends that postpartum checks be done every 15 minutes for the first hour, every 30 minutes for the second hour, and then every 4 hours for the first 24 hours. More frequent assessment should be carried out if indicated. The assessment includes vital signs as well as status of the uterus.

A thorough and systematic newborn assessment must be made and the findings documented. All measurements, vital signs, and assessments are usually performed shortly after birth. Newborn documentation forms can provide a system whereby checkmarks or initials can indicate expected findings and the narrative notes reflect abnormal findings. The newborn physical exam includes assessment of all systems and provides the baseline for serial examinations during the infant's stay in an institution. The nurse must be able to identify normal anomalies related to intrauterine positioning and the birth process from more serious abnormalities that may require early intervention and treatment. A sample newborn assessment form is displayed in Figure 10-5 on pages 157-158.

Postdelivery and postpartum care varies from hours to a few days, depending on early discharge

text continues on page 159

FIGURE 10-2: SAMPLE LABOR AND DELIVERY FLOW SHEET (1 OF 2)

RISK FACTORS: _____

_____

PEDIATRICIAN: _____

ST. JOSEPH HOSPITAL
Living the Mission

Labor-Delivery Flow Sheet

Admit Date / /	Admit Time	Blood Type and Rh	Age	G	T	Pt	A	I	EDD __/__/__ LMP __/__/__	Membranes	☐ Intact ☐ Ruptured SROM AROM ☐ Bulging Date ___/___/___ Time ___		

		Current Date / /	Time →												

VITAL SIGNS

| Blood Pressure |
| Pulse |
| Respirations |
| Temperature |
| Pain Scale 0 - 10 |

INTAKE/OUTPUT — CC's/HR

| IV Fluids |
| P O |
| Running Total |
| Urine |
| Emesis |
| Running Total |

MATERNAL

| Deep Tendon Reflexes |
| Clonus |
| Urine Protein |
| Vaginal Bleeding |
| Breath Sounds |
| Vaginal Exam: Dilation |
| Effacement |
| Station |
| Initials of Examiner: |

UTERINE ACTIVITY

| Monitor Mode |
| Frequency |
| Intensity |
| Duration |
| Resting Tone |
| MVUs |

FETAL ASSESSMENT

| Monitor Mode |
| Baseline (FHR) Range |
| STV |
| LTV |
| Accelerations |
| Decelerations |
| Membranes |
| Fluid |

CONT MEDS

| Pitocin mU/min |
| MgSo4 gms/hr |
| MgSo4 Level |

| Position Change |
| O₂ L/min |
| Epidural |
| PRN Meds: |
| Side Rails/Call Light |
| Initials |

Abbreviations/Key
Pain Scale 0 - 10
0 = No Pain
10 = Worst Pain

STV Short Term Variability
Present +
Absent -

LTV Long Term Variability
Absent 0-2 bpm
Min. 3-5
Avg. 6-10
Mod. 11-25
Marked > 25

S = Sinusoidal 1-10 minute Fluctuations of Long Term Variability, Appearing Wavy, Ominous Regardless of Wave Depth

Monitor Mode Fetal
F = Fetoscope
D = Doppler
E = External
I = Internal (Scalp Electrode)

Accelerations
+ = Present
0 = Absent

Form No. 1900019 Rev. 3/01

FIGURE 10-2: SAMPLE LABOR AND DELIVERY FLOW SHEET (2 OF 2)

Fluid	☐ **Clear** ☐ Foul Smelling	Medication Allergy/Sensitivity	☐ None	☐ Breast	☐ Bottle	
	☐ Meconium ☐ Bloody	(Identity/Reaction) _____				Page _____ of _____

| **Decelerations**
N = None
E = Early
V = Variable
L = Late | **Vaginal Bleeding**
NS = Normal show
ABN = Frank Vaginal
      Bleeding | **Membranes**
I = Intact
B = Bulging
R = Ruptured | **Fluid**
C = Clear
M= Meconium
      Stained
B = Bloody
F = Foul Smelling | **Monitor Mode Uterine Activity**
P = Palpation
E = External
I = Internal | **MVUs Montevideo Units**
The sum of the peak of each
uterine contraction minus
resting tone, in a 10
minute period. | **Side Rails** ↑ up
             ↓ down
Call Light —
    ✓ within Reach | **Pulse Oximeter**
             ✓ = ON
Dermatone Levels
State Level: |

Form No. 1900019   Rev. 3/01

Reprinted with the permission of St. Joseph Hospital, Augusta, GA.

FIGURE 10-3: SAMPLE LABOR AND DELIVERY FORM

ST. JOSEPH HOSPITAL
2260 Wrightsboro Road
AUGUSTA, GEORGIA 30910-3199

LABOR AND DELIVERY DATA

EDC	Admit Date

Date of Del.

Time

Membranes Rupt.

☐ Spont.   ☐ Artif.   Date

☐ Prem.   Time

Onset Labor

Comp. Dilat.

Del. Placenta Time

Hr./Min.

Stage I	/	___
Stage II	/	___
Stage III	/	___
Total Labor	/	___
RH Type RPR		

COMPLICATIONS

MATERNAL

☐ Hypertensive
___Toxemia ___Mild
_____Severe
___Eclampsia
___Anemia
___Diabetes
___Heart Disease
___KUB Disease
___Pulmonary Dis.
___Venereal Dis.
___Gyn. Pathology
___Fever (100.4)
___Other

FETAL

___Cong. Anomalies
___Meconium
___Dec. FHT Var.
___Ext. Fetal Tachy.
___Mult. Late Decel.
___Mult. Var. Decel.

DECEASED

Date_____ Time_____
___Antepartum
___Intrapartum
___Neonatal

LABOR

___Failed Induct.
___Uterine Inertia
___Disproportion
___Multiple Preg.
___Hydramnios
___Amnionitis
___Persist. Occ. Post.
___Deep Trans. Arrest
___Dystocia
___Hemmorrhage
___Uterine Atony
___Shoulder Dyst.
___Failed Forceps
___Other

ANESTHESIA

___Convulsion
___Fetal Brad
___Hypotension
___Other

C-Section — ☐ Repeat

☐ Primary
Reason _____

Comments _____

B/P p Del.

☐ Breast   ☐ Bottle

G	T	P	A	L	M	

MOTHER

ANESTHESIA FOR LABOR & DELIVERY	EPISIOTOMY	LACERATION	DELIVERY

ANESTHESIA FOR LABOR & DELIVERY
☐ Para Cervical   ☐ Spinal
☐ Pudendal   ☐ General
☐ Saddle   ☐ None
☐ Other   ☐ Complication
☐ Local   ☐ Epidural ☐ Labor ☐ Del
   Infiltration   ☐ Caudal ☐ Labor ☐ Del

EPISIOTOMY
☐ None
☐ Mid Line
☐ Med Lat
☐ Episio-
   proctotomy

LACERATION
☐ Uterine
☐ Cervical
☐ Vaginal
☐ Perineal
☐ I°   ☐ II°
☐ III°   ☐ IV°

DELIVERY
☐ Perineal Prep & Drape   Position_____

VAGINAL VERTEX
☐ Spontaneous
☐ Outlet Forceps
☐ Mid Forceps
☐ Rotation:
☐ Silastic Extraction

VAGINAL BREECH
☐ Spontaneous
☐ Assisted Ext.
☐ Total Ext.
☐ Piper

C-SECTION
☐ Low Trans
☐ Low Vert
☐ Classical
☐ C-Section/Hy

NEWBORN

MULT BIRTH
☐ No
☐ Twin
☐ Triplet
☐ A ☐ B ☐ C

CONDITION
☐ Liveborn
☐ Stillborn
☐ Early
   Neonatal
   Death

RESUSCITATION
☐ None
☐ Suction Bulb
☐ Oxygen
☐ Pos Pressure
☐ Endotrach Tube
☐ Suction Cath
☐ Umbil Cath
   ☐ Arter ☐ Ven
☐ Medication
☐ Cardiac
   Massage
☐ Complications

APGAR	0	1	2	1 Min	5 Min
Heart Rate	Absent	100	100		
Resp Effort	Absent	Slow Irreg	Good Cry		
Muscle Tone	Limp	Some Flexion	Active Motion		
Reflex Irritabil	No Response	Grimace	Cry		
Color	Pale/Blu	Body Pink Ext. Blu	All Pink		
TOTAL SCORE					

SEX ☐M ☐F
☐ Undeterm
GEST AGE
   wks

CONGENITAL
ABNORMALITIES
INFANT ☐ Urine   –
PASSED ☐ Stool ☐ None
BAPTIZED
☐ Yes   ☐ No

EYE PROPHYL
Erythro-
mycin
☐ Yes
☐ No
☐ No
☐ Yes

WEIGHT

FHT

TAG #

INFANT NOTE

MED. RECORD #

CORD

☐ Normal
☐ Neck X 1
☐ Or More
☐ PH

☐ 3 Vessels
☐ 2 Vessels
☐ Blood to Lab
☐ Abnormality:

PLACENTA
☐ Spontaneous
☐ Expressed
☐ Manual
☐ Abnormality:
☐ To Lab

☐ Previa
☐ Abruptio _____%
☐ Marginal
   Separation _____%

SCALP PH
☐ Yes
☐ No

UTERINE EXPLORATION
☐ No   ☐ Yes
☐ Abnormality:

BLOOD LOSS
☐ < 500
☐ > 500

MEDICATIONS FOR LABOR		MEDICATIONS FOR DELIVERY						
Medications	Total Dosage	Date	Time	Site	Route	Dose	Medication	Sig.

Time of Last Narcotic

Pediatrician _____

Pediatrician
In Attendance _____   Nurse_____

Obstetrician _____

Obstetrician
In Attendance _____

Reprinted with the permission of St. Joseph Hospital, Augusta, GA.

FIGURE 10-4 : SAMPLE POST DELIVERY RECOVERY RECORD (1 OF 2)

Date _____

RR Nurse _____ Procedure _____

Anesthesia: Epidural / Spinal   Medical Problems _____

ASA _____ Pre-Op BP_____ Pre-Op Medication _____

OR Meds: _____

ADMISSION		Delivery Time: _____	EQUIPMENT
Siderails _____		Sex: _____	EKG Moniter _____ Alarm Setting 140/50
ID Band _____		Breast or Bottle: _____	Oximeter _____ Alarm Settings 85
IV Site _____		with Mom: _____	IV Pump _____
AIRWAY		In Nsy: _____	CADD Pump _____
Natural _____		Significant Other Present: _____	PCA Pump _____
Other _____		Incision: Vert or Trans	X-ray _____
O₂ Therapy		Comments: _____	Others _____
O₂ _____		_____	

TIME	MEDICATIONS / IV FLUIDS	_____ Epidural Infusion of Fentanyl 10mcg/cc
		at _____ ml/hr continuous
		PCA Dosage _____ ml, _____ min, lockout _____ doses / hr
		IV PCA _____ MS 1 mg / cc _____ Demerol 10mg / cc

	PCA ONLY	CONT. ONLY	PCA + CONT
	____MG Q ____MIN		_____MG / HR
		_____MG / HR	PCA____MG Q ____MIN
	4 HR LIMIT_____MG		4 HR LIMIT_____MG

ALDRETE SCORE	A	D	INTAKE OUTPUT	DISMISSAL	DISCHARGED
Able to move 4 extrem. voluntarily or on command 2	‒	‒	**OR** IV____cc URINE____cc	Per Bed_____ Per Stretcher_____	_____ _____
Able to move 2 extrem. voluntarily or on command 1			BLD _____ EBL _____cc	Arrival Time_____ Moved From_____	_____ _____
Unable to move extrem. 0				Stretcher,	_____
Able to deep breathe and cough 2	‒	‒		Self_____	_____
Dyspnea or limited breathing 1					_____
Apneic 0			Total ____cc____cc	Assist_____	_____M.D.
	‒	‒		Roller_____	
BP 20% of PRE ANES LEVEL...............2			**RR**		**TRANSFER TO LDRP**
BP 20%-50% PRE ANES LEVEL.........1					**VITAL SIGNS**
BP 50% of PRE ANES LEVEL..............0	‒	‒	IV____cc URINE____cc	**Call Light in**	
Fully Awake 2				Easy Reach_____	BP_____
Arousable on Calling 1			BLD ____cc____cc	Side Rail Up_____	
Not Responding 0				Bed in Low_____	P_____ R_____
Pink 2	‒	‒	Total ____cc____cc	Position_____	
Pale, dusky, blotchy, jaundice,				Rx _____	Time: _____
Others 1			_____		
Cyanotic...............................0			_____		RN: _____
TOTAL			Total____cc Total____cc	_____	SIGNATURE OF NURSE

FIGURE 10-4: SAMPLE POST DELIVERY RECOVERY RECORD (2 OF 2)

NURSING ASSESSMENTS AND INTERVENTIONS

✔ UNCHANGED
X CHANGED - SEE NOTES

	Admission												Discharge
B/P													
PULSE													
RESP													
TEMP													
O$_2$ SAT													
EKG													
LOC													
FUNDUS													
LOCHIA													
DRESSING													
DERMATOME LEVEL													
PAIN SCALE													
FOLEY URINE COLOR													
PULSES													
BREATH SOUNDS													
WARMING BLANKET													
WARMING LIGHTS													

	NOTES:
	RN SIGNATURE:

FIGURE 10-5: SAMPLE NEWBORN ASSESSMENT FORM (1 OF 2)

ST. JOSEPH HOSPITAL
NEWBORN DELIVERY NOTES
AND PHYSICAL ASSESSMENT

1. **DATE:_____ TIME:_____AM/PM SEX**: Male / Female   Pediatrician:_____
   Attending Pediatrician:_____ Obstetrician:_____
   Maternal History: ❑ GBS+ ❑ Diabetes/ Gestational Diabetes ❑ Other:_____
   EDC:_____   G____T____P____A____L____M_____
2. **PRESENTATION:** ❑ Cephalic   ❑ Breech   ❑ Other _____
3. **MEMBRANE:** Date & Time: _____ ❑ AROM   ❑ SROM   ❑ CLEAR   ❑ Meconium (Light, Moderate, Thick)
4. **METHOD OF DELIVERY:**   ❑ Vaginal ❑ Forceps ❑ Vacuum ❑ C-Section
   Reason for C-Section:_____ APGAR Score: 1 minute_____ 5 minutes_____
5. **CORD:**   ❑ Nuchal   ❑ Knot ❑ Meconium stained   Number of Vessels_____
6. **MATURITY EVALUATIONS**   EGA by date_____wks   EGA by exam_____wks

   ❑ **Pre-term (less than 37 wks.)** ❑ **Term (37 - 42 wks)** ❑ **Post - Term (greater than 42 wks.)**   ❑ **SGA**   ❑ **AGA**   ❑ **LGA**

   Weight:_____ Length:_____   Head Circumference:_____   Chest Circumference:_____
7. **INITIAL STEPS:** Suction on perineum: ❑ Bulb ❑ Delee Color_____   Amount_____
   Suction on warmer: ❑ Bulb ❑ N/G-size _____   Color_____   Amount_____
   Placed on: ❑ Pre-warmed Radiant warmer ❑ Mom's abdomen with warm blankets
   Cords Visualized : ❑ Yes ❑ No   By:_____
   Dried and stimulated: ❑ Yes ❑ No   Heart rate: ❑ > 100 ❑ < 100
   Oxygen: ❑ Blowby with 100% for _____minutes   ❑ PPV with 100% for _____minutes
   Intubation: Size_____ By:_____ Breath Sounds: ❑ Equal   ❑ Bilateral ❑ RT ❑ LT ❑ Clear ❑ Course
   Chemical Resusitation: ❑ Yes   ❑ No ❑ NA (See below for documentation)
8. **GROSS ABNORMALITIES NOTED:** ❑ Yes ❑ No   If yes, please describe:_____
9.

VITAL SIGNS:	ADM	1ST	2ND	3RD	4TH
Time					
Temp					
Pulse					
Resp					
Feeding					
Void					
Stool					
Glucose					
Time MD called:					
Aquamephyton, 1mg IM ❑ RVL ❑ LVL					
Erythromycin Opth Solution OU @					
Neonatal Glucose Whole Blood by Meter Reference Range 40-100 mg					

10. ❑ FOOTPRINTS OF INFANT TAKEN

11. ❑ ID BAND: No_____

    Applied on ankle and wrist of infant in delivery room

12. ❑ Transponder placed: Number_____
    ❑ Entered in Computer

13. ❑ METHOD OF FEEDING: ❑ Breast ❑ Bottle

    Breast fed in L&D? ❑ Yes ❑ No
    L_____   *(See LATCH score tool)*
    A_____
    T_____   Consultation needed ❑ Yes ❑ No
    C_____   Consultant notified (ext 7207) ❑ Yes ❑ No
    H _____
    Total_____

EMERGENCY MEDICATIONS							Birth Time:_____ Weight_____ Apgar: 1_____ 5_____ 10_____
Narcan 0.4mg/cc							**NURSES NOTES:**
Sodium Bicarb. .5mg/cc							
Epinephrine1:10,000							
Atropine 0.1mg/cc							
Calcium Gluc. 10%							
Glucose10%							

Physicians in Attendance:_____   **RN Signature in Attendance:**_____

FIGURE 10-5: SAMPLE NEWBORN ASSESSMENT FORM (2 OF 2)

PHYSICAL ASSESSMENT

CONDITION ON ADMISSION:

Color: Central Pink_____   Cyanosis_____   Acrocyanosis_____   Mottled_____   Pallor_____

               Vasomotor Instability_____   Tongue & Mucous Membranes   Pink_____   Other_____

Heart: Apical Rate_____   Character_____   Murmur_____

Head: Molded_____   Caput_____   Cephalohematoma_____   Bruised_____

               Internal Monitor Scratch_____   Overriding Sutures_____   Fontanels_____

               No Abnormalities   Notes_____

Eyes: Open & Clear_____   Scleral Hemorrhage_____   Cataract_____

               Other_____

Ears   Canals Patent_____   Normal Placement_____   Other_____

Nose: Nares Patent_____   Other_____

Mouth: Hard & Soft Palate Intact_____   Sucking Reflex_____   Other_____

               Cleft Lip_____   Facial Expression Equal_____

Skin: Ecchymosis_____   Petechia_____   Rash_____   Birthmark_____   Vernix_____

               Forcep Mark_____   Turgor_____   No Abnormality   Notes_____

Respirations: Regular_____   Irregular_____   Labored_____   Equal on L&R upon auscultation_____

               Apneic_____   Seesaw_____   Gasping_____   Nasal Flaring_____   Expiratory Grunting_____

               Intercostal Retractions_____   Substernal Retractions_____   Subcostal Retractions_____

               Other_____

Cry: Lusty_____   Weak_____   High Pitched_____

Abdomen: Soft & Flat_____   Distended_____   Scaphoid_____   Hernia_____   Other_____

Muscle tone: Limp_____   Some Flexion_____   Well Flexed_____

Activity: Normal_____   Hypoactive_____   Jittery_____

Genitalia: (Male)   Testes descended_____   (Female) Clitoris & minora completely covered_____

               Any abnormality or Anomaly:_____

Extremities: Full Range of Motion present_____

Date and Time of Exam:_____   Nurse's Signature:_____

Transferred to: _____ By:_____ Report to:_____

Nurses Notes:

_____

_____

_____

_____

_____

_____

_____

_____

_____

status. Continued assessment of the status of the postpartum mother and newborn is performed. The mother's breasts, uterus, bowels, bladder, legs (Homan's sign), and emotional status are evaluated each shift. The weight, vital signs, and eating patterns of the newborn are also evaluated at least once a day or as designated by the hospital. Flow sheets can be used for these evaluation methods that provide quick assessment and identification of any potential problems. Education is a crucial part of the postpartum period and should be carefully documented (see Figures 10-6 and 10-7 on pages 160-164).

No matter what type of documentation method is used, the documentation should provide the record of the nursing care given to the patient during labor, delivery, and recovery and to the newborn following delivery. To help reduce the number of lawsuits, nurses should follow the nursing process, document accurately and appropriately, and know their institutional policies and procedures. Remember: When in doubt, document.

NEONATAL INTENSIVE CARE UNITS DOCUMENTATION

When a newborn is born prematurely, with a congenital anomaly, or is ill, the baby will be placed in a neonatal intensive care unit (NICU). The NICU is designed to facilitate the diagnosis and treatment of infant's immediate and acute, essentially life-threatening problems. Nurses working in the NICU struggle with difficult challenges on a daily basis as they work with parents and other health care professionals to make life-and-death decisions about ill newborns. Proper care can result in a dramatic reduction in the morbidity and mortality rates of these infants. Careful, precise, accurate, and detailed documentation is required in the NICU.

Many patients in the NICU fall into a gray area where it is appropriate for nurses, practitioners, and parents to struggle to determine the neonate's best interest and to proceed accordingly. Many ethicists and health care providers believe that over-treatment, rather than under-treatment, is the major problem in NICU. Fear of legal liability, a failure to understand legal requirements, and the inability to accept the limits of technological medicine contribute to over-treatment.

Intensive care of the ill and immature newborn requires specialized knowledge and skill in a number of areas of expertise. At birth, the newborn is given an assessment to determine any apparent problems and to identify those that need immediate attention. The assessment includes the assignment of an APGAR score (the assessment of immediate adjustment to extrauterine life based on heart rate, respiratory effort, muscle tone, reflex irritability, and color) and an evaluation for any obvious congenital anomalies or evidence of neonatal distress. All of this information must be documented. Maintaining detailed, ongoing records of all activities and observations is an important responsibility of nurses in the intensive care setting. It is not uncommon for nurses to work in pairs with one nurse doing all the charting and the other nurse caring for the newborn. In such an event, the nurse doing the documentation must indicate, by name, who is performing what procedure and then both providers sign the notes.

The NICU normally uses a 24-hour documentation form and begins a new form every day. It is basically a Charting by Exception (CBE) form with a display of frequent observations and vital signs recording format. The Agency for Healthcare Research and Quality (AHRQ) and the AAP has developed clinical guidelines for provision of care and documentation. The National Association of Neonatal Nurses (NANN) and the National Association of Pediatric Nurses Associations and Practitioners (NAPNAP) have developed guidelines to assist in developing procedures and regulations for documentation in the NICU. The neonates'

text continues on page 165

FIGURE 10-6: SAMPLE POSTPARTUM FLOW SHEET (1 OF 2)

ST. JOSEPH HOSPITAL
AUGUSTA, GEORGIA

PATIENT CARE RECORD

O B FLOW SHEET		P1, P2, P3, etc. = Problem documented in Nurses Notes A.S. = ALL SHIFT TOL = Toleration		
DATE:		0700 - 1500	1500 - 2300	2300 - 0700
MENTAL-EMOTIONAL STATUS	Alert & Oriented			
	Confused			
	Lethargic			
	Emotional Affect			
NUTRITION	Diet Type/TOL			
HYGIENE	Oral/Denture Care/cond.			
	AM Care/Type			
	TED - Removed/Reapplied			
	P.M. Care			
	Peri Care			
ACTIVITY	Ambulation: self/assist.			
	Freq./TOL			
	Other: Chair/TOL			
	BRP/BSC			
	Bedrest			
	Turn/Reposition			
SAFE ENVIRON-MENT	Siderail/Bed Position			
	Call Bell Location			
NATURE OF SLEEP	Restful			
	Sleepless			
	Rest measures			
	Results			
BOWEL FUNCTION	B.M.			
	Bowel Sounds			
	Enema/results/TOL			
BLADDER FUNCTION	Voiding/appearance			
	Cath/type			
	Residual			
RESP. FUNCTION	Breath Sounds			
	Pulmonary Care/Type			
	Oxygen			
SKIN/WOUND ASSESSMENT	General Skin Appearance			
	Dressing change/Reinforce			
	Drainage/Amount/Nature			
	Wound Site/Appearance			
	Perineum/Appearance			
	Lochea/Amount/Nature			
	Hemorrhoids			
	Fundus/Level/Location			
	Legs/Homans			
BREASTS	General Appearance/Nipples			
	BRA/Binder			
	pump/Type			
Signature of Principle Care Giver				
	Other Signatures			
		INIT. SIGNATURE	INIT. SIGNATURE	INIT. SIGNATURE

FIGURE 10-6: SAMPLE POSTPARTUM FLOW SHEET (2 OF 2)

IV Prep: (A) Alcohol; (B) Betadine/Alcohol; Tubing Δ: p = primary; s = secondary

DATE:		0700 - 1500	1500 - 2300	2300 - 0700
I.V. THERAPY	1. Site/Appearance			
	pump/tubing Δ (p-s)			
	2. Site/Appearance			
	pump/tubing Δ (p-s)			
	Needle Δ: Size/Type/Prep			
	Site/Appearance			
PAIN INTER-VENTION	Nature/Site			
	Duration			
	Intervention			
	Results			
PRN INTER-VENTION	Nature			
	Duration			
	Intervention			
	Results			
PRO-CEDURES	Sitz bath/TOL			
	Peri light/TOL			
	Heat lamp/TOL			
	Ice/Site/TOL			
	Tucks			
	Creams/Sprays			
	Abdominal Binder			
	Other:			
PHYSICIAN VISITS	Physician(s) Visits			
TRANS-PORTATION	Place/Mode			
	Left/Returned			
PSYCHO-SOCIAL	Support			
	Referrals			
	Infant Bonding			
PATIENT EDUCATION	Topic:			
	Room/Unit Orientation			
	Hygenique/Perilite			
	Tucks/Spray/Pericare			
	Breast Care/Cream			
	Breast Pump			
	Breast Self Exam			
	Post Partum Exercises			
	Incision Care			
	Resp. Care (T, C, DB)			
	Intake/Output			
	PCA Pump			
	Type of Instruction:			
	Evidence of Understanding:			
	Taught To/By Whom			
Signature of Principle Care Giver				
	Other Signatures			
		INIT. / SIGNATURE	INIT. / SIGNATURE	INIT. / SIGNATURE

Reprinted with the permission of St. Joseph Hospital, Augusta, GA.

FIGURE 10-7: SAMPLE NEWBORN CARE RECORD (1 OF 3)

MEDICAL COLLEGE OF GEORGIA
HOSPITALS AND CLINICS   Baby's Blood Type_____
COLLABORATIVE CARE PATHWAY (CCP)   Mom's Blood Type _____
PLAN OF CARE   Type of Delivery _____
Well Baby

DRG: 391   ICD-9 code: 650-659

Date of Birth_____ Time of Birth_____ Time of Arrival to Nursery_____
Sex _____ ID Bands x 2 _____

Care Element/ Focus #	POST DELIVERY 0 – 24 HOURS DATE _____	POST DELIVERY > 24 HOURS DATE _____	AT DISCHARGE DATE _____
Assessment/ Monitor	☐ NB Reassessment ☐ TPR q 30 min x 2 then q 1 hr x 2; then q4 ☐ B/P x 1	☐ NB Reassessment ☐ TPR q8	☐ NB Reassessment ☐ TPR
Procedure/ Test	☐ Capillary Hct @ 12 hrs age	☐ Cord clamp removed ☐ Hearing Screen	☐ Metabolic screens b/f discharge ☐ CIRCUMCISION, if desired
Treatment	☐ Scalp electrode site care per protocol ☐ Bathe per protocol	☐ Scalp electrode site care q 8 hrs with Bacitracin ☐ Bath, prn ☐ Circumcision care, if indicated	☐ Scalp electrode site care ☐ Bath, prn
Meds/IV's	☐ Hep B vaccine IM ordered ☐ Triple dye to cord x 1 ☐ Make sure eye prophylaxis, vitamin K are done in L&D	☐ Alcohol swab to cord ☐ Hep B vaccine IM x1	☐ Alcohol swab to cord ☐ Hep B vaccine IM x1
Nutrition	☐ Breast fed on demand or at least q 3 hr ☐ Non-breast fed per protocol	☐ Breast fed on demand or at least q 3 hrs ☐ Non-breast fed per protocol	☐ Breast fed on demand or at least q 3 hrs ☐ Non-breast fed per protocol
Activity/Self Care	☐ Position on back	☐ Position on back	☐ Position on back
Education & Discharge Coordination	☐ NB feeding ☐ Bulb syringe usage ☐ Positioning ☐ Assess home environment/support ☐ Car seat availability	☐ See Well Baby Teaching Plan: ___ Bath ___ Cord ___ Diapering Care ___ Feeding techniques ___ Positioning ___ Safety/Immunizations	☐ See Well Baby Teaching Plan ☐ Birth Certificate completed ☐ Car seat available ☐ Discharge Instructions given ☐ Lab screens completed
Daily Outcomes	☐ NB vital signs stable ☐ Tolerated bath & first feeding ☐ Parent(s)/family taught feeding positions and use of bulb syringe ☐ Parent(s) showing appropriate bonding behavior ☐ Has car seat & beginning supplies & equipment for baby	☐ NB transitioning and remaining stable ☐ Parent(s)/family receptive to learning & giving care ☐ Discharge instructions begun	☐ Discharge instructions completed ☐ Teaching plan completed

Initials   Name   Title   Initials   Name   Title

_____ _____   _____ _____ _____   _____

_____ _____   _____ _____ _____   _____

_____ _____   _____ _____ _____   _____

_____ _____   _____ _____ _____   _____

FLWSHEET

FIGURE 10-7: SAMPLE NEWBORN CARE RECORD (2 OF 3)

FLWSHEET

MCG H/C
CCP
Well-Baby Flowsheet

Date _____ Time _____ Weight _____

TIME	Vital Signs				Assessment								Nutrition			Elimination			Safety			INITIALS
	TEMP 36.6 - 37.0 (A)	Reg rate & rhythm APICAL PULSE 120-160	Clear & unlabored RESP. 30-60	BP S=50-80 D=25-50	Fontonel - Soft/Flat	Brachial/femoral strong, reg & equal	Skin - dry/intact	Color - Pink, Ruddy, Jaundice	Mucous Membranes - Pink/moist	Activity - quiet, alert, sleeping, crying	Extremities - flexed full ROM	Abd - Soft, Full, BS x 4	FORMULA TYPE	VOLUME CC	FED BY	URINE	STOOL	EMESIS	IV Therapy	Photo Therapy	Blood Glucose	
12ᴹ																						
1																						
2																						
3																						
4																						
5																						
6																						
7																						
8																						
9																						
10																						
11																						
12ᴺ																						
1																						
2																						
3																						
4																						
5																						
6																						
7																						
8																						
9																						
10																						
11																						
24°T																						

Initials _____ Name _____ Title _____ Time _____ Tests/Procedures _____ Initials _____

FIGURE 10-7: SAMPLE NEWBORN CARE RECORD (3 OF 3)

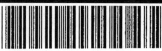

FLWSHEET

LEGEND

SAFETY:	BLOOD GLUCOSE:	FORMULA:	COLOR:	ABDOMEN:	ACTIVITY:	
Write IV amount:	A = Accucheck	E20F = ENFAMIL 20/FE	P = Pink	S = Soft	Q = Quiet	✓ = Normal
B = Bili Mask on	L = Lab	S20F = SIMILAC 20/FE	R = Ruddy	F = Full	A = Alert	X = See Staff Notes
A = Apnea monitor on			J = Jaundice	BS = Bowel Sounds	S = Sleeping C = Crying	

FED BY:		BREASTFEEDING:	STOOL:		EMESIS:
M = MOTHER	F = FATHER	M = MOTHER B = BABY	S = SEEDY	ME = MECONIUM	S = SPIT UP
GP = GRANDPARENT	NS = NURSING STAFF	+ = Behavior Observed	Y = YELLOW	T = TRANSITIONAL	P = PROJECTILE
O = OTHER		O = Behavior not observed	LO = LOOSE	B = BROWN	
		✓ = Help given by another person, i.e. family member, nurse, or L.C.	F = FORMED	G = GREEN	

Breastfeeding

Mother		**Baby**
Step 1 demonstrates readiness, Reads baby's cues	**SIGNALING**	Stirs, moves around, roots
Step 2 Baby held in good alignment, Head & Shoulders supported	**POSITIONING**	Roots, mouth wide open, tongue down
Step 3 Holds breast, brings baby in, may express a few drops of milk	**FIXING**	Latches taking in nipple + 2 cms, demonstrates Burst-pause sucking pattern
Step 4 Mother reports feeling thirst, uterine cramps, breast tingling/ache, relaxation/sleepiness, milk leaks from opposite breast	**MILK TRANSFER**	Change in sucking rhythm (from 2 sucks/second to 1 suck/second), audible swallowing
Step 5 Breast/nipple is comfortable, allows baby to end feeding, breast feels softer	**ENDING**	Baby releases nipple, appears satieated, appears relaxed. May fall asleep

	Date _____		Date _____		Date _____		Date _____	
	M	**B**	**M**	**B**	**M**	**B**	**M**	**B**
Signaling	/	/	/	/	/	/	/	/
Positioning	/	/	/	/	/	/	/	/
Fixing	/	/	/	/	/	/	/	/
Milk Transfer	/	/	/	/	/	/	/	/
Ending	/	/	/	/	/	/	/	/
Total	/	/	/	/	/	/	/	/
Initials	/	/	/	/	/	/	/	/

Initials	Name	Title
_____	_____	_____
_____	_____	_____
_____	_____	_____

Reprinted with the permission of Medical College of Georgia Children's Medical Center, Augusta, GA.

developmental stage must be carefully evaluated and the findings documented. There are not many lawsuits filed against NICU nurses; however, that does not mean NICU nurses can disregard the importance of accurate, clear, and complete documentation (see Figure 10-8 on pages 166-168).

PEDIATRIC UNIT DOCUMENTATION

Pediatric documentation of nursing care is similar to the documentation for nursing care of adults. Many forms appear similar; however, the developmental and psychosocial issues of children must be further explored. Pediatric documentation tools must be flexible enough to accommodate patients from infancy through adolescence. Grant, Skinner, Fleming, and Bean (2002) found that age-specific assessment forms resulted in marked improvement and completeness of the documentation of procedures and assessments carried out with children.

Nurses should document direct quotes from family members or guardians of children in their care. Children who are old enough should also be questioned directly. The history of the present illness is very important and may identify areas that need further investigation. Past medical history of a child is also very important. Topics should include birth history, dietary history, immunizations, and developmental milestones.

If a child is taking medication, the nurse should ask about how the child takes the medication. Such information will help the nurse plan medication administration. A careful diet history can also help indicate developmental milestones, allergies, actual or potential problems, and formula or food preferences.

Information about growth and development is an essential part of a pediatric patient's assessment. Safety issues and normal habits, such as sleep patterns, toileting, and other rituals and routines, can be used to plan the child's care. The admission form must be completed. The nurse should write a note for any missing information.

Flow sheets are frequently used in pediatric units and are very helpful if frequent monitoring is necessary. Other forms may be developed for specific problems or concerns. An example of a pediatric nursing documentation form is found in Figure 10-9 on pages 169-172. Some issues in pediatrics require precise and complete documentation. These issues are listed in Table 10-3 on page 173.

Restraints are often necessary when performing procedures with pediatric patients. They are used for patient protection, such as restriction of body movements to protect a site (such as an IV site) or to keep equipment from being dislodged. The nurse must use good judgment if and when restraints are used and make sure to clearly document the process of following Joint Commission for Accreditation of Healthcare Organizations (JCAHO) and institutional policies.

Injuries from child abuse are one of the leading reasons that children are admitted to hospitals. The Federal Child Abuse Prevention and Treatment Act of 1973 required each state to pass laws for mandatory reporting of suspected child abuse to appropriate county or state social service agencies. Likewise, all states have mechanisms for the removal or suspension of parental custody when child abuse or neglect is suspected or verified. The state has an obligation to protect the health and welfare of children. Failure to report may be a misdemeanor, so nurses should become familiar with their state requirements.

Pediatric patients are legally minors who cannot consent on their own behalf to medical treatments or procedures. The parent or legal guardian must provide written consent for treatment of a child. In emergency situations, verbal consent may be obtained over the telephone until the parent or guardian arrives. Refer to Chapter 11 for information on consent in emergency situations, emancipated minors, and special circumstances under which minors do not

text continues on page 173

FIGURE 10-8: SAMPLE NICU NURSING RECORD (1 OF 3)

DATE _____ AGE _____

TODAY'S WEIGHT _____

YESTERDAY'S WEIGHT _____

WEIGHT DISCREPANCY _____

H.C. _____

**INTENSIVE CARE
NURSERY FLOW SHEET**

TIME	THERMOREGULATION					VITAL SIGNS												OXYGEN		TC	INSPECTION					
	AX	Rectal	ISC	Skin	ISO Temp.	PULSE				RESP.				P. B/P		C. B/P		MET	%	PO₂/PCO₂	Re	Color Perf	BS	BoS	Act
						00	15	30	45	00	15	30	45	00	30	00	30								
12m																									
1A																									
2A																									
3A																									
4A																									
5A																									
6A																									
7A																									
Total																									
8A																									
9A																									
10A																									
11A																									
12N																									
1P																									
2P																									
3P																									
Total																									
4P																									
5P																									
6P																									
7P																									
8P																									
9P																									
10P																									
11P																									
Total																									
24° Total																									

IV FLUIDS:

1. _____

2. _____

3. _____

4. _____

FLUSH _____

Tube Change

*See Nurses Notes

RE - Respirations
  G - Grunting
  F - Flaring
  R - Retracting
  A - All
  √ - Normal
PERF - Perfusion
  P - Poor
  F - Fair
  G - Good

COLOR
  P - Pink
  W - Pale
  D - Dusky
  B - Blue
  J - Jaundice
  M - Mottled
BS - Breath Sounds
  √ - Normal
  * - See Nurses Notes

BOS - Bowel Sounds
  √ - Normal
  * - See Nurses Notes
POSITION
  P - Prone
  S - Supine
  LS - Left Side
  RS - Right Side
TC - Transcutaneous Monitor

FIGURE 10-8: SAMPLE NICU NURSING RECORD (2 OF 3)

Position	Flush or Dilute	Site	1 Rate / Inf	2 Rate / Inf	3 Rate / Inf	4 Rate / Inf	COLLOIDS		ORAL NUTRITION From	Route	Res / In	IN Total	Urine	Stool	Emesis	OG	CHEST CC CTD	CC CTD	OUT Total	BLOOD VOL. WD	Total

ACT - Active
++ Active
+ Active (Stimulated)
- Limp
A Irritable
B Jittery
CTD - Chest Tube Drainage
F - Fluctuating
B - Bubbling
R - Bright Red

COLLOIDS
WB - Whole Blood
PC - Packed Cells
FFP - Fresh Frozen Plasma
PLAS - Plasmanate
ALB - Albumin
PLAT - Platlets

S - Serous
SS - Serosanguineous

STOOLS
B - Brown
Y - Yellow
G - Green
Mc - Meconium
S - Seedy
M - Mushy
F - Formed
Mu - Mucoid
W - Water Ring
Bl - Bloody

IV SITE
√ - All OK
* - See Nurses Notes

FIGURE 10-8: SAMPLE NICU NURSING RECORD (3 OF 3)

DATE ⎯⎯⎯⎯⎯⎯⎯⎯⎯⎯ **LABORATORY DATA**

TIME	URINE							STOOL			DEX	TIME	NA	K	Cl	CO₂	BUN	Glu	Creat	Serum Osmo	++ Ca	Mg	Trig	
	Sp gr	ph	prot	glu	bl	uro	bili	ph	hem	Rs														

	ABGs																							
	Ph	PCO₂	PO₂	HCO₃	CO₂ conc.	O₂ Sat.	Base ex.																	

TIME	Hbg	Hct	RETIC	ph	TSS	Bilirubin		Levels				
						T	D	Gent	Dig	Theo	Dilantin	Phen
TIME												

BACTERIOLOGY   **STATE METABOLIC SCREENING** ⎯⎯⎯⎯⎯⎯⎯⎯⎯

BLOOD: ⎯⎯⎯⎯⎯⎯⎯   OTHER LAB: ⎯⎯⎯⎯⎯⎯⎯⎯⎯⎯⎯⎯⎯⎯

SPINAL: ⎯⎯⎯⎯⎯⎯⎯⎯⎯⎯⎯⎯⎯⎯⎯⎯⎯⎯⎯⎯⎯⎯⎯⎯⎯⎯⎯⎯⎯⎯

OTHER: ⎯⎯⎯⎯⎯⎯⎯⎯⎯⎯⎯⎯⎯⎯⎯⎯⎯⎯⎯⎯⎯⎯⎯⎯⎯⎯⎯⎯⎯⎯

INITIAL AND TIME WHEN COMPLETED:

AM CARE:	PM CARE:	CORD CARE:	11 - 7	7 - 3	3 - 11
PHOTOTHERAPY-EYES PROTECTED:	11 - 7	7 - 3	3 - 11		
MOUTH CARE:	11 - 7	7 - 3	3 - 11		
DRESSING CHANGE:	11 - 7	7 - 3	3 - 11		
TRANSDUCER CHANGE:	OG TUBE CHANGE:	NJ TUBE:			
TYPE MONITOR:	X-RAY (TYPE & TIME):				

CIRCUMCISION: TYPE OF ISOLATION:

SONOGRAM: PARENT INTERACTION:

CONSULTATION: 7 A - 7 P

EKG: 7 P - 7 A

ECHO:

FIGURE 10-9: SAMPLE PEDIATRIC RECORD (1 OF 4)

20302-02

Children's Healthcare of Atlanta

ADMISSION DATA BASE

PATIENT IDENTIFICATION

Name child likes to be called	Admission Date	Time	Age	Gest.	Informant/Relationship to pt.	Language

Emergency Contacts (name / phone): _____

Relationship to pt. _____

VITAL SIGNS/MEASUREMENTS

Temp (O-R-A-Ty)	Pulse	Resp	LOC	BP	WT (kg)

HT (cm)	HC (<24 mos.)	FiO2	Pulse ox.

Is patient in any pain now? ☐ Yes ☐ No ☐ Unable to assess _____ Pain Intensity Rating _____

Pain Scales Used: ☐ Faces ☐ Numeric ☐ OPS ☐ FLACC ☐ CRIES ☐ Other: _____

Frequency _____

Duration _____

Quality _____

ALLERGIES

☐ NKA	Medications/reaction	Foods/reaction	Latex/reaction

Environmental/reaction _____

HEALTH HISTORY

Reason for Hospitalization _____

Past Medical History/Previous Hospitalizations _____

Maternal History _____ Apgar Scores _____

Previous Blood Transfusion? ☐ No ☐ Yes Date: _____ Reaction: _____

Primary Doctor/Clinic _____ Home health agency _____ Phone # _____

Specialty Doctors/Clinics _____

CURRENT MEDICATIONS
Include all prescription, non-prescription, herbal remedies, and supplements.

Child prefers medicine as ☐ pills ☐ crushed pills ☐ mixed in food ☐ chewables ☐ liquid ☐ no previous experience

Was medicine brought to hospital? If yes, ☐ sent home or ☐ contact pharmacy

Medication	☐ Strength ☐ Not Available	Dose	Route	Frequency	Last Dose

Comments: _____

FIGURE 10-9: SAMPLE PEDIATRIC RECORD (2 OF 4)

NUTRITIONAL SCREENING

☐ **Refer to Nutrition Services for further evaluation:** ☐ Yes ☐ No   Date_____   Initials_____

Diet Prior to Admission:

☐ Regular   ☐ Special: _____

    Restrictions/Precautions: _____

☐ Infant   ☐ Formula (type, amt., schedule): _____

        ☐ Breast Fed   ☐ Jar Foods   ☐ Finger Foods

☐ Tube Fed   ☐ NG   ☐ GT   ☐ JT   ☐ OG   ☐ G/J

        Formula/Schedule: _____

☐ TPN/IL Hours/day_____   Schedule _____

☐ NPO since: _____   Last Void: _____   Last BM: _____

Nutrition related risk conditions:
☐ condition or surgery related to admission alters baseline growth or nutrition
☐ excessive weight gain
☐ weight loss
☐ TPN
☐ Tube Feeding
☐ Lactation Concerns

COMMUNICABLE DISEASES

Disease	Had Disease	Exposure/Date
Measles	☐ Yes ☐ No	☐ Yes _____ ☐ No
Chicken Pox	☐ Yes ☐ No	☐ Yes _____ ☐ No
Tuberculosis	☐ Yes ☐ No	☐ Yes _____ ☐ No

Multiply Resistant Organisms: (circle type)

    MRSA   Vancomycin Resistant Enterococcus   Cepacia

Any other exposures? (w/in 3 wks)_____

_____

IMMUNIZATIONS

Child's immunizations are   ☐ up to date   ☐ verbal report
                                                              ☐ record
                            ☐ not sure
                            ☐ missing the following doses

_____

_____

Varicella (chicken pox) Vaccine   ☐ yes   ☐ no

PSYCHOSOCIAL AND CULTURAL SCREENING

☐ **Refer for further evaluation to** ☐ Social Work ☐ Child Life ☐ Chaplain ☐ School

    Date/time notified:_____   by: _____

Pt. lives with: ☐ mother   ☐ father   ☐ grandmother   ☐ grandfather   ☐ foster parent/s   other:_____

No. of siblings_____   Legal Guardian:_____   ☐ carseat   ☐ carseat referral

Pets in home:_____   Smokers in home: ☐ Yes   ☐ No

Visitor Restrictions:_____   Expected mode of transport at discharge:_____

Are there any spiritual or cultural beliefs/practice that might impact your child's treatment?   ☐ Yes   ☐ No   If yes, explain:_____

_____

Are there any emotional or behavioral issues that might impact your child's treatment?   ☐ Yes   ☐ No   If yes, explain:_____

_____

Are you concerned about your safety or the safety of anyone in your home?   ☐ Yes   ☐ No   If yes, explain:_____

_____

For patients 18 and older
Advance Directive
☐ Patient has an Advance Directive   ☐ Living Will   ☐ Durable Power of Attorney for Health Care Decisions
    The patient's Advance Directive was: ☐ available at time of admission and placed in the patient's chart
                                            ☐ not available at admission; requested

☐ No Advance Directive exists
        ☐ Patient/representative has received Advance Directive information
        ☐ Patient requests additional information, Social Worker notified.
        ☐ Patient has received the information and does not want an Advance Directive.

FIGURE 10-9: SAMPLE PEDIATRIC RECORD (3 OF 4)

THIS PAGE TO BE COMPLETED BY A LICENSED STAFF MEMBER

GROWTH AND DEVELOPMENTAL SCREENING

Infant/Toddler (0 - 36 months)	Birth weight: _____ Gestation: _____ Sleep habits: _____ Newborn Metabolic Screen (< 30 d.) _____ Favorite Toy/Comfort Measures: _____ Problems at birth: _____ Day Care: _____ Concerns: _____
Preschool (3 - 5 years)	Toilet Trained: ☐ urine ☐ stool Sleep habits: _____ Concerns: _____ Favorite Toy/Comfort Measures: _____ _____ Day Care/Preschool: _____
School Age (6 - 12 years)	Sports/hobbies: _____ Grade: _____ Drug/alcohol/tobacco use: _____ Concerns: _____
Adolescent/Adult (> 12 years)	Sports/hobbies: _____ Grade: _____ Drug/alcohol/tobacco use: _____ Employment: _____ Sexually Active: ☐ Yes ☐ No Contraceptives: ☐ Yes ☐ No Concerns: _____ Reported by: _____ Female: LMP _____ Problems with menstruation: _____

FUNCTIONAL SCREENING

☐ **Patient meets all indicators for age.**

Note: <u>Mark any indicator not present for child's applicable age.</u> Screening indicators are intended to provide an opportunity for the parent and/or physician to identify the need for intervention or further evaluation.

Functional Area	Feeding/ Swallowing	Gross Motor/ Mobility	Fine Motor ADLs	Communication/ Vision
Neonate/Infant (0 - 12 months)	☐ Eats/drinks without signs of distress	☐ Holds up head (3-4 mo.) ☐ Rolls over (4-6 mo.) ☐ Sits up (6-8 mo.) ☐ Crawls (10-12 mo.)	☐ Reaches for object (5-8 mo.) ☐ Picks up small objects (10-14 mo.)	☐ Startles to sound (2-3 mo.) ☐ Coos/babbles (3-6 mo.) ☐ Eyes focus on object (1-3 mo.)
Infant/Toddler (12 - 36 months)	☐ Eats/drinks without choking/coughing ☐ Eats finger foods	☐ Stands alone (10-15 mo.) ☐ Walks (12-18 mo.) ☐ Catches ball (36 mo.)	☐ Unbuttons large buttons (36 mo.)	☐ Says one word (12-15 mo.) ☐ Follows simple directions ☐ Speech is understandable (24-36 mo.)
Preschool (3 - 5 years)	☐ Drinks from cup ☐ Eats/drinks without choking/coughing	☐ Runs (3 yr.) ☐ Rides tricycle (4 yr.)	☐ Dresses self (3 yr.) ☐ Feeds self (3 yr.)	☐ Speaks understandable sentences (4-6 yr.) ☐ Sits > 4 ft from television
School Age (6 - 12 years)	☐ Eats/drinks without choking/coughing	☐ Rides bike (6-8 yrs.) ☐ Age appropriate independent mobility and strength	☐ Buttons and zips clothing ☐ Prints name	☐ Reads at grade level
Adolescent (> 12 years)	☐ Eats/drinks without choking/coughing	☐ Age appropriate independent mobility and strength	☐ Independent in all ADL's	☐ Reads at grade level

- No referral necessary:
  - ☐ Rehab Services order is already present.
  - ☐ Parent feels current therapy/services are appropriate.
  - ☐ Defer intervention at this time due to medical status or other treatment priorities. Review functional screening prior to discharge.

- Contact Rehab Services for further evaluation and/or consultation **(MD order required):**
  - ☐ Screening indicates possible functional problem *(for concerns related to vision, contact attending MD)*
  - ☐ Condition or surgery related to admission alters baseline in any functional area (i.e.: new neurological impairment, surgery or trauma to upper or lower extremity, tracheostomy limits ability to speak)
  - ☐ Parent reports other difficulties in hearing, speech, mobility, or ADL's. Specify: _____

Rehab Services notified: (date/time) _____ **by:** _____

FIGURE 10-9: SAMPLE PEDIATRIC RECORD (4 OF 4)

ADAPTIVE EQUIPMENT (USED AT HOME)

☐ No Adaptive Equipment

☐ Wheelchair ☐ Augmentative Communication Device ☐ Hearing Aid(s) ☐ Glasses ☐ Contact Lenses

☐ Feeding Equipment: _____ ☐ Splints ☐ Braces ☐ Prosthesis: _____ ☐ Other (specify): _____

Problems noted with equipment: _____

Equipment brought from home: _____

Biomed. Eng. Notified: _____

ORIENTATION CHECKLIST

Equipment: ☐ TV; CCTV
☐ Telephone
☐ Bed controls/Siderails
☐ Nurse call system
☐ Medical devices

Services: ☐ Family library
☐ School program
☐ Parking
☐ Cafeteria/vending areas
☐ Activity Center

Policies: ☐ Unit specific
☐ Isolation
☐ Visiting
☐ Smoking

Other: ☐ ID/allergy band RA LA RL LL
☐ Parent's role during hospitalization
☐ Patient/family rights and responsibilities

Comments: _____

Data collector: _____

Reviewed by: _____ RN Date: _____

FACES Scale

0	2	4	6	8	10
No Hurt	Hurts little bit	Hurts little more	Hurts even more	Hurts whole lot	Hurts worst

(From Wong D.L., Hockenberry-Eaton M., Wilson D., Winkelstein M.L., Schwartz P.: Wong's Essentials of Pediatric Nursing, ed. 6, St. Louis, 2001, p. 1301. Copyrighted by Mosby, Inc. Reprinted with permission.)

NUMERIC SCALE

No Pain .... Worst Possible Pain

0 1 2 3 4 5 6 7 8 9 10

OBJECTIVE PAIN SCALE (OPS)

Observation	Criteria	Points
Blood Pressure	+ 10% Baseline	0
	> 20% Baseline	1
	> 30% Baseline	2
Crying?	Not Crying	0
	Crying but responds to tender loving care (TLC)	1
	Crying and does not respond to TLC	2
Movement	None	0
	Restless	1
	Thrashing	2
Agitation	Patient asleep or calm	0
	Mild	1
	Hysterical	2
Verbal Evaluation	Patient asleep or states no pain	0
	Mild pain (cannot localize)	1
	Moderate pain (can localize) verbally or by pointing	2

FLACC (Face-Legs-Activity-Cry-Consolability) Behavioral Scale

This scale can be used for children 0-5 years of age who cannot self-report pain.

Points	FACE	LEGS	ACTIVITY	CRY	CONSOLABILITY
0	smiling or relaxed	relaxed	lying quietly	not crying	content, relaxed
1	occasional grimace	squirming	squirming and shifting back and forth	moans and whimpers	reassured by occasional touching, hugging, distractible
2	clenched jaw and quivering chin	kicking	arched, rigid or jerking	crying steadily, screams or sobs	difficult to console or comfort

Level of Consciousness (LOC) Scale

S Asleep

0 Unresponsive/unarousable
1 Somnolent/difficult to arouse
2 Sleepy/responds appropriately to speech/touch
3 Awake/alert/oriented or baseline

CRIES Neonatal Pain Measurement Score

	0	1	2
Crying	No	High pitched	Inconsolable
Requires O2 for sat ≥ 95	No	<30 % O2	>30 % O2
Increased VS	HR & BP ≤ baseline	HR or BP ↑ <20 % OF baseline	HR or BP ↑ >20 % of baseline
Expression	None	Grimace	Grimace/grunt
Sleepless	No	Wakes at frequent intervals	Constantly awake

Reprinted with the permission of Children's Healthcare of Atlanta, Inc.

TABLE 10-3: PEDIATRIC CONCERNS
• Use of restraints
• Child abuse and neglect
• Consent and privacy issues
(Hamlin & Coplein, 1999)

need parental consent. Nurses should refer to state legislation for rules and regulations governing minors and situations in which they can give consent.

Like adults, minors also have privacy rights. A nurse should remember to discuss the child's condition and care with only the legal parents or guardian. If the child is old enough, the nurse may want to discuss concerns with the child and ask whether the parents or guardians should be informed. Some state laws allow health care providers to inform the parents, guardians, or minor's spouse even though the minor has expressed the information should not be given out. All nurses working in pediatric units must know the laws involved with disclosing information to or about a minor.

Astute monitoring and documentation are essential aspects of pediatrics that help protect pediatric patients from injury and minimize liability risks for nurses in pediatric settings. Using the previously discussed documentation techniques can help the nurse make chart notes that are accurate, complete, and timely, thus providing evidence to avoid a lawsuit.

CRITICAL CARE AND INTENSIVE CARE UNIT DOCUMENTATION

The American Association of Critical Care Nurses (AACCN) in 1989 stated that critical care nursing involves the diagnosis and treatment of human responses to actual or potentially life-threatening illnesses. The scope of critical care nursing practice is defined by the interaction of the nurse, the critically ill patient, and the environment that provides adequate resources for the provision of care.

The acuity of the patient dictates staffing patterns in the intensive care unit (ICU) and supports a nurse to patient ratio of 1:2, depending on patient needs. One nurse may care for three patients and, occasionally, a patient may require the assistance of more than one nurse. The support and treatment of ICU patients requires a highly technical environment.

Documentation challenges in critical care are related to the intensity of nursing care; the performance of highly repetitive, technical skills at frequent intervals; and complex patient problems. Timely, comprehensive, and meaningful documentation is a challenge for even the most competent and experienced ICU nurse.

Most ICU documentation systems consist of manual medical records; however, some facilities have computerized, automated bedside records. Computers that interface with bedside equipment can provide continuous data flow that eliminates the need for some continuous manual documentation. These systems are very expensive and have not been widely implemented. Numerous patient monitoring systems used with ICU patients provide printed strips of information. Nurses often use the printouts in addition to flow sheet charting. As a result, a review of nursing documentation may include a mix of manual and printed information.

A well-constructed, comprehensive flow sheet is the basis of ICU documentation. It should be based on the standards of the American Nurses Association (ANA) and the AACCN. The flow sheet should reflect the standard of care for the primary patient population being served, organized so that assessments and routine interventions are predetermined, and should address all essential areas of nursing intervention.

Flow sheet design varies by institution and unit. Some are folded to provide a landscape style form, whereas others continue with single pages. Regardless of the style adopted, information such as vital signs, medication administration, laboratory results, and other ongoing assessment and intervention data should be easily identified. Many forms represent the 24-hour style of documentation. Documentation is done as events unfold to provide an ongoing, continuous record of the patient's status.

Using flow sheets can lead to sources of liability. They can cause casual charting, with a nurse simply checking the same criteria as the previous nurse did without truly doing an assessment. Likewise, a nurse may rely too heavily on the flow sheet and not include any other nursing documentation. ICU-related liability cases found insufficient or lack of documentation, as well as the issues listed in Table 10-4, to be problematic.

TABLE 10-4: SOURCES OF ICU LIABILITY
• Omission of critical thinking
• Inadequate evaluation of patient status
• Missing or incomplete documentation of changes in patient condition before an arrest and resuscitation
• Insufficient documentation of physician notification regarding changes in patient status
(Santarelli-Kretovics, 1999)

Flow sheets require passive judgment and, unless the nurse documents some narrative or progress notes, little if any critical thinking on the nurse's part (see Figure 10-10 on pages 175-180). If critical care nurses are expected to form judgments, then a failure to record those judgments could be viewed as providing less than the standard of care.

One of the leading areas in litigation is the failure to document a patient's progress and response to treatment. The practice of documenting nursing judgments provides ongoing evaluation of the patient's progress or deterioration and helps explain the rationales for any treatments or interventions that were carried out.

Documentation of arrests and resuscitations present a challenge to the ICU nurse. The nurse has to be able to anticipate and recognize deteriorating conditions and to document very specific details in very rapid succession in an extremely stressful situ-

ation. To accomplish this task, another form may be used during arrest and resuscitation, a code sheet. The code sheet, progress notes, monitor strips, and flow sheet must demonstrate consistent recording of timed events to accurately reflect the care provided (see Figure 10-11 on page 181).

Timely notification to the physician is a critical liability issue in all areas of an institution. In ICUs, it is not uncommon for numerous physicians to be involved in a patient's care. The nurse must coordinate and organize the implementation of prescribed treatments and ensure that information is communicated to the appropriate physicians. A nurse's failure to notify a physician can be an act of omission resulting in liability.

Developing a system to make timely documentation entries is very important in an ICU. The nurse who keeps the flow sheet up-to-date, links activities to patient outcomes, ensures consistency of all components of the chart, and documents every communication with health care providers can protect the staff and the institution and present a defensible patient medical record.

EMERGENCY DEPARTMENT DOCUMENTATION

The fast-paced, intense nature of the emergency department (ED) presents many challenges to nurses working in this area and for their documentation. The 1983 ENA standards of care for ED nurses remain the foundation for nursing practice today. These standards serve as the reference point for determining nursing negligence in adverse outcomes. Along with EMTALA (discussed in the L&D section), these standards guide the ED and the practice of nurses working in that area.

The 1985 Consolidated Omnibus Budget Reconciliation Act requires that any hospital receiving Medicare funds evaluate all patients who come

text continues on page 182

FIGURE 10-10: SAMPLE CRITICAL CARE FLOW SHEET (1 OF 6)

F1

WELLSTAR
Health System
CRITICAL CARE FLOW SHEET

DATES: _____ TO: _____

ALLERGIES: _____

_____

			0700	0800	0900	1000	1100	1200	1300	1400	
HEMODYNAMICS	Temp/Mode		/	/	/	/	/	/	/	/	
	Pulse										
	Respirations										
	Blood	00 / 30									
	Pressure	15 / 45									
	PAS	PCWP									
	PAD	CVP									
	CO	SVR									
	ICP	CI									

PAIN ASSESS

Pain Level
0 No Pain
1-2 Mild Pain
3-4
5-6 Distressing
7-8
9
10 Unbearable

Comfort	0700	0800	0900	1000	1100	1200	1300	1400
Times								
Location								
Pain Level								
Intervention								
Pain Level after intervention								

Interventions
M Medication
AM Alternative Measures

MISC.

Safety	7a - 7p	7p - 7a
Alarms On		
Siderails		
Call Light		
ID Bands On		

Turn / Reposition								

INTAKE

SITE	MEDS/CC	0700	0800	0900	1000	1100	1200	1300	1400
	1.								
	2.								
	3.								
	4.								
	5.								
	6.								
	7.								
	8.								
	9.								
	10.								

OUTPUT

	0700	0800	0900	1000	1100	1200	1300	1400
1. URINE								
2.								
3.								
4.								
Cumulative								
Stool								

VENTILATION

		0700	0800	0900	1000	1100	1200	1300	1400
O₂ METHOD									
MODE	F₁O₂								
RATE	TV								
PEEP/CPAP	PS								
Pulse Ox %									

SX / Mouth Care

ABG TIME	SITE	ALLEN TEST	0700	0800	0900	1000	1100	1200	1300	1400
			/ /	/ /	/ /	/ /	/ /	/ /	/ /	/ /
pH	B.E.									
PO₂	HCO₃ Content									
PCO₂	O₂ SAT									

	0700	0800	0900	1000	1100	1200	1300	1400

FIGURE 10-10: SAMPLE CRITICAL CARE FLOW SHEET (2 OF 6)

WELLSTAR
Health System

F2

DATES: _____ TO: _____
DAYS ON UNIT: _____
DIAGNOSIS: _____

CRITICAL CARE FLOW SHEET

1500	1600	1700	1800	TOTAL	1900	2000	2100	2200	2300	0000	0100
/	/	/	/	12HOUR	/	/	/	/	/	/	/

				TOTAL							
				1.							
				2.							
				3.							
				4.							
				5.							
				6.							
				7.							
				8.							
				9.							
				10.							
			12 hr.								
				1.							
				2.							
				3.							
				4.							
			12 hr.								

/ /	/ /	/ /	/ /		/ /	/ /	/ /	/ /	/ /	/ /	/ /

1500	1600	1700	1800		1900	2000	2100	2200	2300	0000	0100

FIGURE 10-10: SAMPLE CRITICAL CARE FLOW SHEET (2 OF 6)

FIGURE 10-10: SAMPLE CRITICAL CARE FLOW SHEET (3 OF 6)

WELLSTAR Health System

F3

DATES: _____ TO: _____

CRITICAL CARE FLOW SHEET

0200	0300	0400	0500	0600	Temp/Mode	Name/Title		Initials	Shift
/	/	/	/	/	Pulse				
					Resp				
					Blood Pressure				
					00 | 30				
					15 | 45				

IV DOCUMENTATION

Codes
✓ = site ck (no redness or swelling or pain; site intact)
* See IV documentation

		7A-7P	7P-7A
Site A	Size/type		
Started			
Cond.			
Tubing Δ			
Location			
Site B	Size/type		
Started			
Cond.			
Tubing Δ			
Location			
Site C	Size/type		
Started			
Cond.			
Tubing Δ			
Location			
Arterial Access			
Started			
Cond.			
Site Care			
Location			

Weight
_____
Today

Adm	Prior
12 Hour	24 Hours
1.	
2.	
3.	
4.	
5.	
6.	
7.	
8.	
9.	
10.	
1.	
2.	
3.	
4.	

Central Access: _____ type
Insertion _____ Site _____
Site Care _____ Location _____
Marking _____

VASCULAR ACCESS

O₂ Method		Site _____	Site _____
Mode	F₁O₂	7A-7P _____	7P-7A _____
Rate	TV	Bruit _____	Bruit _____
Peep/C/pap	Ps	Thrill _____	Thrill _____
Pulse Ox%			

DIETARY INTAKE

Bag + Sx

B _____ % L _____ % D _____ %

/ /	/ /	/ /	/ /	/ /	ABG	SITE	ALLEN

I/O

pH	B.E.
PO₂	HCO₃ Content
PCO₂	O₂ Sat

24° Previous Day Balance: _____
24° Balance: _____
Cum. Balance: _____

| 0200 | 0300 | 0400 | 0500 | 0600 | | | |

FIGURE 10-10: SAMPLE CRITICAL CARE FLOW SHEET (4 OF 6)

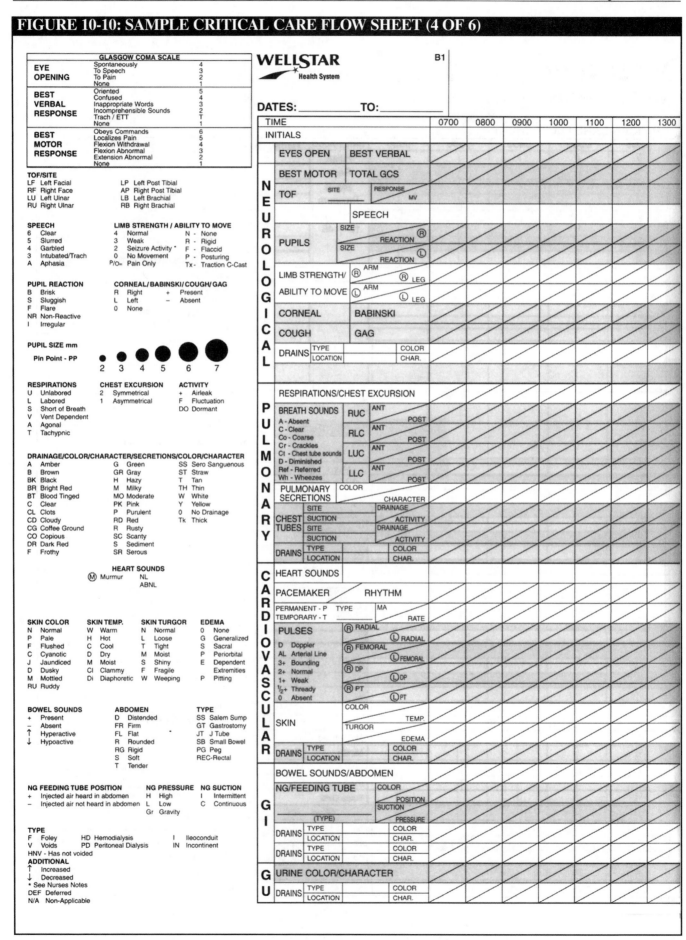

FIGURE 10-10: SAMPLE CRITICAL CARE FLOW SHEET (5 OF 6)

WELLSTAR Health System

B2

DATES: _____ TO: _____

1400	1500	1600	1700	1800	1900	2000	2100	2200	2300	0000	0100	0200	0300	0400	0500	0600	

NEUROLOGICAL

PULMONARY

CARDIOVASCULAR

GI

GU

FIGURE 10-10: SAMPLE CRITICAL CARE FLOW SHEET (6 OF 6)

WELLSTAR
Health System

☐ WELLSTAR Paulding Hospital   ☐ WELLSTAR Windy Hill Hospital   **B3**
☐ WELLSTAR Douglas Hospital   ☐ WELLSTAR Kennestone Hospital
☐ WELLSTAR Cobb Hospital

DATES: _____ **TO:** _____   **Plan of Care:**

R   L   L   R

Goals:

7A 7P _____   ☐ Met
                                                ☐ Not Met

7P-7A _____   ☐ Met
                                                ☐ Not Met

OUTCOME DOCUMENTATION

SKIN ASSESSMENT

A	Abrasion	E	Ecchymosis	R	Rash
B	Burn	H	Hematoma	S	Scar
C	Casts	I	Incision	SQ	Sub Q Air
Ct	Contusions	L	Laceration	SU	Sutures
D	Decubitus	P	Petechia	DR	Drain
		ST	Staples	DG	Dressing

SKIN ASSESSMENT/ DOCUMENTATION

7A-7P:
SKIN INTACT ☐
SKIN IMPAIRED ☐
location: _____
(see diagram above)
type: wound ☐ skin tear ☐
      laceration ☐ abrasion ☐
      decubitus ☐ stage _____
      incision ☐ intact Y N
      other _____
dressing change/wound care:
      time: _____ initial: _____
      per ET protocols (see chart)
      addt'l documentation: _____
      _____
      _____
      _____

7P-7A:
SKIN INTACT ☐
SKIN IMPAIRED ☐
location: _____
(see diagram above)
type: wound ☐ skin tear ☐
      laceration ☐ abrasion ☐
      decubitus ☐ stage _____
      incision ☐ intact Y N
      other _____
dressing change/wound care:
      time: _____ initials: _____
      per ET protocols (see chart)
      addt'l documentation: _____
      _____
      _____
      _____

FIGURE 10-11: SAMPLE CODE SHEET

CPR Record (page 1 of 2)

Date: _____ Time of Arrest: _____ Location: _____ Admitting Diagnosis: _____

Time CPR Initiated: _____ By: _____

Initial Assessment: Cardiac: ☐ VF ☐ VT ☐ PEA ☐ Asystole ☐ Other: _____

Respiratory: ☐ Spont resp. ☐ Apnea ☐ Intubated

Time Concluded: _____ Reason stopped: _____ Pt status: _____

Pt Disposition: _____ Complications: _____

M.D. Attending Code: _____ Time arrived: _____ Primary M.D. _____

Time notified _____

Family Notified: _____ Time: _____

ET Intubation: Time: _____ Site: _____   Chest Tube   site: _____ by: _____

Size: _____ By: _____   IV line   time: _____ by: _____

Blood Gases:

Time	Site	By	Fi02	pH	pO2	pCO2

site: _____ size: _____

NG Tube   time: _____ by: _____

Site: _____ size: _____

Other: _____

Time	P	R	BP	Rhythm	Epinephrine	Atropine	Amiodorone	Lidocaine	Procainamide	Sodium Bicarb	Vasopressin		Lidocaine Gtt	Dopamine Gtt		Defib (joules)	By	Site	Notes

Code member / initials _____ / _____   Code member / initials _____ / _____

Code member / initials _____ / _____   Code member / initials _____ / _____

RN Signature _____   MD Signature _____

Code Critique complete ☐

to the ED (AHA, 1992b). This legislation put a stop to "dumping" indigent patients. Laws such as EMTALA require that a patient be stabilized or a pregnant woman's active labor be managed before the patient can be transferred to another facility. The receiving facility must agree to accept the patient and have enough space and staff to care for the patient. A copy of the initial treating institution's medical records must be sent to the receiving institution with the patient.

Accurate documenting in an emergency situation can prove challenging. Charting must demonstrate that the ED nurse assessed, communicated, planned, collaborated, implemented, and evaluated the care given and reported important findings to the health care provider as often as necessary during a serious situation. Likewise, the documentation must demonstrate that the ED nurse acted as the patient's advocate when disruptions of the standards of care threatened the patient's safety or a positive outcome (see Figure 10-12).

The ENA practice standards require that every patient who comes to the ED be triaged by a nurse to determine priorities. Triage enables the nurse to evaluate the urgency of a patient's symptoms and rapidly determine who needs the most-immediate attention.

The complexity of ED nursing responsibilities and the pace in the department necessitates the use of flow sheets for documenting nursing activities. In many cases, more than one nurse is assigned to a patient, so one nurse becomes the patient care provider, one the recorder, and the third the runner. The nurses must coordinate the care provided to the patient and communicate clearly with each other. This method facilitates timeliness and accuracy of the patient's medical record.

Patient education is an important part of ED nursing, and ENA standards indicate that the nurse must keep the patient and family informed. On discharge from the ED, the patient needs precise verbal and written discharge instructions, which should be clearly documented in the medical record.

The ED nurse is important in coordinating care in emergency situations. Few areas other than the ED experience the range of disastrous patient outcomes that result from not following standards of practice. Very precise documentation is necessary, especially with telephone orders because ED nurses frequently communicate with physicians in this way. ED nurses who follow the standards of care and use good documentation techniques can present a very defensible patient medical record.

PERIOPERATIVE DOCUMENTATION

Successful surgery requires quality clinical and technical skills of a surgical team and effective preoperative assessment, treatment, and diagnostic testing to get the patient ready for surgery. Nursing documentation in the perioperative setting is as dynamic as the technologic advances in surgery. Complete, clear, and consistent documentation must occur in the hospital operating room (OR), surgical center setting, endoscopy suite, and physician's office surgical suite.

The pace of the perioperative setting requires that documentation be timely, precise, and concise. The forms used to collect all the required information must be easy to use, consistent, and comprehensive. Checklists are commonly used, with significant space provided for interventions, nurse's notes, and important communications. All forms should have specific guidelines and instructions for use that facilitate clear documentation.

With elective surgeries, the patient may report for preadmission testing and education prior to the surgery. This should be done early enough for all laboratory reports to be on the patient's chart at the time of surgery. In case of an emergency, the nurse should work diligently to complete as much of the patient's record as possible and should document why areas may not be complete. It is critical that the

text continues on page 185

FIGURE 10-12: SAMPLE ED DOCUMENTATION FORM (1 OF 2)

Wellstar Emergency Services   **Initial Nursing Documentation**

Name	Date	DOB	Age	SSN	PCP	To Rm@	Room No.
		If no sign-in sheet completed		If no sign-in sheet completed			

Chief Complaint

Time	☐WS ER/hosp ≤ 24°	Non-English? ☐ Spanish Other _____
	☐Other ER/hosp ≤ 24°	☐ Hearing Impaired ☐ Interpreter Requested

Potential Threat	Infectious Threat	Assessment ☐NAD	Skin	Pulse Ox		
☐ None apparent ☐ Life ☐ Vision ☐ Limb ☐ Infant/Child is _NOT_ appropriate for age	☐ ? TB ☐ ? SARS ☐ ?Meningitis ☐ ?ChickenPox/Measles ☐ ?Immune suppressed	☐Resp distress ☐Chest Pain ☐ Altered LOC ☐Abnormal drooling ☐ Stroke sx w/ onset <8hrs ☐Suicidal ☐OD ☐Violent ☐Hemorrhage ☐Obvious fracture ☐Severe Pain ☐Severe burn ☐Contamination -chemical, biological, nuclear	☐ WNL ☐Flushed ☐Pale ☐Cyanotic ☐ Diaphoretic		I Red II Yellow III Green IV Orange (FT)	

Appearance	Arrival	Disposition	Signature
☐ Alert ☐ Uncooperative ☐Cooperative ☐Unresponsive	☐ Ambulatory ☐ WC ☐Assisted ☐ Police ☐Carried ☐EMS ☐ Alone	☐ Exam ☐ Assess ☐ Registration ☐ WR ☐ LBS ☐ Peds ER	Sign at bottom when you complete entire assessment.

Time	Allergies ☐NKDA ☐Tape ☐Latex ☐ Food ☐ Environmental (pollen/bees)	Wt _____ ☐ Measured **Peds weight in kilograms** Ht _____ Asthma > 6yrs	Tetanus ☐≤5yrs ☐ > 5 yrs ☐ Peds Immunizations UTD (Info discussed if not current) ☐ Chooses not to immunize

Limb/Position	Blood Pressure	Pulse ☐Irreg	Resp	Temp	Pulse Ox	Oxygen Therapy	BBG	Pain Scale 0 – 10 (Numbers/Faces > 3 yrs). Circle the appropriate value or describe behavior for those ≤ 3 years.				
RA LA LL RL → ☒ ↑ ☐ Manual						☐Room Air ☐Oxygen @ ____lpm @		0	1 / 2	3 / 4	5 / 6	7 / 8 9 / 10
RA LA LL RL → ☒ ↑ ☐Manual				**Visual Acuity** ☐Glasses ☐Contacts ☐Implant ☐Blind L____ R____ Both____ Corrected____ ☐ Deferred d/t chemical contamination								

Safety Equip: ☐Denies ☐Seatbelt ☐Airbag ☐Child Safety Seat ☐Helmet ☐Goggles ☐Pads ☐Unk
Treatment PTA: ☐ Denies ☐ See EMS sheet ☐ Immobilized ☐ IV access ☐ Medications
PPMH: ☐Denies ☐Diabetes ☐Cardiac _____ ☐HTN ☐Asthma ☐COPD ☐Infect Dx
☐TB ☐Seizure ☐Stroke ☐GI ____ ☐Cancer ____ ☐ RF/Dialysis____ ☐Depression ☐Migraine
Past Surgical History: ☐CABG ☐Cholecystectomy ☐Appendectomy ☐Angioplasty/PCI
Other:
CURRENT MEDS (OTC, Rx, Herbal): ☐ See Medication Sheet if multiple medications reported

LMP_____ ☐ Birth Control Pills
NA → ☐Menopausal ☐Hysterectomy ☐ Depo-Provera
Pregnant? Y N UNK FHT____ Due Date ____
Social History: ☐ Assessed and none reported
☐ ETOH _____ (Occ QD) ☐ Drugs
☐ Cigarettes/cigar/pipe ____ ppd ☐ Smoker in home
Cultural/Religious/Spiritual/Psychosocial/Learning Needs:
None identified
List:

Mark only those systems that apply to complaint or presenting symptoms.

Neurologic	Y	N	Respiratory	Y	N	Cardiac	Y	N	Skin	Y	N	Surface Problems		WR Reassess	
Alert			Able to speak			Chest pain			Warm/Dry			☐ Laceration ☐Abrasion		Time	Status/VS
Oriented X 3			Retractions			Epigastric Substernal			Diaphoretic			☐ Bruises ☐ Deformity			
+ LOC			Cough Prod			Sharp Pressure Dull			Hot Cool Cold			☐ Amputation ☐ Rash			
Dizzy			Nasal flaring			Radiates to:			Pale Flushed			Where			
Headache			Dyspnea DOE			Palpitations			Cyanotic Jaundice						
Slurred speech			Shallow Stridor			Murmur heard			Cap Refill ≤3 sec >3 sec			Size/Appearance			
Face Asymmetry			Breath Sound R L			Risk factors present			**GYN/GU**	Y	N				
MAE			Clear			Positive family history			Itching						
Weakness			Crackles			**EENT**	Y	N	VB ____ pds in last hr			Pulses: NL ↓ ↑ Ø			
RA LA RL LL			Wheezes			Hoarse			Dischg V P			Sensory/ROM			
Blurred vision			Decreased			Sore throat			Frequency Dysuria						
Photophobia			Abnormal			Nosebleed Drainage			Hematuria			NL ↓ ↑ Ø			
Pupils PERL			Absent			Earache			**Gastrointestinal**	Y	N				
Triage Medications:						Eyes: Red Drainage			N V D			*Updated Acuity @*			
						FB_____			Stools: Bldy Tarry			☐ I/Red ☐ II/Yellow ☐ III/Green			

Patient Sticker

☐C-collar ☐Ice ☐Elevate
☐Pressure drsg ☐Splint

Assessed by

FIGURE 10-12: SAMPLE ED DOCUMENTATION FORM (2 OF 2)

NARRATIVE PAGE   **Date**

	Time	BP	Pulse	RR	Temp	Intls	Signature/Title	Intls	Signature/Title

Patient Sticker

PROTOCOLS: ☐Chest Pain ☐Resp ☐FeverAdult ☐FeverPeds ☐ UTI ☐Tetanus ☐Sprain ☐Obv Fracture ☐Amputation ☐IVP ☐Eye Injury
EXCLUDED: ☐Age ☐Preg ☐Other

PATIENT EDUCATION : Oriented to Room/Call light in reach   Medications   Procedures   Diagnosis   Other

Time	INT/IVF Amt/ Rate/Cath/Site	Intls	Dn @	Amt	Time	Medications – Dose/Route/	Site	Intls

☐Monitor	NS SB ST Other:		
☐ECG	O2 _____ lpm Via: ☐Cannula ☐NRMask Other:		

Time	Narrative ▼ ▼ ▼ ▼ Include Response to Medication and Treatment

☐ *NOTES CONTINUED - SEE ATTACHED*

Disposition of Valuables:		Admit Rm _____ Report called to _____ @ _____
		☐ Surgery ☐ L&D Other:
IV/INT DC'd ☐ Site OK	**Discharge** ☐ Home ☐ Other _____	**Transferred to** _____ ☐Form Completed
☐ Red ☐ Swelling	☐ Amb ☐WC ☐STR ☐ Carried ☐ EMS	Time / **Discharge Nurse Signature and Title**
☐ Bruise ☐ Infiltrated	☐ AMA ☐ LBS ☐ EXPIRED	
Discharge Instructions Given	*See DC/Aftercare Sheet*	

WS 0220 ITEM #61527 (10/02)

Reprinted with the permission of WellStar Health System, Marietta, GA.

nurse document attempts to contact family members or significant others.

On the day of surgery, preoperative checklists may be used to ensure the standard items are discussed with the patient and that all forms are included in the chart. It is important that the signed informed consent form be included in the patient's record and that a written description of surgery be correct for the procedure to be performed.

In 1996, the Association of PeriOperative Registered Nurses (AORN) recommended standards for perioperative nurses. The standards recommended that perioperative nursing documentation should reflect the patient's plan of care, which includes assessment, diagnosis, outcomes, planning, implementation, and evaluation. The AORN standards are frequently used for development of perioperative documentation forms.

Like many other specialty areas, the OR is also governed by organizational standards of practice (AORN, 2000). These standards reflect approved nursing diagnoses and provide firm nursing actions with measurable parameters for evaluating patient care. Although the method of documenting perioperative nursing care varies among practice settings, documentation forms should include, but not be limited to, the forms listed in Table 10-5.

There are some specific OR sources of liability that require specific documentation. These areas include skin assessment; patient positioning and

TABLE 10-5: PERIOPERATIVE FORMS
• Operative record
• Perioperative patient checklist
• Informed consent form
• Nurse's notes
• Laboratory reports
• Flow sheets
• Care plans
• Initial history assessment
• Implant records
• Laser logs
• Other specific forms
(AORN, 2000)

patient safety; use of assistive and electrical devices; needle, instrument, and sponge counts; medication administration; and any implant insertion. One of the most frequent causes of OR liability is the loss of a sponge, needle, or instrument in the patient. The injuries incurred often result in large financial settlements for these patients. Therefore, it is critical to perform and document accurate or inaccurate counts.

Specialty areas in the OR often require highly specific equipment and procedures, which must be recorded. Such areas are listed in Table 10-6, with at least one specific documentation requirement noted.

All perioperative emergencies must be documented. The most common emergencies are shock and hemorrhage. Risk management should be notified of all unusual occurrences in surgical patients and the OR. Such occurrences might include

TABLE 10-6: SURGICAL AREAS REQUIRING ADDITIONAL DOCUMENTATION
• Neurosurgery: cotton ball and cottonoid sponge count
• Cardiac, thoracic, and vascular surgery: vessel clamps and time on and time off
• Gastrointestinal endoscopic procedures: use of video camera
• Genitourinary surgery: nonhemolytic isotonic or nonelectrolytic solutions
• Caesarean section birth: deposition of placenta
• Orthopedic surgery: tourniquet time on and time off
• Conscious sedation: continuous monitoring of vital signs
• Local anesthesia procedures: evaluation of patient on discharge
(Cairone, 1999)

surgery on the wrong patient, performance of the wrong procedure or operating on the wrong side of the patient, medication errors, patient return to surgery for repair or removal of an organ or body part damaged in surgery or following surgery, and unexpected patient return to surgery or unplanned readmission to the hospital. No operation or procedure should be performed for which the surgeon does not have clinical privileges.

A perioperative documentation form using a checklist or short fill-in-the-blank format with space provided for further evaluation comments is an easy method to use. It is very important that time-in and time-out of the OR be documented, along with patient demographic data and vital signs. Verification of the patient's identification; the procedure to be performed; the side of the body to be operated on, if applicable; and the patient's consent form must correlate with the scheduled procedure. Additionally, the nurse has the responsibility of assessing and periodically reassessing the patient and recording all nursing interventions. When the nursing process is used in perioperative practice settings, it demonstrates the critical thinking skills practiced by the nurse in caring for the surgical patient. Documentation of the surgical care provides useful data for the nurse who provides postoperative patient care (see Figure 10-13 on pages 187-189).

POSTANESTHESIA CARE DOCUMENTATION

Postanesthesia care units (PACUs) no longer restrict their scope of care to postsurgical patients but have become specialized critical care units. PACUs provide care to patients who have undergone various complex, sedation-related procedures, such as epidural blocks, elective cardioversion, electroconvulsive therapy, and angiogram procedures. The PACU may focus on specific patient populations, such as pediatrics, or be very broad in services offered.

The primary role of a PACU nurse is to ensure safe patient recovery from anesthesia. Compliance with nursing standards of care for PACU patients can only be validated by timely, factual, and accurate documentation. Regardless of the documentation method used, the documentation should relay the message that the patient was cared for by a knowledgeable PACU nurse.

Typically, a flow sheet type of documentation is used in a PACU. By checking an assessment section, the nurse implies that the task, procedure, or assessment was carried out in accordance to standards of care. Narrative documentation should be used to describe any actual or potential problems and the patient's outcomes. The nursing process includes a review of all patient systems.

Many PACU flow sheets include a postanesthesia scoring system as part of the patient's assessment. Once such system is the Alderete system that incorporates objective data about the patient's movements, respiration, circulation, consciousness, and skin color. If a scoring system is not used, the nurse's narrative notes must clearly describe the patient's recovery from the anesthesia (see Figure 10-14 on pages 190-192).

The American Society of PeriAnesthesia Nurses and the AORN have developed guidelines and standards of practice for PACU nurses. When a patient arrives in a PACU, the nurse immediately takes the patient's vital signs and receives a report from the surgical nurse. The standards of care require the PACU nurse to review the anesthesia record, admission history and physical, preadmission records, and preoperative checklist. These forms may provide important information that could influence a patient's recovery and care needed in the PACU.

Because the status of a PACU patient may rapidly change, the standards recommend the patient's vital signs be monitored closely and documented every 10 to 15 minutes for the first hour. If the patient is unstable, more-frequent documentation may be

text continues on page 193

FIGURE 10-13: SAMPLE OPERATING ROOM FORMS (1 OF 3)

St. Joseph Hospital
Augusta, Georgia

PERIOPERATIVE RECORD

PRE-OP ASSESSMENT (Check all applicable boxes)

Mode of Transportation

☐ Stretcher   ☐ Wheelchair
☐ Safety strap on   ☐ Arms
☐ Siderails up   ☐ Other: _____
☐ Bed

Surgical Site Verification

Surgical Site Verification
☐ N/A (Policy Exceptions)
Site Initialing Consistent with:
☐ Informed Consent   ☐ Patient Statement
☐ History & Physical ☐ Surgical Schedule
☐ Imaging Studies
Final Verification in OR Room Prior to Incision:
☐ Correct Patient   ☐ Correct Surgical Site
☐ Correct Procedure

Following Present   ☐ none

☐ Oxygen @ _____ liters ☐ Ambu
☐ IV   ☐ IV Pump   ☐ IV portal
☐ Arterial line ☐ CVP   ☐ Swan-ganz
☐ Foley catheter   ☐ Colostomy
☐ Nasogastric Tube   ☐ Chest tube
☐ Tracheostomy   ☐ Endotracheal tube

Emotional Status

☐ Alert   ☐ Sedated ☐ Nonresponsive
☐ Oriented   ☐ Calm   ☐ Anxious
☐ Disoriented ☐ Crying

Physical Limitations   ☐ none

☐ Language   ☐ Prosthesis
☐ Auditory   ☐ Other: _____
☐ Visual _____
☐ Mobility _____

Allergies: ☐ none

List: _____
_____
_____
_____

Delay Factors

☐ No delay   ☐ Pt Not Ready
☐ Prior case late   ☐ Pt X-Ray
☐ Bumped   ☐ Pt EKG
☐ Surgeon   ☐ Pt Lab
☐ Anesthesia   ☐ Unknown
☐ Nurses   ☐ H & P
☐ Other _____   ☐ Consent
_____

Nursing Diagnosis: Potential for anxiety related to surgical intervention   Goal: patient displays decreased anxiety

Plan and Implementation:

☐ Introduce perioperative staff
☐ Communicate patient concerns to other healthcare members
☐ Give clear, concise explanations
☐ Provide comfort measures: ☐ warm blankets
☐ Remain with patient during anesthesia delivery

Patient/Procedure Verification – Chart Reviewed

☐ Armband   ☐ History & Physical ☐ Blood/Blood Products
☐ Pre-op meds   ☐ Lab Report   ☐ Autologous _____ units
☐ Hosp Tx Consent ☐ EKG Report   ☐ Designated _____ units
☐ Informed Consent ☐ X-Ray Chest Report ☐ Type/hold ☐ Type/cross
☐ Special Permits ☐ NPO   ☐ Type/screen Blood Bank # ____
☐ Data Base Reviewed

Outcome: Demonstrates adaptive coping abilities ☐ Yes ☐ No _____   Initials: _____

Nursing Diagnosis: .Potential for injury   Goal: Patient will remain injury free   Plan and Implementation

Transfer to OR Table
☐ Assisted ☐ Manually
☐ Roller

OR Table Used
☐ Regular   ☐ Cysto
☐ Eye/Stretcher ☐ Jackson
☐ Fracture   ☐ Other: ____

Patient Position
☐ Supine   ☐ Prone
☐ Left lateral ☐ Right lateral
☐ Lithotomy ☐ Frog-legged
☐ Jack knife ☐ Sitting
☐ Other _____

Positioning/Protection
☐ Sheets / Towels _____   ☐ Shoulder Table w/Helmet
☐ Foam Headrest ☐ Pillow _____ ☐ Roll _____
☐ Safety strap ☐ Stirrups _____
☐ Right arm: ☐ padded armboard ☐ at side ☐ hand table ☐ airplane splint
☐ Left arm: ☐ padded armboard ☐ at side ☐ hand table ☐ airplane splint
☐ Wilson Frame ☐ Beanbag (Vac-pac)   ☐ Sand bag _____
☐ Other

Electrocautery   ☐ none

SETTINGS: Coag _____
Type   Cutting _____
_____ Blend _____
Pad Site _____
Applied By: _____
Pad Lot _____
Pad Exp. _____
ECU Hosp. # _____
Post-Op Pad Site Clear: ☐ Yes   ☐ No

Compression Device   ☐ none

☐ Thigh Sleeves   ☐ Foot Cuff
☐ Knee Sleeves

Setting: _____   Hosp. # _____

Harmonic Scalpel   ☐ none
Setting _____
Hosp. # _____

Bipolar ☐   ☐ none
Arthrowand ☐
Setting _____
Hosp. # _____

Tourniquet 1 ☐ None Type _____
Tested by: _____ Hosp. # _____
Applied by: _____
Site: _____
Pressure _____
Time Up _____
Time Down _____
Post-Op Site Clear: ☐ Yes   ☐ No
Circulation Intact: ☐ Yes   ☐ No

Warming Device   ☐ none

K-Thermia   ☐
Bair Hugger   ☐
CO$_2$ Warmer ☐

Setting _____
Hosp. # _____

Tourniquet 2 ☐ None Type _____
Tested by: _____ Hosp. # _____
Applied by: _____
Site: _____
Pressure _____
Time Up _____
Time Down _____
Post-Op Site Clear: ☐ Yes   ☐ No
Circulation Intact: ☐ Yes   ☐ No

Outcome: Patient tolerated procedure with no apparent injury   ☐ Yes ☐ No _____   Initials: _____

Pre-Operative Comments:

RN Signature: _____   **Date:** _____

FIGURE 10-13: SAMPLE OPERATING ROOM FORMS (2 OF 3)

OR Rm # _____   Emergency ☐ Yes ☐ No
General   M.A.C.   Spinal   Epidural   Mod Sed
Block _____   Local _____
Endotracheal Tube   ☐ Yes   ☐ No
Surgeon: Primary _____
Assistant: _____
Anesthesiologist: _____
CRNA: _____   PSN _____

TIME IN	ANESTHESIA	PREP	INCISION	CLOSURE	TIME OUT
OR: _____	START TIME: _____	TIME: _____	TIME: _____	COMPLETION: _____	OR _____
		PREP	INCISION	CLOSURE	TIME IN
		TIME: _____	TIME: _____	COMPLETION: _____	POST OP _____

Fill in appropriate boxes

Scrub Nurse	IN / OUT	IN / OUT	IN / OUT
Circulator/ Laser Op.	IN / OUT	IN / OUT	IN / OUT
Relief Scrub	IN / OUT	IN / OUT	IN / OUT
Relief Circulator	IN / OUT	IN / OUT	IN / OUT

Additional Personnel

Pediatrician _____
NICU Staff _____
EEG _____
SSEP _____
Cell Saver _____
Other: _____

Preoperative Diagnosis: _____

Postoperative Diagnosis: _____

Operative Procedure: _____

Pre-Op Shave   ☐ None
☐ Wet   ☐ Dry   ☐ Razor
☐ Clipper·
Shaved by: _____
Site _____

Operative Prep   ☐ None
Site(s) _____
Solution(s) _____
Time (min.) _____
By Whom: _____

Irrigation

Type of Irrigation	Amount	Site	☐ None

Implants   ☐ None   Site: _____

Type	Serial #	Lot #	Model	Size

Medications: (Not given by Anesthesia) ☐ None

Type	Dosage	Method	Time

RN Signature: _____   **Date:** _____

FIGURE 10-13: SAMPLE OPERATING ROOM FORMS (3 OF 3)

COUNTS: ☐ Correct   ☐ Incorrect   ☐ NA

Sponges _____	Adenoid sponges _____	Plastic bags _____
Lap tapes ____ _____	Tonsil Sponges _____	Safety Pins _____
Needles _____	Cottonoids _____	Hypo Needle _____
Pushers _____	Hydrajaw _____	Snare Wires _____
Blades _____	Umb. Tapes _____	Hemovac needle _____
Appendix tapes _____	Surgiwall _____	Instruments _____
Bovie Tips _____	Booties _____	Reels _____
Bovie Scrapper _____	Weck sponge _____	Others _____
2x2 sponges _____	Vessel loop _____	Tech _____
3x3 sponges _____	Penrose Drain _____	RN _____

Nursing Diagnosis: Potential for Infection   Goal: Avoidance of Patient Infection   Plan and Implementation

Specimen / ORC   ☐ None
  ☐ Surgeon Requests No Pathology

_____
_____
_____

Cytology   ☐ None

_____
_____

Cultures 1:   ☐ None
  ☐ Anaerobic   ☐ AFB   Site: _____
  ☐ Aerobic   ☐ TB   _____
  ☐ Fungus   ☐ Other   _____

Cultures 2:   ☐ None
  ☐ Anaerobic   ☐ AFB   Site: _____
  ☐ Aerobic   ☐ TB   _____
  ☐ Fungus   ☐ Other   _____

Catheters: ☐ None
  ☐ In on arrival   Amt. _____
  ☐ Foley size _____   ☐ Suprapubic size _____
  ☐ Straight size _____   Total OR Output _____
  Inserted by _____   D/C'd in OR   Y / N

Laser: ☐ None   ☐ Safety Precautions observed per standards
        ☐ KTP   ☐ CO$_2$ _____
  ☐ Videotape Done: ☐ Yes ☐ No ☐ N/A

Drains 1:   ☐ None ☐ Other _____
  ☐ Penrose   ☐ Chest Tube   Site: _____
  ☐ Hemovac   ☐ Jackson-Pratt
  ☐ Salem Sump ☐ T-Tube ☐ Autovac   _____

Drains 2:   ☐ None ☐ Other _____
  ☐ Penrose   ☐ Chest Tube   Site: _____
  ☐ Hemovac   ☐ Jackson-Pratt
  ☐ Salem Sump ☐ T-Tube ☐ Autovac   _____

Packing: ☐ None
_____
_____

Dressing/Immobilization 1:   ☐ None
  Type _____
  Location _____

Dressing/Immobilization 2:   ☐ None
  Type _____
  Location _____

Wound Classification: ☐ Class I   ☐ Class II   ☐ Class III   ☐ Class IV

Outcome: Infection Control Measures Implemented   ☐ Yes   ☐ No   Initials: _____

X-Rays - Intraoperative: ☐ None
C-arm   **Flat plate**
☐ Yes   ☐ No   ☐ Yes   ☐ No
Total time _____   Number of films taken:
Site: _____   _____
Radiologist to read: _____

Skin Post-Op   ☐ Unchanged   ☐ Other: _____

Post-Op Comments:

Patient Transfer: Condition: ☐ Satisfactory   ☐ Fair   ☐ Other _____

Method of Transfer	**Receiving Unit**	**Level of Consciousness**	**Transfer Device** ☐ None
☐ Stretcher ☐ Bed	☐ Day Surgery ☐ ER	☐ Under Anesthesia Care	☐ EKG ☐ AMBU
☐ Wheelchair ☐ Crib	☐ PACU ☐ Pt Room	☐ Awake Responsive to Deep Stimuli	☐ IV ☐ IV Pump
☐ Arms	☐ SICU / CCU	☐ Awake Responsive to Verbal Stimuli	☐ Oximeter ☐ Oxygen
	☐ Other _____	☐ Awake & Unsedated	☐ Arterial Monitor

Report given to: _____

  ☐ **Report given by Anesthesiologist / CRNA / Circ RN**

  RN Signature: _____   **Date:** _____

Reprinted with the permission of St. Joseph Hospital, Augusta, GA.

FIGURE 10-14: SAMPLE PACU FORM (1 OF 3)

WELLSTAR

Kennestone Hospital
Marietta, Georgia

PACU RECORD

ROOM # _____

DATE: _____ SURGEON: _____ ANESTH: _____ ANESTH: GEN   SP   EPID   BLK   MAC

PROCEDURE: _____

HISTORY: _____ ALLERGIES: _____

ADM ASSESSMENT TIME: _____		DISCHARGE ASSESSMENT TIME: _____	
AIRWAY:	Natural ☐ Oral ☐ Nasal ☐ ET ☐ Trach ☐	Natural ☐ Oral ☐ Nasal ☐ ET ☐ Trach ☐	
LOC:	Awake ☐ Oriented ☐ Drowsy ☐ Confused ☐ Unresponsive ☐	Awake ☐ Oriented ☐ Drowsy ☐ Confused ☐ Unresponsive ☐	
RESP:	Equal ☐ Full ☐ Shallow ☐ Labored ☐ Apneic ☐	Equal ☐ Full ☐ Shallow ☐ Labored ☐ Apneic ☐	
O₂	Nebulizer ☐ Cannula ☐ T-piece ☐ Vent ☐ Trach Collar ☐	Nebulizer ☐ Cannula ☐ T-piece ☐ Vent ☐ Trach Collar ☐	
	% / Liters / √ Settings:	% / Liters / √ Settings:	
BREATH SOUNDS	Clear ☐ Rhonchi ☐ Wheezes ☐ Crackles ☐	Clear ☐ Rhonchi ☐ Wheezes ☐ Crackles ☐ SaO₂: _____ RR: _____	

O_2: O₂

	SaO₂: _____ RR: _____	**NURSING DIAGNOSIS**	**EXPECTED OUTCOME**	Comments:
Comments:		Potential alteration in ventilation related to effects of anesthesia IV sedation (i.e. decreased respiratory drive muscle relaxation altered level of consciousness)	1. Patent / clear airway maintained. 2. Adequate ventilation maintained.	

ADM	DISCHARGE
BP: _____ Pulse: _____ Card Rhythm: _____	BP: _____ Pulse: _____ Card Rhythm: _____
Temp: _____ Skin: Warm ☐ Cool ☐ Dry ☐ Moist ☐	Temp: _____ Skin: Warm ☐ Cool ☐ Dry ☐ Moist ☐
Color: Pale ☐ Pink ☐ Cyanotic ☐	Color: Pale ☐ Pink ☐ Cyanotic ☐
Peripheral Pulses: Radial L _____ R _____ ☐ NA	Peripheral Pulses: Radial L _____ R _____ Pedal L _____ R _____ NA ☐
Pedal LDP _____ LPT _____ RDP _____ RPT _____	Other: _____
TEDS: Y ☐ N ☐ SCD: Y ☐ N ☐	TEDS: Y ☐ N ☐ SCD: Y ☐ N ☐
Capillary Refill: Brisk ☐ Sluggish ☐ NA ☐	Capillary Refill: Brisk ☐ Sluggish ☐ NA ☐
Sensation: Normal ☐ Dull ☐ Absent ☐ NA ☐	Sensation: Normal ☐ Dull ☐ Absent ☐ NA ☐
Spinal Level _____ NA Discharge @ _____	Spinal Level _____ NA Discharge @ _____

Comments:	**NURSING DIAGNOSIS**	**EXPECTED OUTCOME**	Comments:
	Potential alteration in cardiovascular function and tissue perfusion related to surgical intervention and effects of anesthesia.	1. Vital Signs within acceptable limits 2. Cardiac rhythm within acceptable limits 3. No evidence of excessive bleeding 4. A-line patent. Distal extremity / pink and warm with adq. capillary refill and sensation.	

Comments:	**NURSING DIAGNOSIS**	**EXPECTED OUTCOME**	Comments:
	Pain / anxiety due to surgical procedure.	1. Effect of comfort measure noted. 2. Verbal or non verbal expression of reasonable comfort	

Pt. arrived with Personal Effects Bag: Y ☐ N ☐	PT. CLASS I II III IV Pt. discharged with Personal Effects Bag: Y ☐ N ☐
PAR Score:	PAR Score: _____ (If < 8 ok by _____ M.D.)
Dsg D/I Y ☐ N ☐ NA ☐ Surg Site WNL Y ☐ N ☐	Floor notified of special needs: NA ☐
Comments:	☐ O₂ _____ ☐ Suction Other:
	☐ PCA ms / demerol ☐ Traction
IV(s) / A-Line Site: WNL Y ☐ N ☐ Patent Y ☐ N ☐	Drain(s) / Line(s) / IV'(s) Patent + WNL Yes ☐ No ☐
Comment:	Dgs / Surg site WNL Yes ☐ No ☐
Drain(s) Patent Y ☐ N ☐ NA ☐	Transported c̄ : O₂; Monitors:
Comment:	Report to:
	Comments:
ADMITTING RN:	DISCHARGE RN:

K2951 ITEM #207

(Rev. 6/96)

FIGURE 10-14: SAMPLE PACU FORM (2 OF 3)

ON GOING ASSESSMENT																							
TIME	Adm																						
ACTIVITY																							
RESPIRATIONS																							
CIRCULATION Pre-op:																							
CONSCIOUSNESS																							
COLOR																							
PAR SCORE																							
BP CUFF / A-LINE																							
PULSE																							
RESPIRATIONS																							
O2 SAT																							
TEMP / ICP																							
O2 (L = Cannula, % = Nebulizer, V = Vent, T-Piece)																							
TV:																							
FiO2																							
RATE / PEEP																							
CO2 / PA																							
WEDGE / CVP																							
Requires Mand. Supp																							
Requires ETT / Oral / Nasal																							
Initials																							

PAR SCORE:

2 ABLE TO MOVE 4 EXTREMITIES VOLUNTARY OR ON COMMAND
1 ABLE TO MOVE 2 EXTREMITIES VOLUNTARY OR ON COMMAND
0 ABLE TO MOVE 0 EXTREMITIES VOLUNTARY OR ON COMMAND

2 ABLE TO DEEP BREATHE AND COUGH FREELY
1 DYSPNEA OR LIMITED BREATHING
0 APNEIC

2 BP +/- 20% OF PREANESTHETIC LEVEL
1 BP +/- 20-50% OF PREANESTHETIC LEVEL
0 BP +/- 50% OF PREANESTHETIC LEVEL

2 FULLY AWAKE
1 AROUSABLE ON CALLING
0 NOT RESPONDING

2 PINK OR NORMAL
1 PALE OR DUSKY
0 CYANOTIC

(√) YES   (–) NO   (N/A) NOT APPLICABLE

*SEE NOTE

INT.	SIGNATURE

FIGURE 10-14: SAMPLE PACU FORM (3 OF 3)

INTAKE OR:					OUTPUT OR:			MEDICATIONS:			
TIME	SITE	PACU	IN	LTC	TIME	URINE:	AMOUNT	TIME	ROUTE	MEDICATION	INT
						OTHER:					
						OTHER:					
						OTHER:					

PACU TOTALS	CRYSTALLOIDS	OTHER:	URINE	OTHER:	OTHER:	OTHER:			

TIME	LAB / X-RAY / CONSULT	REASON	TIME	RESULTS / INTERVENTION	INT

NOTES:

K2951

(Rev. 6/96)

Reprinted with the permission of WellStar Health System, Marietta, GA.

TABLE 10-7: PACU FREQUENT OBSERVATION AREAS

- Airway: Check breathing and patent airway every 10 to 15 minutes for first hour
- Circulation: Check the following areas every 10 to 15 minutes for first hour:
    - Pulses
    - Color and temperature
    - Electrocardiogram
    - Hemodynamics
    - IV fluids
- Level of consciousness: Check ability to move, pupil size, and reaction to painful stimuli.
- Renal assessment: Check amount of output.
- Areas specific to the surgery: For example, check neurological status or status of uterus with caesarean section.

(Kuc, 1999)

necessary. The patient's airway is a very critical system that needs close observation and documentation because the greatest risk of general anesthesia is respiratory compromise. The areas in need of frequent observation and documentation are listed in Table 10-7. The use of bedside monitors assists with frequent assessments.

A PACU nurse must always be alert to potential complications associated with specific surgeries. This requires constant, vigilant observations, documentation of changes in patient status, timely notification of physicians or anesthetists, proper interventions, and accurate documentation of all activities. Areas of great concern that require extravigilant documentation are listed in Table 10-8.

When a patient is ready for discharge from the PACU, it is usually the responsibility of the anesthesia personnel. However, some facilities permit the nursing staff to use discharge criteria protocols. These protocols are developed through joint efforts of anesthesia, surgical, and nursing staff and should be approved by the institution's medical board. The PACU nurse and an assistant will then transfer the patient to the appropriate unit for further care. Patients rarely remember the PACU nurse or the care they received there; however, the PACU is considered a high-risk environment. Adverse outcomes do occur, but they can be minimized with close

TABLE 10-8: COMMON PACU PATIENT PROBLEMS

- Hypotension
- Laryngospasms
- Respiratory distress syndrome
- Hyperthermia or hypothermia
- Anaphylaxis

(Kuc, 1999)

patient monitoring, prompt reporting of deviations from baseline data, and defensive documentation.

PSYCHIATRIC DOCUMENTATION

Psychiatric conditions pose unique and diverse issues for health care providers and for the institution providing mental health services. These services may be rendered in a specialty facility, in a small unit in a general hospital, in scattered ambulatory centers, or in private offices.

Numerous regulatory agencies oversee psychiatric services and care. Confidentiality is a major concern in this area. The stigma of mental illness places special emphasis on the need for confidentiality. There is a great need to protect information received from the patient. Nursing documentation is also an important factor in psychiatric nursing.

Generally, nurses use the nursing process to document patient behaviors. Sometimes patients are unable to verbalize their plans or concerns; some patients become outwardly violent. The nurse must assess and document any indicators or signs that the patient could progress to suicidal or violent behavior.

After assessing the patient's risk, the nurse should plan, implement, and document interventions to reduce the risk of injury to the patient or others. If an event occurs and a lawsuit develops, the nurse will be evaluated on whether the incident could have been predicted and whether the nurse followed hospital policy.

The best method for documenting potential crises is to write direct quotes. Direct quotes added to the documentation of the nurse's follow-up actions provide a sound defense. A description in simple, concrete terms of the behavior or comment that posed a threat to the patient or others should be noted along with notification of the health care provider, the safety precautions ordered, and the time the precautions were started.

If a patient is placed in seclusion, a form representing the frequent checks, behaviors, and treatments may be used for documentation. This form facilitates charting, and the findings are clearly spelled out so anyone can easily identify the patient's behaviors (see Figure 10-15 on pages 195-196).

Nurses are challenged to provide the safest, most therapeutic care possible to the patient while minimizing obvious and not-so-obvious risks. There are areas of concern in psychiatric practice that require astute observation and clear precise documentation. These concerns are listed in Table 10-9 on page 198.

In psychiatric settings, protection of communication between a patient and health care provider is very important. However, when a patient presents a danger to self or to others, it is necessary to report this information in order to obtain assistance in caring for the patient. Institutions need legal definitions in their policies and procedures to guide nurses' practice.

Many medications used in psychiatry cause side effects; these side effects must be carefully observed and documented. The Abnormal Involuntary Movement Scale (AIMS) may be used in psychiatric facilities to document medication side effects. It is set up in checklist format for ease of use. If AIMS is not available, the nurse should accurately, carefully, and completely document the side effects observed after a medication is administered. Therefore, it is necessary for each nurse to be aware of medication side effects.

Even though a patient is admitted for a mental health problem, there may be other concerns to which the nurse must pay attention. Many psychiatric patients have medical problems as well as mental health problems. Therefore, a nurse must be knowledgeable in both medical and psychiatric care management. Documentation is required for both the medical and psychiatric conditions. Blood tests are run to check for therapeutic medication levels as well as routine blood work to analyze the patient's status. Institutionalization increases a patient's exposure to and risk of infection. Nursing standards of practice require nurses to use appropriate nursing measures for infection control and to provide proper documentation if an infection occurs.

Basically, documentation in a psychiatric facility follows the nursing process. Additional forms or requirements might be necessary in the documentation; however, the overall process is the same as for any other area. Being knowledgeable about risk liabilities and concerns about the mental health patient protects practitioners and institutions while they provide care to patients. Effective documentation is essential to minimize the risks of liability. Another form used for psychiatric documentation can be found in Figure 10-16 on page 197.

FIGURE 10-15: SAMPLE SECLUSION FORM (1 OF 2)

WELLSTAR HEALTH SYSTEM   **RESTRAINT/SECLUSION FLOWSHEET**

☐ CH ☐ DH ☐ KH ☐ PH ☐ WHH Other_____
Date_____

I. Type: ☐Roll/lap belt ☐Vest ☐Mittens #_____ ☐Soft Limb (RU__LU__RL__LL__) ☐Seclusion Other_____

II. Alternatives attempted and ineffective: (note daily)
☐ Family involvement   ☐ Fall Prevention Protocol implem.   ☐ Review/remind of necessity of medical therapies
☐ Wrapping IV site, etc.   ☐ Frequent pt √/needs assessment   ☐ Patient relocated for closer observation
☐ Psychosocial interventions   ☐ Medications reviewed/revised   ☐ Bed/chair alarms   ☐ Other

Hour	Safety/Comfort q 15-30 min.** Observations q15'- 4 pt restraint Initials=pt. √'ed .00 :15 :30 :45	Behavior Assessed Q 2 hr **refer to codes	*Toileting offered q 2 hrs. T=toileted R=refused F=Foley	*Fluids/nourishment offered q 2 hrs. A=accepted R=refused	*Limb restraint released q 2 hrs. √ = done N/A if vest	Circ-√'s q 2 hr (Limb rst) A=adeq C=comp	*Promote ROM, activity q 2 hrs. √ = done	Assess need for continued use of restraint (RN - √ q 8 hrs & initial)	Comments (must include restraints off/on, family with pt, trial release, restraint d/c'ed, RN d/c'ing) Initials/signature/Title (RN/LPN/NCA/Security - any initials require signature/title)
2400								
0100								
0200								
0300								
0400								
0500								
0600								
0700								
0800								
0900								
1000								
1100								
1200								
1300								
1400								
1500								
1600								
1700								
1800								
1900								
2000								
2100								
2200								
2300								

Item # 2597   * = while awake   ** Codes: Refer to back of flowsheet   1 - Patient record   2 - Nurse Manager/Resource Nurse   10/00

FIGURE 10-15: SAMPLE SECLUSION FORM (2 OF 2)

RESTRAINT/SECLUSION FLOWSHEET

Instructions: Restraint/Seclusion Flowsheet to be completed by nursing staff at specified intervals. RN to be responsible for evaluating continued need for restraint (document reassessments every 8 hrs) and verifying pt. monitoring and physician orders are appropriate. When restraint is released, this, as well as reapplication of restraint if necessary, must be documented under comments and include name of RN d/c'ing. Initials and abbreviation codes are to be used as indicated; initials/signature/title should be documented under comments at least once/24 hrs

Safety and Comfort
q 15-30 mins
(minimum of q 15 mins for pt. in 4 point restraint and/or for Mental Health pt.)
Initial to indicate visual observation for:
restraint applied properly, no respiratory difficulty or pt. safety issues - verify pt. comfort if awake. Initials indicate that pt. observed to be safe/comfortable
Note: If pt. agitated or in 4 point restraint, more frequent observations, continuous to q 15 mins, as indicated

Circulation checks
q 2 hrs
(for limb restraints only)

Document as follows:
adequate = extremity warm with adeq. pulse present
comp = compromised with cool extremity, loss of palpable pulse
(notify RN/MD)

Behavior assessed

Document q 2 hrs. as follows:
a = agitated
c = calm
d = disoriented
o = oriented
r = resting quietly
s = sleeping

Limb Restraint Release
q 2 hrs while awake
(for limb restraints only)

Document restraint released by initialing.
If not able to release, document reason, i.e., pt agitated. threat to self or others, under comments

Toileting
offered q 2 hrs while awake

Document as follows:
T = toileted
R = refused
F=Foley
S = sleeping
If foley/indwelling catheter present, document this.

Range of Motion
q 2 hrs as indicated while awake
(for limb restraints only)

ROM to be performed on pt who needs assistance/unable to do active ROM independently

Fluids/nourishment
offered q 2 hrs while awake

Document as follows:
A = accepted
R = refused
S = sleeping
Note: If not taking p.o. fluids, document presence of IV

Assess need for continued use of restraint
q 8 hrs
(by RN)

RN to assess pt. at least once q 8 hrs to determine that continued use of restraint is appropriate. Initials indicate that pt. was reassessed. If trial release of restraint felt appropriate, document this under comments.

Restraint/Seclusion Flowsheet

page 2 of 2

FIGURE 10-16: SAMPLE PSYCHIATRIC DOCUMENTATION FORM

WellStar
Health System

☐Cobb ☐Douglas ☐Kennestone
☐Paulding ☐Windy Hill

Group Progress Note

DATE: _____/_____/_____   **(Place bar code label above)**

GROUP TYPE: _____PROCESS (S.W.) _____MEDICATION _____ACTIVITY _____EDUCATION _____FOCUS _____GROUP TOPIC

Attendance:	( ) Attended	( ) Came Late	( ) Left Early	( ) Absent	
Cognition:	( ) Oriented x 3	( ) Psychotic Thinking	( ) Hallucinating	( ) Delusional	( ) Preoccuppied
Affect:	( ) Flat	( ) Bright	( ) Angry	( ) Labile	( ) Appropriate
Mood:	( ) Depressed	( ) Angry	( ) Anxious	( ) Normal	
Patricipation:	( ) Active	( ) Passive			

COMMENTS: _____
_____
_____

Signature _____   Discipline _____

DATE: _____/_____/_____

GROUP TYPE: _____PROCESS (S.W.) _____MEDICATION _____ACTIVITY _____EDUCATION _____FOCUS _____GROUP TOPIC

Attendance:	( ) Attended	( ) Came Late	( ) Left Early	( ) Absent	
Cognition:	( ) Oriented x 3	( ) Psychotic Thinking	( ) Hallucinating	( ) Delusional	( ) Preoccuppied
Affect:	( ) Flat	( ) Bright	( ) Angry	( ) Labile	( ) Appropriate
Mood:	( ) Depressed	( ) Angry	( ) Anxious	( ) Normal	
Patricipation:	( ) Active	( ) Passive			

COMMENTS: _____
_____
_____

Signature _____   Discipline _____

DATE: _____/_____/_____

GROUP TYPE: _____PROCESS (S.W.) _____MEDICATION _____ACTIVITY _____EDUCATION _____FOCUS _____GROUP TOPIC

Attendance:	( ) Attended	( ) Came Late	( ) Left Early	( ) Absent	
Cognition:	( ) Oriented x 3	( ) Psychotic Thinking	( ) Hallucinating	( ) Delusional	( ) Preoccuppied
Affect:	( ) Flat	( ) Bright	( ) Angry	( ) Labile	( ) Appropriate
Mood:	( ) Depressed	( ) Angry	( ) Anxious	( ) Normal	
Patricipation:	( ) Active	( ) Passive			

COMMENTS: _____
_____
_____

Signature _____   Discipline _____

Pg. 1 of 1   GROUP PROGRESS NOTE

Reprinted with the permission of WellStar Health System, Marietta, GA.

TABLE 10-9: PSYCHIATRIC AREAS OF CONCERN
• Informed consent
• Right to treatment
• Psychopharmacology
• Electroconvulsive therapy
• Suicide
• Seclusion and restraints
• Elopement and wandering
• Discharge and aftercare planning
• Child and adolescent psychiatry
• Confidentiality and stigma
• High-risk incidents: violence, illicit substance abuse, and sexual misconduct
(Oldham & Meyer-Tulledge, 1999; Wysoker, 1997)

HOME HEALTH CARE DOCUMENTATION

Home health care is one of the fastest growing areas of health care. Home health care meets the nursing needs of a large number of generally elderly people with disabilities and chronic illnesses who do not need acute hospital care or who have recently been discharged from a hospital. Home health care includes professional and paraprofessional services and equipment for the purposes of health promotion and maintenance, patient and family education, illness prevention, diagnosis and treatment of diseases, palliation, and rehabilitation.

Home health care requires coordination of care by the entire health care team. Documentation of care has different implications than in other areas of nursing. Documenting quality patient care within the constraints imposed by regulations, resources, and finances is a challenge. The ideal documentation system should provide comprehensive patient information, address standards of practice and patient outcomes, facilitate reimbursement from government and insurance company payers, and serve as a legal document.

The home health care field has many public and voluntary regulators that ensure the quality of home health care services. Agencies providing home care services must be licensed by the individual states and may be certified by Medicare or Medicaid; the Community Health Accreditation Program, part of the National League for Nursing (NLN); and JCAHO.

Additional regulators have also emerged. In 1986, the ANA published standards for home health nursing practice. In 1988, JCAHO issued standards and began accrediting home health care organizations that volunteered. In 1995, JCAHO published revised standards. At the same time, the federal Centers for Medicare & Medicaid Services (CMS) [previously Health Care Financing Administration (HCFA)] indicated that individual home health agencies accredited by the NLN and hospital-based agencies accredited by JCAHO met Medicare certification requirements (Peters, 1999; Singleton, 1997).

Quality control regulations are increasing, which may lead to a greater risk of exposure. Up to this time, there have not been a large number of negligence claims against home health care agencies. This may change as more regulations come into play.

Even though documentation in home health care does not differ much from acute care settings, there are still concerns. Home health care providers have minimal direct supervision, tend to be transient in their employment patterns, and may become bored and lax with documentation when involved with long-term patients. The continuity of patient care can be recognized in well-organized patient charts. Therefore, home health care documentation should be simplified yet complete and meet legal requirements and the standards for accreditation.

The purpose of home health care documentation is to establish the need for services, present a legal document, and communicate care provided. Today, because of increased pressure for efficiency and accountability, documentation has become a decision-making and informational tool. Home health care documentation must contain accurate information about nursing interventions as well as a way to track all parts of care and the analysis of outcomes.

A comprehensive documentation system for organizing a nurse's charting known as the Omaha Classification System has been developed. This system is composed of the Problem Classification Scheme (PCS), the Rating Scale for Outcomes (RSO), and the Intervention Scheme (IS).

The PCS is an orderly, nonexhaustive, mutually exclusive list of nursing diagnoses used for data collection and problem identification. The RSO is presented in a five-point response-scale form that measures patient progress in three areas: knowledge, behavior, and status. The response scale is used with each nursing diagnosis in the PCS section. Evaluation of the patient's progress should be performed periodically throughout the time of providing care. The IS section provides information that is helpful in developing plans of care. The Omaha System can easily be used so the patient can be mutually involved in identifying problems.

The Omaha System does not include an acuity scale, so the Community Health Intensity Rating Scale may also be used. This comprehensive assessment form has 15 parameters that fully describe the scope of home care services. It can be used to determine the skill level of the care provider prior to assignment.

Many forms are used in home health care. A complete home and patient assessment must be conducted. Some of the forms used in home health care are listed in Table 10-10. Other forms may also be included, depending on requirements by insurers, if the agency is to be reimbursed for services.

A recently required form is the Physician's Recommendation Concerning Nursing Facility Care or Intermediate Care for the Mentally

---

TABLE 10-10: HOME HEALTH CARE DOCUMENTATION FORMS

- Patient assessment
- Referral source information/intake form
- Home and environment assessment
- Discipline-specific (e.g., nurse, therapist, aid, social worker) care plans.
- Physician's plan of treatment
- Medication sheet
- Clinical progress notes (narrative, flow sheets, or both).
- Miscellaneous (e.g., conference notes, verbal order forms, telephone calls)
- Discharge summary
- Reports to third-party payers

(Borchers, 1999; Peters, 1999)

Retarded, which replaces CMS forms 485 and 486. The form requires Medicare certification and plan of treatment and must be signed by the physician. It becomes a mandatory part of the patient's chart (see Figure 10-17 on page 200).

Home health care providers may have problems accessing patients' medical records. Because many different providers need the record, documentation may become fragmented. Frequently, information is recorded on more than one form. It is challenging to accurately, completely, consistently, clearly, quickly, and concisely document simultaneously provided care.

Computerized patient records may solve some of these problems. The nurse providing home health care may use a laptop computer, which can be taken into the patient's home. If the patient's records are integrated, all information can be sent to a central location and additional care needed may be easily identified (Triplett, 2002). The information is more accurate, can be easily retrieved, and can be presented in ways to help measure outcomes, show trends, and identify problems.

Home health care documentation is challenging. The documentation can be time-consuming because of the numerous forms required by regulating bodies

FIGURE 10-17: SAMPLE PHYSICIAN'S RECOMMENDATION CONCERNING NURSING FACILITY CARE OR INTERMEDIATE CARE FOR THE MENTALLY RETARDED

Section A – Identifying Information

1. Facility's Name and Address

County _____

2. Medicaid Number

3. Social Security Number

— — — — — — — — — —

4. Sex | Age | 4A. Birthdate

7. Patient's Name (Last, First, Middle Initial)

5. Type of Facility (Check One)
1. ☐ Nursing Facility
2. ☐ ICF/MR

6. Type of Recommendation
1. ☐ Initial
2. ☐ Level Change
3. ☐ Continued Placement

8. Date of Nursing Facility Admission
/   /

9. Patient Transferred from: (check one)
☐ Hospital   ☐ Home   ☐ Another Nurs. Home
☐ Private Pay   ☐ Medicare

Member's Home Address _____
Member's Telephone Number _____
Mother's Maiden Name:

Date of Medicaid Application
/   /

9A. State Authority (MH & MR Screening)

Level I/II

This is to certify that the facility or attending physician is hereby authorized to provide the Dept. of Community Health, Division of Medical Assistance and the Dept. of Human Resources, Division of Family and Children Services with necessary information including medical data.

10. Signed _____
(Patient, Spouse, Parent, or other Relative or Legal Representative)

11. Date _____

Restricted Auth. Code   Date

9B. This is not a re-admission for OBRA purposes

Restricted Auth. Code   Date

Section B – Physician's Examination Report and Recommendation

1. ICD | 2. ICD | 3. ICD

12. Diagnosis on Admission to Facility (Hospital Transfer Record May Be Attached)

1. Primary _____   2. Secondary _____   3. Other _____

13. Treatment Plan (Attach copy of order sheet if more convenient)

Hospital Dates: _____ to _____

Hospital Diagnosis 1. Primary _____ 2. Secondary _____ 3. Other _____

Medications				Diagnostic and Treatment Procedures	
Name	Dosage	Route	Frequency	Type	Frequency

14. Recommendation Regarding Level of Care Considered Necessary
1. ☐ Skilled 2. ☐ Intermediate 3. ☐ Intermediate care for the Mentally Retarded

15. Length of Time Care Needed   Months
1. ☐ Permanent   2. ☐ Temporary _____ estimated

16. Is Patient free of communicable diseases? 1. ☐ Yes 2. ☐ No

17. This patient's condition ☐ could ☐ could not be managed by provision of ☐ Community Care or ☐ Home Health Services.

18. I certify that this patient requires the level of care provided by a nursing facility or an intermediate care facility for the mentally retarded.

Physician's Signature

19. Physician's Name (Print)

Physician's Address (Print)

20. Date Signed By Physician
/   /

21. Physician's Licensure No.

Physician's Phone No.
(   )

Section C – Evaluation of Nursing Care Needed (check appropriate box only)

22. Diet
☐ Regular
☐ Diabetic
☐ Formula
☐ Low Sodium
☐ Tube Feeding
☐ Other

23. Bowel
☐ Continent
☐ Occas. Incontinent
☐ Incontinent
☐ Colostomy

24. Overall Cond.
☐ Improving
☐ Stable
☐ Fluctuating
☐ Deteriorating
☐ Critical
☐ Terminal

25. Restorative Pot.
☐ Good
☐ Fair
☐ Poor
☐ Questionable
☐ None

26. Mental & Behavioral Status
☐ Agitated   ☐ Noisy   ☐ Dependent
☐ Confused   ☐ Nonresponsive ☐ Independent
☐ Cooperative ☐ Vacillating   ☐ Anxious
☐ Depressed   ☐ Violent   ☐ Well Adjusted
☐ Forgetful   ☐ Wanders   ☐ Disoriented
☐ Alert   ☐ Withdrawn   ☐ Inappropriate Reaction

27. Decubiti
☐ Yes   ☐ Surgery
☐ No   Date
☐ Infected
☐ On Admission

28. Bladder
☐ Continent
☐ Occas. Incontinent
☐ Incontinent
☐ Catheter

29. Hours Out of Bed Per Day ☐ IV
☐ Intake
☐ Output ☐ Bedfast

☐ Catheter Care
☐ Colostomy Care
☐ Sterile Dressings
☐ Suctioning

30. Indicate Frequency Per Week

	Physical Therapy	Occupational Therapy	Remotive Therapy	Reality Orientation	Speech Therapy	Bowel and Bladder Retrain	Activities Program
Received							
Needed							

31. Record Appropriate Legend
1. Severe
2. Moderate
3. Mild
4. None

IMPAIRMENTS

Sight	Hear	Speech	Ltd. Motion	Paralysis
☐	☐	☐	☐	☐

1. Dependent
2. Needs Asst.
3. Independent
4. Not App.

ACTIVITIES OF DAILY LIVING

Eats	Wheel chair	Transfers	Bath	Ambulation	Dressing
☐	☐	☐	☐	☐	☐

32. Remarks

33. Pre-Admission Certification Number

34. Signed

35. Date Signed
/   /

Do Not Write Below This Line

Continued Stay Review Date: _____

Payment Date _____ Approved For _____ Days Only!

36. Level of Care Recommended

LOS

37. Signature

Date
/   /

38. Attachments
1. ☐ Yes 2. ☐ No

and the need for several different health care providers to have access to the patient's record. Computerized documentation can be an effective method for home health care documentation. Other forms commonly used in home health care are displayed in Figure 10-18 on pages 202-204.

LONG-TERM CARE DOCUMENTATION

Long-term care (LTC) facilities are licensed by the states in which they are located. Each state that has established its definition of a LTC facility has its own licensing requirements and regulations. In 1987, the Federal Nursing Home Reform Act, a part of the Consolidated Omnibus Budget Reconciliation Act (COBRA) of 1987, made significant changes in how LTC facilities were to be operated and evaluated to conform to Medicare and Medicaid reimbursement requirements. COBRA '87 requires that each state adopt regulations that specify a minimum number of staff who are registered and licensed nurses. The law also requires additional training for certified nursing assistants (Singleton, 1997).

LTC facilities are highly regulated, and the focus of evaluation now centers on the caring process, residents' feelings, and patient care outcomes. Each regulatory body makes its own on-site visit and reviews administrative policies, operations, finances, and medical and nursing care services. Credentials of professionals, minutes of meetings, patient care conferences, nursing documentation, and all aspects of the facilities' activities and functions are reviewed. If a facility is identified as having deficiencies, it has a chance to correct them. The most commonly cited deficiencies are presented in Table 10-11 on page 205.

If standards are not met, licensure may be revoked or reimbursement to the facility may be delayed. Compliance with multiple government regulations, federal Medicare and Medicaid requirements, state licensure specifications, and JCAHO rules is important to maintaining the facility's existence. A list of possible LTC facility regulators is provided in Table 10-12 on page 205.

The basic documentation techniques previously discussed also apply to documentation in LTC settings. The patient's progress notes are the primary way to communicate care provided. Careful, precise documentation is critical in LTC facilities because LTC patients typically are of advanced age, have chronic health problems, and are generally in poor health. The patient is in a LTC facility because of the great need of skilled nursing care.

The frequency of documentation may vary according to state requirements. Some states require daily summaries the first 5 days after admission, then once a week for 4 weeks, and then monthly after that. Summaries are required in addition to regular nursing notes. Worksheets may be helpful to alert nurses as to when summaries are due. Any time an incident occurs, more frequent documentation is required.

The COBRA and CMS developed a Resident Assessment Instrument (RAI), a standardized way for planning and delivering care focused on assessing, planning, and providing individualized care. The RAI consists of a Minimum Data Set (MDS) of elements, common definitions, and coding categories needed to perform comprehensive assessment of a LTC facility resident. The RAI is composed of three parts: the MDS, resident assessment protocols (RAPs), and utilization guidelines. The RAI is designed to produce comprehensive, accurate, standardized, reproducible assessment of each LTC facility resident's functional capacity.

Since June of 1998, computerized reporting of the RAI is required. LTC facilities must enter information from the RAI in accordance with CMS-specified formats. The facility sends the data about each resident's assessment to the state every month (Cavallaro, Newman, & Iyer, 1999).

text continues on page 205

FIGURE 10-18: OTHER HOME HEALTH CARE FORMS (1 OF 3)

NURSING VISIT NOTE

DATE_____ TIME IN _____ TIME OUT_____

TYPE OF VISIT: ☐ **Skilled** Planned / PRN ☐ **Skilled & Supervisory** ☐ **Supervisory Only** ☐ **Other**_____

Homebound reason:_____
Reason for visit:_____
_____

Vital Signs: Temperature:_____ ☐ Oral ☐ Axillary ☐ Tympanic ☐ Rectal   Pulse:_____ ☐ Radial ☐ Apical ☐ Brachial
☐ Regular ☐ Irregular

Respirations:_____ ☐ Regular ☐ Irregular   Blood Pressure: Right_____/_____ Left_____/_____ ☐ Lying ☐ Standing ☐ Sitting

Weight:_____ ☐ Actual ☐ Reported

Pain: ☐ None ☐ Same ☐ Improved ☐ Worse   Origin_____ Location(s)_____
Duration_____ Intensity 0-10_____ Other_____ Relief measures_____

NURSING ASSESSMENT AND OBSERVATION SIGNS/SYMPTOMS
(Mark all applicable with an "X". Circle appropriate item(s) separated by "/".)

CARDIOPULMONARY

Lung Sounds ☐ Clear ☐ Crackles/Rales Location_____
☐ Rhonchi/Wheeze Location_____
☐ Diminished ☐ Absent ☐ Other_____
Cough ☐ None ☐ Dry/acute/chronic
☐ Non-productive/Productive Amount: ☐ Small ☐ Medium ☐ Large
☐ Hemoptysis frequency_____ Amount_____
☐ Able/unable to cough up secretions Suction: ☐ Yes ☐ No
Respiratory Status ☐ Accessory muscles used ☐ Orthopnea
☐ Dyspnea: ☐ At rest ☐ With exertion/activity
☐ Stridor/retractions ☐ O₂_____ LPM ☐ PRN ☐ Continuous
☐ O₂ saturation _____%
Chest Pain ☐ Denies ☐ Anginal ☐ Postural ☐ Localized
☐ Substernal ☐ Radiating ☐ Dull ☐ Aching ☐ Sharp/stabbing
☐ Viselike ☐ Other_____
Associated with: ☐ Shortness of breath ☐ Activity ☐ Rest
☐ Frequency/duration_____
Heart Sounds ☐ Normal ☐ Regular/Irregular ☐ Murmur
☐ Abnormal (explain)_____
Other
☐ Fatigued ☐ Edema ☐ Pedal: Right_____ Left_____
☐ Pitting +1/+2/+3/+4 ☐ Non-pitting site:_____
☐ Cramps/claudication
☐ Capillary refill: Greater than 3 seconds/Less than 3 seconds

NEUROMUSCULAR

☐ Alert/oriented to person/place/time ☐ Disoriented ☐ Syncope
☐ Headache
Grasp Right ☐ Equal ☐ Unequal ☐ Other_____
Left ☐ Equal ☐ Unequal ☐ Other_____
Pupils ☐ PERRLA ☐ Right ☐ Left ☐ Both ☐ Other_____
Impairment ☐ Speech ☐ Hearing ☐ Visual
☐ Decreased sensitivity ☐ Tremors
☐ Numbness/tingling ☐ Vertigo/Ataxia
☐ Falls (explain):_____
☐ Balance WNL ☐ Unsteady gait
☐ Weakness (describe)_____
☐ Change in ADL (explain)_____

GASTROINTESTINAL

Appetite ☐ Good ☐ Fair ☐ Poor ☐ NPO
☐ Anorexia ☐ Nausea/vomiting
☐ Difficulty swallowing Oral intake_____
☐ Tube feeding (specify)_____ ☐ Cont. ☐ Intermittent
Bowel Sounds ☐ Active/absent/hypoactive/hyperactive x___quadrants
☐ Abdominal pain/distention/flatulence
☐ Last BM_____
☐ Incontinence ☐ Diarrhea ☐ Constipation ☐ Impaction
☐ Enema administered (results)_____
☐ Patient tolerated procedure well
☐ Other_____

GENITOURINARY

Urine color:_____ ☐ Odor: ☐ Burning ☐ Hesitancy
☐ Nocturia ☐ Oliguria/anuria ☐ Retention ☐ Incontinence occurs_____
Urinary Catheter Type (specify)_____ French_____
Bulb inflated_____mL sterile water Date changed_____
Irrigated with (specify)_____ amt _____mL
☐ Other_____

ENDOCRINE

Blood sugar range_____
☐ Hyperglycemia: glycosuria / polyuria / polydipsia
☐ Hypoglycemia: sweats / polyphagia / weak / faint / stupor
Monitored by: ☐ Self ☐ Caregiver ☐ Nurse ☐ Other_____

MEDICATIONS

(New or changed since last visit) ☐ None ☐ Update Medication Profile
Drug(s)_____
Dosage/frequency_____
Effective ☐ Yes ☐ No ☐ Other_____
☐ Orders obtained
Instructed on:
☐ Medication(s) names   ☐ Pill count (if applicable)_____
☐ S/S allergic reaction   ☐ S/E contraindications
☐ Drug/food interactions   ☐ Ample supply
☐ Drug/drug interactions   ☐ Proper disposal of sharps
☐ Expiration dates   ☐ Duration of therapy
☐ Prescription refill by_____ ☐ Other_____
☐ Missed doses/what to do
☐ Administered by: ☐ Self ☐ Family/Caregiver ☐ Nurse
☐ Other:_____
☐ Medication administered this visit (document in narrative on back page)

Type of line: ☐ Peripheral ☐ PICC ☐ Central (type) _____
☐ Implanted port Location (specify)_____
Site (if appropriate)_____ Site (describe) _____
Catheter length _____cm Arm circumference _____cm
☐ No evidence of infection
☐ Dressing change performed by: ☐ Self ☐ Family/caregiver ☐ Nurse
☐ Other_____
☐ Cap change performed by: ☐ Self ☐ Family/caregiver ☐ Nurse
☐ Other_____
☐ Extension/tubing changed by: ☐ Self ☐ Family/caregiver ☐ Nurse
☐ Other_____
☐ Line flushed _____mL saline/sterile water
☐ Heparin _____unit/mL _____mL
☐ Instructed patient/family/caregiver on infusion therapy
☐ Patient/family/caregiver demonstrates/verbalizes proper
management of infusion(s)
Comments: _____
_____

Lab: ☐ None ☐ Blood drawn from _____ for_____
☐ Other_____ Delivered to_____

PATIENT NAME – Last, First, Middle Initial   ID#

Form 3489P © BRIGGS, Des Moines, IA 50306 (800) 247-2343 www.BriggsCorp.com
R1203   PRINTED IN U.S.A.

NURSING VISIT NOTE

FIGURE 10-18: OTHER HOME HEALTH CARE FORMS (2 OF 3)

EMOTIONAL STATUS

❏ Coping ❏ Lethargic ❏ Agitated
❏ Forgetful ❏ Confused ❏ Depressed
❏ Other_____
_____

SKIN

Color:_____ Turgor:_____
Temperature:_____
Access site (describe)_____

❏ Rash/itching/dry
❏ Incision clean - healing/approximating
❏ Other_____

WOUND CARE PROVIDED

❏ Soiled dressing removed/disposed of properly
❏ Wound cleaned (specify)_____
❏ Wound irrigated (specify)_____
❏ Type of dressing(s) used_____
❏ Wound debridement
❏ Drainage collection container emptied. Volume _____
❏ Patient tolerated procedure well
❏ Medicated prior to wound care
❏ Wound care/dressing change performed by: ❏ Self ❏ Nurse
   ❏ Family/caregiver ❏ Other_____
❏ Patient/family/caregiver instructed on wound care/disposal
   of soiled dressing
❏ Patient/family/caregiver to perform wound care/dressing
   change

Denote Location / Size of Wounds / Pressure Sores / Measure Ext. Edema Bil.

Anterior   Posterior

	#1	#2	#3	#4
Length				
Width				
Depth				
Drainage				
Tunneling				
Odor				
Sur. Tis.				
Edema				
Stoma				

INTERVENTIONS/INSTRUCTIONS
(Mark all applicable with an "X". Circle appropriate item(s) separated by "/".)

❏ Skilled observation & assessment (A1)
❏ Foley care (A2)
❏ Urine testing
❏ Wound care/dressing
❏ Decubitus care
❏ Venipuncture (A6)
❏ Post-cataract care (A8)
❏ Bowel/Bladder training (A9)
❏ Digital exam with manual removal/Enema
❏ Chest physio./Postural drainage (A10)
❏ Change NG/G tube (A17)
❏ Admin. of vitamin B$_{12}$ (A11)

❏ Prep./Admin. insulin (A12)
❏ Teach/Admin. IVs/Clysis (A14)
❏ Teach ostomy/ileo. conduit care (A15)
❏ Teach/Admin. tube feedings (A16)
❏ Teach/Admin. care of trach. (A20/A21)
❏ Teach/Admin. Inhalation Rx (A22/A23)
❏ Teach care - terminally ill
❏ IM injection (A13)
❏ Psych. intervention
❏ Observe S/S infection
❏ Diabetic observation

❏ Teach diabetic care (A25)
❏ Observe/Teach medication (N or C) effects/side effects
❏ Physiology/Disease process teaching
❏ Observe ADLs
❏ Evaluate diet/fluid intake
❏ Diet teaching
❏ Safety factors
❏ Prenatal assessment
❏ Post-partum assessment
❏ Teach infant/child care
❏ Pain Management
❏ Other:_____
_____

ANALYSIS/INTERVENTIONS/INSTRUCTIONS/PATIENT RESPONSE

_____
_____
_____
_____
_____
_____
_____
_____
_____

SUMMARY CHECKLIST

CARE PLAN: ❏ Reviewed/Revised with patient involvement
   ❏ Outcome achieved ❏ PRN order obtained
PLAN FOR NEXT VISIT: _____

NEXT PHYSICIAN VISIT: _____
APPROXIMATE NEXT VISIT DATE: _____/_____/_____
DISCHARGE PLANNING DISCUSSED? ❏ Yes ❏ No ❏ N/A
BILLABLE SUPPLIES RECORDED? ❏ Yes ❏ No
CARE COORDINATION: ❏ Physician ❏ PT ❏ OT ❏ ST
   ❏ MSW ❏ SN ❏ Other (specify)_____

AIDE SUPERVISORY VISIT (Complete if applicable)

AIDE: ❏ Present ❏ Not present
SUPERVISORY VISIT: ❏ Scheduled ❏ Unscheduled
IS PATIENT/FAMILY SATISFIED? ❏ Yes ❏ No Explain:_____
_____

AIDE CARE PLAN UPDATED? ❏ Yes ❏ No
OBSERVATION OF:_____
_____

TEACHING/TRAINING OF:_____
_____

NEXT SCHEDULED SUPERVISORY VISIT _____/_____/_____

SIGNATURE/DATE–Complete **TIME OUT** (on front) prior to signing below.

X_____   _____/_____/_____
Nurse (signature/title)   Date

Patient Signature (optional)_____

NURSING VISIT NOTE

FIGURE 10-18: OTHER HOME HEALTH CARE FORMS (3 OF 3)

SKILLED NURSING VISIT NOTE

DATE OF VISIT_____

TIME IN _____ OUT _____

HOMEBOUND REASON: ❏ Needs assistance for all activities ❏ Residual weakness ❏ Requires assistance to ambula ❏ Confusion, unable to go out of home alone ❏ Unable to safely leave home unassisted ❏ Severe SOB, SOB upon exertion ❏ Dependent upon adaptive device(s) ❏ Medical restrictions ❏ Other (specify)_____

NURSING DIAGNOSIS/PROBLEM _____

TYPE OF VISIT: ❏ SN ❏ SN & Supervisory ❏ Supervisory Only ❏ Other

VITALS

T°_____ Wt._____
Resp. _____ ❏ Reg. ❏ Irreg.
Pulse: A _____ R _____
❏ Regular ❏ Irregular

B/P	LYING	SITTING	STANDING
Right			
Left			

Denote Location / Size of Wounds / Pressure Sores / Measure Ext. Edema Bil.

NURSING ASSESSMENT AND OBSERVATION SIGNS/SYMPTOMS
(Mark all applicable with an "X". Circle appropriate item(s) separated by "/".)

CARDIOVASCULAR
- Fluid retention
- Chest pain
- Neck vein distension
- Edema (specify)-
  - ❏ RUE ❏ LUE
  - ❏ RLE ❏ LLE
- Peripheral pulses
- Other:

RESPIRATORY
- Rales/Rhonchi/Wheeze
- Cough
- Dyspnea/SOB
- Orthopnea
- Other:

DIGESTIVE
- Bowel sounds
- Nausea/Vomiting
- Anorexia
- Epigastric distress
- Difficulty swallowing
- Abdominal distension
- Colostomy
- Diarrhea
- Constipation/Impaction
- Bowel incontinence
- Other:

GENITOURINARY
- Burning
- Distension/Retention
- Frequency/Urgency
- Hesitancy
- Hematuria
- Bladder incontinence
- Catheter
- Urine-
  - Color: _____
  - Consistency: _____
  - Odor: _____
- Pain
- Discharge
- Diabetic urine testing
- Other:

SKIN
- Color:
- Jaundiced
- Temperature
- Chills
- Decubitus/Wound
- Rash/Itching
- Turgor
- Other:

PAIN
- Origin:
- Location:
- Duration:
- Intensity (0-10):
- Other:

MUSCULOSKELETAL
- Balance/Unsteady gait
- Weakness
- Other:

NEUROSENSORY
- Syncope
- Headache
- Grasp-
  - Right:
  - Left:
- Movement-
  - ❏ RUE ❏ LUE
  - ❏ RLE ❏ LLE
- Pupil reaction-
  - Right: Left:
- Tremors
- Vertigo
- Speech impairment
- Hearing impairment
- Visual impairment
- Decreased sensitivity
- Other:

EMOTIONAL STATUS
- Disoriented
- Lethargic
- Agitated
- Oriented
- Comatose
- Forgetful
- Depressed
- Other:

	#1	#2	#3	#4
Length				
Width				
Depth				
Drainage				
Tunneling				
Odor				
Sur. Tis.				
Edema				
Stoma				

Anterior Posterior

INTERVENTIONS/INSTRUCTIONS (Mark all applicable with an "X". Circle appropriate item(s) separated by "/".)

Skilled observation & assessment (A1)	Chest physio./Postural drainage (A10)	IM injection (A13)	Evaluate diet/fluid intake
Foley care (A2)	Change NG/G tube (A17)	Psych. intervention	Diet teaching
Urine testing	Admin. of vitamin B12 (A11)	Observe S/S infection	Safety factors
Wound care/dressing	Prep./Admin. insulin (A12)	Diabetic observation	Prenatal assessment
Decubitus care	Teach/Admin. IVs/Clysis (A14)	Teach diabetic care (A25)	Post-partum assessment
Venipuncture (A6)	Teach ostomy/ileo. conduit care (A15)	Observe/Teach medication (N or C) effects/side effects	Teach infant/child care
Post-cataract care (A8)	Teach/Admin. tube feedings (A16)		Pain Management
Bowel/Bladder training (A9)	Teach/Admin. care of trach. (A20/A21)	Physiology/Disease process teaching	Other:
Digital exam with manual removal/ Enema	Teach/Admin. Inhalation Rx (A22/A23)		
	Teach care - terminally ill	Observe ADLs	

ANALYSIS/INTERVENTIONS/INSTRUCTIONS/PATIENT RESPONSE _____
_____
_____

CARE PLAN: ❏ Reviewed/Revised with patient involvement
❏ Outcome achieved ❏ PRN order obtained
PLAN FOR NEXT VISIT _____
APPROXIMATE NEXT VISIT DATE _____/_____/_____
MEDICATION STATUS: ❏ No change ❏ Order obtained
DISCHARGE PLANNING DISCUSSED? ❏ Yes ❏ No ❏ N/A
BILLABLE SUPPLIES RECORDED? ❏ Yes ❏ No
CARE COORDINATION: ❏ Physician ❏ PT ❏ OT ❏ ST ❏ SS
❏ SN ❏ Other (specify) _____

SIGNATURE/DATE—Complete **TIME OUT** (above) prior to signing below.
X _____ _____/_____/_____
Nurse (signature/title)   *Date*

Patient Signature (optional) _____

AIDE SUPERVISORY VISIT (Complete if applicable.)
AIDE: ❏ Present ❏ Not present
SUPERVISORY VISIT: ❏ Scheduled ❏ Unscheduled
AIDE CARE PLAN UPDATED? ❏ Yes ❏ No
OBSERVATION OF _____
_____
_____
TEACHING/TRAINING OF _____
_____
NEXT SCHEDULED SUPERVISORY VISIT _____/_____/_____

PART 1 – Clinical Record   **PART 2 – Care Coordination**

PATIENT NAME – Last, First, Middle Initial   ID#

Form 3570/2P © 1994 Briggs Corporation, Des Moines, IA 50306 www.BriggsCorp.com
103   To order, phone 1-800-247-2343 PRINTED IN U.S.A

SKILLED NURSING VISIT NOTE

TABLE 10-11: THE 10 MOST COMMONLY CITED DEFICIENCIES IN LONG-TERM CARE FACILITIES

1. Failure to provide the necessary care and services to attain or maintain the highest practicable physical, mental, and psychosocial well-being

2. Failure to provide the housekeeping and maintenance services necessary to maintain a sanitary, orderly, and comfortable interior

3. Failure to ensure that a resident who enters the facility without pressure sores does not develop pressure sores, unless they are unavoidable; a resident who has pressure sores must receive necessary treatment and services to promote healing, prevent infection, and prevent new sores from developing

4. Failure to store, prepare, distribute, and serve food under sanitary conditions

5. Failure to establish an infection-control program that investigates, controls, and prevents infections in the facility

6. Failure to ensure that the resident environment remains as free from accident hazards as possible

7. Failure to provide pharmaceutical services to meet the needs of all residents

8. Failure to ensure that nurse aides are able to demonstrate competency in skills and techniques necessary to care for residents' needs

9. Failure to ensure that residents receive adequate supervision and assistance devices to prevent accidents

10. Failure to provide the necessary services to maintain good nutrition, grooming, and personal and oral hygiene for residents dependent on the facility for activities of daily living

(Texas Department of Human Services, 2003)

TABLE 10-12: LTC FACILITY REGULATORS

- Occupational Safety and Health Organization
- U.S. Department of Health and Human Services
- JCAHO
- CMS

The CMS sets strict standards about who can assess the resident and how often the resident must be assessed. The assessment includes information necessary to complete the MDS and establish a plan of care addressing the resident's characteristics, strengths, and needs. This form requires multidisciplinary input, so social workers, recreational therapists, and dietitians must also complete part of the assessment. RAIs and care plans are to be kept in a resident's chart for 15 months. These standards apply to all Medicare and Medicaid facilities.

The MDS assessment form contains 500 assessment items and is several pages long. A new resident must be assessed within 7 days of admission. Policies should be clearly spelled out as to which discipline completes which section. Every item on the assessment form must be answered in order to develop a comprehensive plan of care. The MDS does have universal language, and nurses must translate nursing diagnoses into the MDS language. See Figure 10-19 on pages 206-212 for a sample of part of the MDS form.

RAPs are problem-oriented frameworks used for additional assessment and problem identification. RAPs form the last part to informing decisions about the plan of care. The CMS manual contains the RAPs and covers about 90% to 95% of a typical nursing resident's plan of care. CMS guidelines specify that RAPs should be used to determine if a problem exists, to identify relevant causal factors, and to develop an individualized care plan in relation to the resident's needs. All areas identified as problems must have an individualized plans of care developed. Assessment and care plans must be interdisciplinary, just like the assessment.

text continues on page 213

FIGURE 10-19: MDS FORM (1 OF 7)

MINIMUM DATA SET (MDS) - *VERSION 2.0*
FOR NURSING HOME RESIDENT ASSESSMENT AND CARE SCREENING

BASIC ASSESSMENT TRACKING FORM

SECTION AA. IDENTIFICATION INFORMATION

1.	RESIDENT NAME	a. (First) b. (Middle Initial) c. (Last) d. (Jr./Sr.)

2. GENDER — 1. Male   2. Female

3. BIRTHDATE — Month — Day — Year

4. RACE/ETHNICITY
1. American Indian/Alaskan Native
2. Asian/Pacific Islander
3. Black, not of Hispanic origin
4. Hispanic
5. White, not of Hispanic origin

5. SOCIAL SECURITY AND MEDICARE NUMBERS
a. Social Security Number
b. Medicare Number (or comparable railroad insurance number)

6. FACILITY PROVIDER NO.
a. State No.
b. Federal No.

7. MEDICAID NO. ["+" if pending, "N" if not a Medicaid recipient]

8. REASONS FOR ASSESSMENT
(Note-Other codes do not apply to this form)
a. Primary reason for assessment
1. Admission assessment (required by day 14)
2. Annual assessment
3. Significant change in status assessment
4. Significant correction of prior full assessment
5. Quarterly review assessment
10. Significant correction of prior quarterly assessment
0. *NONE OF ABOVE*
b. *Codes for assessments required for Medicare PPS or the State*
1. *Medicare 5 day assessment*
2. *Medicare 30 day assessment*
3. *Medicare 60 day assessment*
4. *Medicare 90 day assessment*
5. *Medicare readmission/return assessment*
6. *Other state required assessment*
7. *Medicare 14 day assessmenttnt*
8. *Other Medicare required assessment*

9. Signatures of Persons who Completed a Portion of the Accompanying Assessment or Tracking Form

I certify that the accompanying information accurately reflects resident assessment or tracking information for this resident and that I collected or coordinated collection of this information on the dates specified. To the best of my knowledge, this information was collected in accordance with applicable Medicare and Medicaid requirements. I understand that this information is used as a basis for ensuring that residents receive appropriate and quality care, and as a basis for payment from federal funds. I further understand that payment of such federal funds and continued partici- pation in the government-funded health care programs is conditioned on the accuracy and truthful- ness of this information, and that I may be personally subject to or may subject my organization to substantial criminal, civil, and/or administrative penalties for submitting false information. I also certify that I am authorized to submit this information by this facility on its behalf.

Signature and Title	Sections	Date
a.		
b.		
c.		
d.		
e.		
f.		
g.		
h.		
i.		
j.		
k.		
l.		

▦ = When box blank, must enter number or letter

a. = When letter in box, check if condition applies

GENERAL INSTRUCTIONS

Complete this information for submission with all full and quarterly assessments (Admission, Annual, Significant Change, State or Medicare required assessments, or Quarterly Reviews, etc.).

FIGURE 10-19: MDS FORM (2 OF 7)

Resident _____ Numeric Identifier _____

MINIMUM DATA SET (MDS)-   *VERSION 2.0*
FOR NURSING HOME RESIDENT ASSESSMENT AND CARE SCREENING
BACKGROUND (FACE SHEET) INFORMATION AT ADMISSION

SECTION AB. DEMOGRAPHIC INFORMATION

1.	DATE OF ENTRY	*Date the stay began. Note - Does not include readmission if record was closed at time of temporary discharge to hospital, etc. In such cases, use prior admission date.* [ ] [ ] — [ ] [ ] — [ ] [ ] [ ] [ ] Month Day Year
2.	ADMITTED FROM (at entry)	1. Private home/apt. with no home health services 2. Private home/apt. with home health services 3. Board and care/assisted living/group home 4. Nursing home 5. Acute care hospital 6. Psychiatric hospital, MR/DD facility 7. Rehabilitation hospital 8. Other
3.	LIVED ALONE (PRIOR TO ENTRY)	0. No 1. Yes 2. In other facility
4.	ZIP CODE OF PRIOR PRIMARY RESIDENCE	[ ] [ ] [ ] [ ] [ ]
5.	RESIDEN-TIAL HISTORY 5 YEARS PRIOR TO ENTRY	*(Check all settings resident lived in during 5 years prior to date of entry given in item AB1 above.)* Prior stay at this nursing home — a. Stay in other nursing home — b. Other residential facility - board and care home, assisted living, group home — c. MH/psychiatric setting — d. MR/DD setting — e. *NONE OF ABOVE* — f.
6.	LIFETIME OCCUPA-TION(S) *(Put "/" between two occupations)*	
7.	EDUCATION *(Highest level completed)*	1. No schooling 5. Technical or trade school 2. 8th grade/less 6. Some college 3. 9-11 grades 7. Bachelor's degree 4. High School 8. Graduate degree
8.	LANGUAGE	*(Code for correct response)* a. Primary language 0. English 1. Spanish 2. French 3. Other b. If other, specify [ ][ ][ ][ ][ ][ ][ ][ ]
9.	MENTAL HEALTH HISTORY	Does resident's RECORD indicate any history of mental retardation, mental illness, or developmental disability problem? 0. No 1. Yes

10.	CONDITIONS RELATED TO MR/DD STATUS	*(Check all conditions that are related to MR/DD status that were manifested before age 22, and are likely to continue indefinitely.)*
		Not applicable- no MR/DD (Skip to AB11) — a.
		MR/DD with organic condition
		    Down's syndrome — b.
		    Autism — c.
		    Epilepsy — d.
		    Other organic condition related to MR/DD — e.
		MR/DD with no organic condition — f.

11.	DATE BACK-GROUND INFORMA-TION COMPLETED	[ ] [ ] — [ ] [ ] — [ ] [ ] [ ] [ ] Month Day Year

[shaded box] =When box blank, must enter number or letter

[a.] =When letter in box, check if condition applies

SECTION AC. CUSTOMARY ROUTINE

1.	CUSTOMARY ROUTINE *(In year prior to DATE OF ENTRY to this nursing home, or year last in community if now being admitted from another nursing home)*	*(Check all that apply. If all information UNKNOWN, check last box only)* **CYCLE OF DAILY EVENTS** Stays up late at night (e.g. after 9 pm) — a. Naps regularly during day (at least 1 hour) — b. Goes out 1+ days a week — c. Stays busy with hobbies, reading, or fixed daily routine — d. Spends most of time alone or watching TV — e. Moves independently indoors (with appliances, if used) — f. Use of tobacco products at least daily — g. *NONE OF ABOVE* — h. **EATING PATTERNS** Distinct food preferences — i. Eats between meals all or most days — j. Use of alcoholic beverage(s) at least weekly — k. *NONE OF ABOVE* — l. **ADL PATTERNS** In bedclothes much of day — m. Wakens to toilet all or most nights — n. Has irregular bowel movement pattern — o. Showers for bathing — p. Bathing in PM — q. *NONE OF ABOVE* — r. **INVOLVEMENT PATTERNS** Daily contact with relatives/close friends — s. Usually attends church, temple, synagogue (etc.) — t. Finds strength in faith — u. Daily animal companion/presence — v. Involved in group activities — w. *NONE OF ABOVE* — x. **UNKNOWN** -Resident/family unable to provide information — y.

[END]

SECTION AD. FACE SHEET SIGNATURES

SIGNATURES OF PERSONS COMPLETING FACE SHEET:

a. Signature of RN Assessment Coordinator	Date

I certify that the accompanying information accurately reflects resident assessment or tracking information for this resident and that I collected or coordinated collection of this information on the dates specified. To the best of my knowledge, this information was collected in accordance with applicable Medicare and Medicaid requirements. I understand that this information is used as a basis for ensuring that residents receive appropriate and quality care, and as a basis for payment from federal funds. I further understand that payment of such federal funds and continued partici-pation in the government-funded health care programs is conditioned on the accuracy and truthful-ness of this information, and that I may be personally subject to or may subject my organization to substantial criminal, civil, and/or administrative penalties for submitting false information. I also certify that I am authorized to submit this information by this facility on its behalf.

Signature and Title	Sections	Date
b.		
c.		
d.		
e.		
f.		
g.		

FIGURE 10-19: MDS FORM (3 OF 7)

Resident _____   Numeric Identifier _____

MINIMUM DATA SET (MDS)- *VERSION 2.0*
FOR NURSING HOME RESIDENT ASSESSMENT AND CARE SCREENING
FULL ASSESSMENT FORM
(Status in last 7 days, unless other time frame indicated)

SECTION A. IDENTIFICATION AND BACKGROUND INFORMATION

1. RESIDENT NAME
a. (First)   b. (Middle Initial)   c. (Last)   d. (Jr./Sr.)

2. ROOM NUMBER

3. ASSESSMENT REFERENCE DATE
a. Last day of MDS observation period
Month — Day — Year
b. Original (0) or corrected copy of form (enter number of correction)

4a. DATE OF REENTRY
Date of reentry from most recent temporary discharge to a hospital in last 90 days (or since last assessment or admission if less than 90 days)
Month — Day — Year

5. MARITAL STATUS
1. Never Married   3. Widowed   5. Divorced
2. Married   4. Separated

6. MEDICAL RECORD NO.

7. CURRENT PAYMENT SOURCES FOR N.H. STAY
(Billing Office to indicate; check all that apply in last 30 days)
Medicaid per diem — a.
Medicare per diem — b.
Medicare ancillary part A — c.
Medicare ancillary part B — d.
CHAMPUS per diem — e.
VA per diem — f.
Self or family pays for full per diem — g.
Medicaid resident liability or Medicare co-payment — h.
Private insurance per diem (including co-payment) — i.
Other per diem — j.

8. REASONS FOR ASSESSMENT
[Note-if this is a discharge or reentry assessment, only a limited subset of MDS items need be completed]
a. Primary reason for assessment
1. Admission assessment (required by day 14)
2. Annual assessment
3. Significant change in status assessment
4. Significant correction of prior full assessment
5. Quarterly review assessment
6. Discharged-return not anticipated
7. Discharged-return anticipated
8. Discharged prior to completing initial assessment
9. Reentry
0. Significant correction of prior quarterly assessment
0. NONE OF ABOVE
b. Codes for assessments required for Medicare PPS or the State
1. Medicare 5 day assessment
2. Medicare 30 day assessment
3. Medicare 60 day assessment
4. Medicare 90 day assessment
5. Medicare readmission/return assessment
6. Other state required assessment
7. Medicare 14 day assessment
8. Other Medicare required assessment

9. RESPONSIBILITY/ LEGAL GUARDIAN
(Check all that apply)
Legal guardian — a.
Other legal oversight — b.
Durable power of attorney/health care — c.
Durable power of attorney/ financial — d.
Family member responsible — e.
Patient responsible for self — f.
NONE OF ABOVE — g.

10. ADVANCED DIRECTIVES
(For those items with supporting documentation in the medical record, check all that apply)
Living will — a.
Do not resuscitate — b.
Do not hospitalize — c.
Organ donation — d.
Autopsy request — e.
Feeding restrictions — f.
Medication restrictions — g.
Other treatment restrictions — h.
NONE OF ABOVE — i.

SECTION B. COGNITIVE PATTERNS

1. COMATOSE
(Persistent vegetative state/no discernible consciousness)
0. No   1. Yes (If yes, skip to section G)

2. MEMORY
(Recall of what was learned or known)
a. Short-term memory OK-seems/appears to recall after 5 minutes
0. Memory OK   1. Memory problem
b. Long term memory OK-seems/appears to recall long past
0. Memory OK   1. Memory problem

▢ = When box blank, must enter number or letter

a. ▢ = When letter in box, check if condition applies

3. MEMORY RECALL ABILITY
(Check all that resident was normally able to recall during last 7 days)
Current season — a.
Location of own room — b.
Staff names/faces — c.
That he/she is in a nursing home — d.
NONE OF ABOVE are recalled — e.

4. COGNITIVE SKILLS FOR DAILY DECISION-MAKING
(Made decisions regarding tasks of daily life)
0. INDEPENDENT-decisions consistent/reasonable
1. MODIFIED INDEPENDENCE-some difficulty in new situations only
2. MODERATELY IMPAIRED-decisions poor; cues/ supervision required
3. SEVERELY IMPAIRED- never/rarely made decisions

5. INDICATORS OF DELIRIUM- PERIODIC DISORDERED THINKING/ AWARENESS
(Code for behavior in the last 7 days.) [Note: Accurate assessment requires conversations with staff and family who have direct knowledge of resident's behavior over this time.)
0. Behavior not present
1. Behavior present, not of recent onset
2. Behavior present, over last 7 days appears different from resident's usual functioning (e.g., new onset or worsening)
a. EASILY DISTRACTED-(e.g., difficulty paying attention; gets sidetracked)
b. PERIODS OF ALTERED PERCEPTION OR AWARENESS OF SURROUNDINGS-(e.g., moves lips or talks to someone not present; believes he/she is somewhere else; confuses night and day)
c. EPISODES OF DISORGANIZED SPEECH-(e.g., speech is incoherent, nonsensical, irrelevant, or rambling from subject to subject; loses train of thought)
d. PERIODS OF RESTLESSNESS-(e.g., fidgeting or picking at skin, clothing, napkins, etc.; frequent position changes; repetitive physical movements or calling out)
e. PERIODS OF LETHARGY-(e.g., sluggishness; staring into space; difficult to arouse; little body movement)
f. MENTAL FUNCTION VARIES OVER THE COURSE OF THE DAY-(e.g., sometimes better, sometimes worse; behaviors sometimes present, sometimes not)

6. CHANGE IN COGNITIVE STATUS
Resident's cognitive status, skills, or abilities have changed as compared to status of 90 days ago (or since assessment if less than 90 days)
0. No change   1. Improved   2. Deteriorated

SECTION C. COMMUNICATION/HEARING PATTERNS

1. HEARING
(With hearing appliance, if used)
0. HEARS ADEQUATELY-normal talk, TV, phone
1. MINIMAL DIFFICULTY when not in quiet setting
2. HEARS IN SPECIAL SITUATIONS ONLY- speaker has to adjust tonal quality and speak distinctly
3. HIGHLY IMPAIRED/absence of useful hearing

2. COMMUNICATION DEVICES/ TECHNIQUES
(Check all that apply during last 7 days)
Hearing aid, present and used — a.
Hearing aid, present and not used regularly — b.
Other receptive comm. techniques used (e.g., lip reading) — c.
NONE OF ABOVE — d.

3. MODES OF EXPRESSION
(Check all used by resident to make needs known)
Speech — a.
Writing messages to express or clarify needs — b.
American sign or Braille — c.
Signs/gestures/sounds — d.
Communication board — e.
Other — f.
NONE OF ABOVE — g.

4. MAKING SELF UNDERSTOOD
(Expressing information content-however able)
0. UNDERSTOOD
1. USUALLY UNDERSTOOD-difficulty finding words finishing thoughts
2. SOMETIMES UNDERSTOOD-ability is limited to making concrete requests
3. RARELY/NEVER UNDERSTOOD

5. SPEECH CLARITY
(Code for speech in the last 7 days)
0. CLEAR SPEECH-distinct, intelligible words
1. UNCLEAR SPEECH-slurred, mumbled words
2. NO SPEECH-absence of spoken words

6. ABILITY TO UNDERSTAND OTHERS
(Understanding verbal information content- however able)
0. UNDERSTANDS
1. USUALLY UNDERSTANDS- may miss some part/ intent of message
2. SOMETIMES UNDERSTANDS-responds adequately to simple, direct communication
3. RARELY/NEVER UNDERSTANDS

7. CHANGE IN COMMUNICATION HEARING
Resident's ability to express, understand, or hear information has changed as compared to status of 90 days ago (or since last assessment if less than 90 days)
0. No change   1. Improved   2. Deteriorated

Resident _____   Numeric Identifier _____

SECTION D. VISION PATTERNS

1.	VISION	(Ability to see in adequate light and with glasses if used)	
		0. *ADEQUATE*- sees fine detail, including regular print in newspapers/books	
		1. *IMPAIRED*- sees large print, but not regular print in news-papers/books	
		2. *MODERATELY IMPAIRED*- limited vision; not able to see newspaper headlines, but can identify objects	
		3. *HIGHLY IMPAIRED*-object identification in question, but eyes appear to follow objects	
		4.*SEVERELY IMPAIRED*-no vision or sees only light, colors, or shapes; eyes do not appear to follow objects	
2.	VISUAL LIMITATIONS/ DIFFICULTIES	Side vision problems-decreased peripheral vision (e.g., leaves food on one side of tray, difficulty traveling, bumps into people and objects, misjudges placement of chair when seating self)	a.
		Experiences any of following: sees halos or rings around lights; sees flashes of light; sees "curtains" over eyes	b.
		NONE OF ABOVE	c.
3.	VISUAL APPLIANCES	Glasses; contact lenses; magnifying glass	
		0. No 1. Yes	

SECTION E. MOOD AND BEHAVIOR PATTERNS

1.	INDICATORS OF DEPRES-SION, ANXIETY, SAD MOOD	(Code for indicators observed in last 30 days, irrespective of the assumed cause)
		0. Indicator not exhibited in last 30 days
		1. Indicator of this type exhibited up to five days a week
		2. Indicator of this type exhibited daily or almost daily (6,7 days a week)

VERBAL EXPRESSIONS OF DISTRESS
a. Resident made negative statements-e.g., *"Nothing matters; Would rather be dead; What's the use; Regrets having lived so long; Let me die"*
b. Repetitive questions-e.g.,*"Where do I go; What do I do?"*
c. Repetitive verbal-izations- e. g., calling out for help ("God help me")
d. Persistent anger with self or others-e.g., easily annoyed, anger at placement in nursing home; anger at care received
e. Self deprecation-e.g., *"I am nothing; I am of no use to anyone"*
f. Expressions of what appear to be unreal-istic fears-e.g., fear of being abandoned, left alone, being with others
g. Recurrent statements that something terrible is about to happen-e.g., believes he or she is about to die, have a heart attack

h. Repetitive health complaints-e.g., persistently seeks medical attention, obsessive concern with body functions
i. Repetitive anxious complaints/concerns (non-health related) e. g., persistently seeks attention/reassurance regarding schedules, meals,laundry/clothing, relationship issues

SLEEP-CYCLE ISSUES
j. Unpleasant mood in morning
k. Insomnia/change in usual sleep pattern

SAD, APATHETIC, ANXIOUS APPEARANCE
l. Sad, pained, worried facial expressions-e.g., furrowed brows
m. Crying, tearfulness
n. Repetitive physical movements-e.g., pacing, hand wringing, restless-ness, fidgeting, picking

LOSS OF INTEREST
o. Withdrawal from activities of interest-e.g., no interest in longstanding activities or being with family/ friends
p. Reduced social inter-action

2.	MOOD PERSIS-TENCE	One or more indicators of depressed, sad or anxious mood were not easily altered by attempts to "cheer up", console, or reassure the resident over last 7 days
		0. No mood 1. Indicators present, 2. Indicators present, indicators easily altered not easily altered
3.	CHANGE IN MOOD	Resident's mood status has changed as compared to status of 90 days ago (or since last assessment if less than 90 days)
		0. No change 1. Improved 2. Deteriorated
4.	BEHAVIORAL SYMPTOMS	(A) *Behavioral symptom frequency in last 7 days*
		0. Behavior not exhibited in last 7 days
		1. Behavior of this type occurred 1 to 3 days in last 7 days
		2. Behavior of this type occurred 4 to 6 days, but less than daily
		3. Behavior of this type occurred daily
		(B) *Behavioral symptom alterability in last 7 days*
		0. Behavior not present OR behavior was easily altered
		1. Behavior was not easily altered (A) (B)

a.WANDERING (moved with no rational purpose, seemingly oblivious to needs or safety)
b.VERBALLY ABUSIVE BEHAVIORAL SYMPTOMS (others were threatened, screamed at, cursed at)
c.PHYSICALLY ABUSIVE BEHAVIORAL SYMPTOMS (others were hit, shoved, scratched, sexually abused)
d.SOCIALLY INAPPROPRIATE/DISRUPTIVE BEHAVIORAL SYMPTOMS (made disruptive sounds, noisiness screaming, self-abusive acts, sexual behavior or disrobing in public, smeared/threw food/feces, hoarding, rummaged through others' belongings)
e.RESISTS CARE (resisted taking medications/injections, ADL assistance, or eating)

5.	CHANGE IN BEHAVIORAL SYMPTOMS	Resident's behavior status has changed as compared to status of 90 days ago (or since last assessment if less than 90 days)
		0. No change 1. Improved 2. Deteriorated

SECTION F. PSYCHOSOCIAL WELL-BEING

1.	SENSE OF INITIATIVE/ INVOLVE-MENT	At ease interacting with others	a.
		At ease doing planned or structured activities	b.
		At ease doing self-initiated activities	c.
		Establishes own goals	d.
		Pursues involvement in life of facility (e.g., makes/keeps friends; involved in group activities; responds positively to new activities; assists at religious services)	e.
		Accepts invitations into most group activities	f.
		NONE OF ABOVE	g.
2.	UNSETTLED RELATION-SHIPS	Covert/open conflict with or repeated criticism of staff	a.
		Unhappy with roommate	b.
		Unhappy with residents other than roommate	c.
		Openly expresses conflict/anger with family/friends	d.
		Absence of personal contact with family/friends	e.
		Recent loss of close family member/friend	f.
		Does not adjust easily to change in routines	g.
		NONE OF ABOVE	h.
3.	PAST ROLES	Strong identification with past roles and life status	a.
		Expresses sadness/anger/empty feeling over lost roles/ status	b.
		Resident perceives that daily routine (customary routine, activities) is very different from prior pattern in the community	c.
		NONE OF ABOVE	d.

SECTION G. PHYSICAL FUNCTIONING AND STRUCTURAL PROBLEMS

1. (A) ADL SELF-PERFORMANCE-(Code for resident's *PERFORMANCE OVER ALL SHIFTS* during last 7 days- Not including setup)
   0. *INDEPENDENT*- No help or oversight-OR-Help/oversight provided only 1 or 2 times during the last 7 days
   1. *SUPERVISION* Oversight, encouragement or cueing provided 3 or more times during last 7 days-OR-Supervision (3 or more times) plus physical assistance provided only 1 or 2 times during last 7 days
   2. *LIMITED ASSISTANCE*- Resident highly involved in activity; received physical help in guided maneuvering of limbs or other nonweight bearing assistance 3 or more times-OR-More help provided only 1 or 2 times during last 7 days
   3. *EXTENSIVE ASSISTANCE*-While resident performed part of activity, over last 7-day period, help of following type(s) provided 3 or more times:
   -Weight-bearing support
   -Full staff performance during part (but not all) of last 7 days
   4. *TOTAL DEPENDENCE*-Full staff performance of activity during entire 7 days
   8. *ACTIVITY DID NOT OCCUR* during entire 7 days

   (B) ADL SUPPORT-(Code for *MOST SUPPORT PROVIDED OVER ALL SHIFTS* during last 7 days; code regardless of resident's self-performance classification)
   0. No setup or physical help from staff   3. Two+ persons physical assist
   1. Setup help only   8. ADL activity itself did not
   2. One person physical assist   occur during entire 7 days

			(A) SELF-PER	(B) SUPPORT
a.	BED MOBILITY	How resident moves to and from lying position, turns side to side, and positions body while in bed		
b.	TRANSFER	How resident moves between surfaces-to/from: bed, chair, wheelchair, standing position (EXCLUDE to/from bath/toilet)		
c.	WALK IN ROOM	How resident walks between locations in his/her room		
d.	WALK IN CORRIDOR	How resident walks in corridor on unit		
e.	LOCOMO-TION ON UNIT	How resident moves between locations in his/her room and adjacent corridor on same floor. If in wheelchair, self-sufficiency once in chair		
f.	LOCOMO-TION OFF UNIT	How resident moves to and from off unit locations (e.g., areas set aside for dining, activities, or treatments). If facility has only one floor,how resident moves to and from distant areas on the floor. If in wheelchair, self-sufficiency once in chair		
g.	DRESSING	How resident puts on, fastens, and takes off all items of street clothing,including donning/removing prosthesis		
h.	EATING	How resident eats and drinks (regardless of skill). Includes intake of nourishment by other means (e.g., tube feeding, total parenteral nutrition)		
i.	TOILET USE	How resident uses the toilet room (or commode, bedpan, urinal); transfers on/off toilet, cleanses, changes pad, manages ostomy or catheter, adjusts clothes		
j.	PERSONAL HYGIENE	How resident maintains personal hygiene, including combing hair, brushing teeth, shaving, applying makeup, washing/ drying face, hands, and perineum (EXCLUDE baths and showers)		

FIGURE 10-19: MDS FORM (5 OF 7)

Resident _____   Numeric Identifier _____

2.	BATHING	How resident takes full-body bath/shower, sponge bath, and transfers in/out of tub/shower (EXCLUDE washing of back and hair). *Code for most dependent in self-performance and support.* (A) BATHING SELF-PERFORMANCE codes appear below. 0. Independent-No help provided 1. Supervision-Oversight help only 2. Physical help limited to transfer only 3. Physical help in part of bathing activity 4. Total dependence 8. Activity itself did not occur during entire 7 days *(Bathing support codes are as defined in Item 1, code B above)* (A) (B)

3.	TEST FOR BALANCE (see training manual)	*(Code for ability during test in the last 7 days)* 0. Maintained position as required in test 1. Unsteady, but able to rebalance self without physical support 2. Partial physical support during test; or stands (sits) but does not follow directions for test 3. Not able to attempt test without physical help
		a. Balance while standing
		b. Balance while sitting-position, trunk control

4.	FUNCTIONAL LIMITATION IN RANGE OF MOTION (see training manual)	*(Code for limitations during last 7 days that interfered with daily functions or placed resident at risk of injury)* (A) RANGE OF MOTION (B) VOLUNTARY MOVEMENT 0. No limitation 0. No loss 1. Limitation on one side 1. Partial loss 2. Limitation on both sides 2. Full loss (A) (B)
		a. Neck
		b. Arm-Including shoulder or elbow
		c. Hand-Including wrist or fingers
		d. Leg-Including hip or knee
		e. Foot-Including ankle or toes
		f. Other limitation or loss

5.	MODES OF LOCOMOTION	*(Check all that apply during last 7 days)*
		Cane/walker/crutch — a.
		Wheeled self — b.	Wheelchair primary mode of locomotion — d.
		Other person wheeled — c.	NONE OF ABOVE — e.

6.	MODES OF TRANSFER	*(Check all that apply during last 7 days)*
		Bedfast all or most of time — a.	Lifted mechanically — d.
		Bed rails used for bed mobility or transfer — b.	Transfer aid (e.g., slide board, trapeze, cane, walker, brace) — e.
		Lifted manually — c.	NONE OF ABOVE — f.

7.	TASK SEGMENTATION	Some or all of ADL activities were broken into subtasks during **last 7 days** so that resident could perform them 0. No 1. Yes

8.	ADL FUNCTIONAL REHABILITATION POTENTIAL	Resident believes he/she is capable of increased independence in at least some ADLs — a.
		Direct care staff believe resident is capable of increased independence in at least some ADLs — b.
		Resident able to perform tasks/activity but is very slow — c.
		Difference in ADL Self-Performance or ADL Support, comparing mornings to evenings — d.
		NONE OF ABOVE — e.

9.	CHANGE IN ADL FUNCTION	Resident's ADL self-performance status has changed as compared to status of **90 days ago** (or since last assessment if less than 90 days) 0. No change 1. Improved 2. Deteriorated

SECTION H. CONTINENCE IN LAST 14 DAYS

1.	CONTINENCE SELF-CONTROL CATEGORIES *(Code for the resident's PERFORMANCE OVER ALL SHIFTS)* 0. *CONTINENT*- Complete control *(includes use of indwelling urinary catheter or ostomy device that does not leak urine or stool)* 1. *USUALLY CONTINENT*- BLADDER, incontinent episodes once a week or less; BOWEL, less than weekly 2. *OCCASIONALLY INCONTINENT*- BLADDER, 2 or more times a week but not daily; BOWEL, once a week 3. *FREQUENTLY INCONTINENT*-BLADDER, tended to be incontinent daily, but some control present (e.g., on day shift), BOWEL, 2-3 times a week 4. *INCONTINENT*- Had inadequate control. BLADDER, multiple daily episodes; BOWEL, all (or almost all) of the time
a.	BOWEL CONTINENCE	Control of bowel movement, with appliance or bowel continence programs, if employed
b.	BLADDER CONTINENCE	Control of urinary bladder function (if dribbles, volume insufficient to soak through underpants), with appliances (e.g, foley) or continence programs, if employed

2.	BOWEL ELIMINATION PATTERN	Bowel elimination pattern regular-at least one movement every three days — a.	Diarrhea — c.
		Constipation — b.	Fecal impaction — d.
			NONE OF ABOVE — e.

3.	APPLIANCES AND PROGRAMS	Any scheduled toileting plan — a.	Did not use toilet room/ commode/urinal — f.
		Bladder retraining program — b.	Pads/briefs used — g.
		External (condom) catheter — c.	Enemas/irrigation — h.
		Indwelling catheter — d.	Ostomy present — i.
		Intermittent catheter — e.	NONE OF ABOVE — j.

4.	CHANGE IN URINARY CONTINENCE	Resident's urinary continence has changed as compared to status of **90 days ago** (or since last assessment if less than 90 days) 0. No change 1. Improved 2. Deteriorated

SECTION I. DISEASE DIAGNOSES

Check only those diseases that have a relationship current ADL status, cognitive status, mood and behavior status, medical treatments, nursing monitoring, or risk of death. (Do not list inactive diagnoses)

1.	DISEASES	*(If none apply, Check the NONE OF ABOVE box)*
		ENDOCRINE/METABOLIC/ NUTRITIONAL	Hemiplegia/Hemiparesis — v.
		Diabetes mellitus — a.	Multiple sclerosis — w.
		Hyperthyroidism — b.	Paraplegia — x.
		Hypothyroidism — c.	Parkinson's disease — y.
		HEART/CIRCULATION	Quadriplegia — z.
		Arteriosclerotic heart disease (ASHD) — d.	Seizure disorder — aa.
		Cardiac dysrhythmias — e.	Transient ischemic attack (TIA) — bb.
		Congestive heart failure — f.	Traumatic brain injury — cc.
		Deep vein thrombosis — g.	**PSYCHIATRIC/MOOD**
		Hypertension — h.	Anxiety disorder — dd.
		Hypotension — i.	Depression — ee.
		Peripheral vascular disease — j.	Manic depression (bipolar disease) — ff.
		Other cardiovascular disease — k.	Schizophrenia — gg.
		MUSCULOSKELETAL	**PULMONARY**
		Arthritis — l.	Asthma — hh.
		Hip fracture — m.	Emphysema/COPD — ii.
		Missing limb (e.g., amputation) — n.	**SENSORY**
		Osteoporosis — o.	Cataracts — jj.
		Pathological bone fracture — p.	Diabetic retinopathy — kk.
		NEUROLOGICAL	Glaucoma — ll.
		Alzheimer's disease — q.	Macular degeneration — mm.
		Aphasia — r.	**OTHER**
		Cerebral palsy — s.	Allergies — nn.
		Cerebrovascular accident (stroke) — t.	Anemia — oo.
		Dementia other than Alzheimer's disease — u.	Cancer — pp.
			Renal failure — qq.
			NONE OF ABOVE — rr.

2.	INFECTIONS	*(If none apply, CHECK the NONE OF ABOVE box)*
		Antibiotic resistant infection (e.g., Methicillin resistant staph) — a.	Septicemia — g.
			Sexually transmitted diseases — h.
		Clostridium difficile (c. diff) — b.	Tuberculosis — i.
		Conjunctivitis — c.	Urinary tract infection In **last 30 days** — j.
		HIV infection — d.	Viral hepatitis — k.
		Pneumonia — e.	Wound infection — l.
		Respiratory infection — f.	NONE OF ABOVE — m.

3.	OTHER CURRENT OR MORE DETAILED DIAGNOSES AND ICD-9 CODES	a. _____ •
		b. _____ •
		c. _____ •
		d. _____ •
		e. _____ •

SECTION J. HEALTH CONDITIONS

1.	PROBLEM CONDITIONS	*(Check all problems present in last 7 days unless other time frame is indicated)*
		INDICATORS OF FLUID STATUS	Dizziness/vertigo — f.
		Weight gain or loss of 3 or more pounds within a 7 day period — a.	Edema — g.
			Fever — h.
		Inability to lie flat due to shortness of breath — b.	Hallucinations — i.
			Internal bleeding — j.
		Dehydrated; output exceeds input — c.	Recurrent lung aspirations in **last 90 days** — k.
		Insufficient fluid; did NOT consume all/almost all liquids provided during **last 3 days** — d.	Shortness of breath — l.
			Syncope (fainting) — m.
		OTHER	Unsteady gait — n.
		Delusions — e.	Vomiting — o.
			NONE OF ABOVE — p.

FIGURE 10-19: MDS FORM (6 OF 7)

Resident_____   Numeric Identifier _____

2.	PAIN SYMPTOMS	*(Code the highest level of pain present in the last 7 days)*

a. FREQUENCY with which resident complains or shows evidence of pain
0. No Pain *(skip to J4)*
1. Pain less than daily
2. Pain daily

b. INTENSITY of pain
1. Mild pain
2. Moderate pain
3. Times when pain is horrible or excruciating

3.	PAIN SITE	*(If pain present, check all sites that apply in last 7 days)*	
		Back pain	a.
		Bone pain	b.
		Chest pain while doing usual activities	c.
		Headache	d.
		Hip pain	e.
		Incisional pain	f.
		Joint pain (other than hip)	g.
		Soft tissue pain (e.g., lesion, muscle)	h.
		Stomach pain	i.
		Other	j.

4.	ACCIDENTS	*(Check all that apply)*			
		Fell in **past 30 days**	a.	Hip fracture in **last 180 days**	c
		Fell in **last 31-180 days**	b.	Other fracture in **last 180 days**	d.
				NONE OF ABOVE	e.

5.	STABILITY OF CONDITIONS	Conditions/diseases make resident's cognitive, ADL, mood or behavior patterns unstable-(fluctuating, precarious, or deteriorating)	a.
		Resident experiencing an acute episode or a flare-up of a recurrent or chronic problem	b.
		End-stage disease, 6 or fewer months to live	c.
		NONE OF ABOVE	d.

SECTION K. ORAL/NUTRITIONAL STATUS

1.	ORAL PROBLEMS	Chewing problem	a.
		Swallowing problem	b.
		Mouth pain	c.
		NONE OF ABOVE	d.

2.	HEIGHT AND WEIGHT	*Record (a.) height in inches and (b.) weight in pounds. Base weight on most recent measure in last 30 days; measure weight consistently in accord with standard facility practice-e.g., in a.m. after voiding, before meal, with shoes off, and in nightclothes.*

a. HT (in.)   **b. WT (lb.)**

3.	WEIGHT CHANGE	**a. Weight loss**-5% or more in **last 30 days**; or 10% or more in **last 180 days** 0. No 1. Yes	
		b. Weight gain-5% or more in **last 30 days**; or 10% or more in **last 180 days** 0. No 1. Yes	

4.	NUTRITIONAL PROBLEMS	Complains about the taste of many foods	a.	Leaves 25% or more of food uneaten at most meals	c.
		Regular or repetitive complaints of hunger	b.	NONE OF ABOVE	d.

5.	NUTRITIONAL APPROACHES	*(Check all that apply in last 7 days)*				
		Parenteral/IV	a.	Dietary supplement between meals	f.
		Feeding tube	b.	Plate guard, stabilized built-up utensil, etc.	g.
		Mechanically altered diet	c.	On a planned weight change program	h.
		Syringe (oral feeding)	d.	NONE OF ABOVE	i.
		Therapeutic diet	e.		

6.	PARENTERAL OR ENTERAL INTAKE	*(Skip to Section L if neither 5a nor 5b is checked)*

a. Code the proportion of **total calories** the resident received through parenteral or tube feedings in the **last 7 days**
0. None
1. 1% to 25%
2. 26% to 50%
3. 51% to 75%
4. 76% to 100%

b. Code the average fluid intake per day by IV or tube in **last 7 days**
0. None
1. 1 to 500 cc/day
2. 501 to 1000 cc/day
3. 1001 to 1500 cc/day
4. 1501 to 2000 cc/day
5. 2001 or more cc/day

SECTION L. ORAL/DENTAL STATUS

1.	ORAL STATUS AND DISEASE PREVENTION	Debris (soft, easily movable substances) present in mouth prior to going to bed at night	a.
		Has dentures or removable bridge	b.
		Some/all natural teeth lost-does not have or does not use dentures (or partial plates)	c.
		Broken, loose, or carious teeth	d.
		Inflamed gums (gingiva); swollen or bleeding gums; oral abscesses; ulcers or rashes	e.
		Daily cleaning of teeth/dentures or daily mouth care-by resident or staff	f.
		NONE OF ABOVE	g.

SECTION M. SKIN CONDITION

1.	ULCERS (Due to any cause)	*(Record the number of ulcers at each ulcer stage- regardless of cause. If none present at a stage, record "0" (zero). Code all that apply during last 7 days. Code 9=9 or more.)* *[Requires full body exam.]*	No. at Stage
		a. Stage 1. A persistent area of skin redness (without a break in the skin) that does not disappear when pressure is relieved	
		b. Stage 2. A partial thickness loss of skin layers that presents clinically as an abrasion, blister, or shallow crater.	
		c. Stage 3. A full thickness of skin is lost, exposing the sub-cutaneous tissues-presents as a deep crater with or without undermining adjacent tissue.	
		d. Stage 4. A full thickness of skin and subcutaneous tissue is lost, exposing muscle or bone.	

2.	TYPE OF ULCER	*(For each type of ulcer, code for the highest stage in the last 7 days using scale in item M1-i.e., 0=none; stages 1,2,3,4)*
		a. Pressure ulcer-any lesion caused by pressure resulting in damage of underlying tissue	
		b. Stasis ulcer-open lesion caused by poor circulation in the lower extremities	

3.	HISTORY OF RESOLVED ULCERS	Resident had an ulcer that was resolved or cured in **LAST 90 DAYS** 0. No 1. Yes	

4.	OTHER SKIN PROBLEMS OR LESIONS PRESENT	*(Check all that apply during last 7 days)*	
		Abrasions, bruises	a.
		Burns (second or third degree)	b.
		Open lesions other than ulcers, rashes, cuts (e.g., cancer lesions)	c.
		Rashes-e.g., intertrigo, eczema, drug rash, heat rash, herpes zoster	d.
		Skin desensitized to pain or pressure	e.
		Skin tears or cuts (other than surgery)	f.
		Surgical wounds	g.
		NONE OF ABOVE	h.

5.	SKIN TREATMENTS	*(Check all that apply during last 7 days)*	
		Pressure relieving device(s) for chair	a.
		Pressure relieving device(s) for bed	b.
		Turning/repositioning program	c.
		Nutrition or hydration intervention to manage skin problems	d.
		Ulcer care	e.
		Surgical wound care	f.
		Application of dressings (with or without topical medications) other than to feet	g.
		Application of ointments/medications (other than to feet)	h.
		Other preventative or protective skin care (other than to feet)	i.
		NONE OF ABOVE	j.

6.	FOOT PROBLEMS AND CARE	*(Check all that apply during last 7 days)*	
		Resident has one or more foot problems-e.g., corns, calluses, bunions, hammer toes, overlapping toes, pain, structural problems	a.
		Infection of the foot-e.g., cellulitis, purulent drainage	b.
		Open lesions on the foot	c.
		Nails/calluses trimmed during **last 90 days**	d.
		Received preventative or protective foot care (e.g., used special shoes, inserts, pads, toe separators)	e.
		Application of dressings (with or without topical medications)	f.
		NONE OF ABOVE	g.

SECTION N. ACTIVITY PURSUIT PATTERNS

1.	TIME AWAKE	*(Check appropriate time periods over last 7 days)* Resident awake all or most of time (i.e., naps no more than one hour per time period) in the:	
		Morning	a.
		Afternoon	b.
		Evening	c.
		NONE OF ABOVE	d.

(IF RESIDENT IS COMATOSE, SKIP TO SECTION O)

2.	AVERAGE TIME INVOLVED IN ACTIVITIES	*(When awake and not receiving treatments or ADL care)*

0. Most-more than 2/3 of time
1. Some-from 1/3 to 2/3 of time
2. Little-less than 1/3 of time
3. None

3.	PREFERRED ACTIVITIES SETTINGS	*(Check all settings in which activities are preferred)*	
		Own room	a.
		Day/activity room	b.
		Inside NH/off unit	c.
		Outside facility	d.
		NONE OF ABOVE	e.

4.	GENERAL ACTIVITY PREFERENCES (Adapted to resident's current abilities)	*(Check all PREFERENCES whether or not activity is currently available to resident)*			
		Cards/other games	a.	Trips/shopping	g.
		Crafts/arts	b.	Walking/wheeling outdoors	h.
		Exercise/sports	c.	Watching TV	i.
		Music	d.	Gardening or plants	j.
		Reading/writing	e.	Talking or conversing	k.
		Spiritual/religious activities	f.	Helping others	l.
				NONE OF ABOVE	m.

FIGURE 10-19: MDS FORM (7 OF 7)

Resident _____

Numeric Identifier _____

5.	PREFERS CHANGE IN DAILY ROUTINE	Code for resident preferences in daily routines
		0. No change 1. Slight change 2. Major change
		a. Type of activities in which resident is currently involved
		b. Extent of resident involvement in activities

SECTION O. MEDICATIONS

1.	NUMBER OF MEDICATIONS	(Record the number of different medications used in the last 7 days; enter "0" if none used)
2.	NEW MEDICA-TIONS	(Resident currently receiving medications that were initiated during the last 90 days)
		0. No 1. Yes
3.	INJECTIONS	(Record the number of DAYS injections of any type received during the last 7 days; enter "0" if none used)
4.	DAYS RECEIVED THE FOLLOWING MEDICATION	(Record the number of DAYS during last 7 days; enter "0" if not used. Note-enter "1" for long-acting meds used less than weekly)
		a. Antipsychotic d. Hypnotic
		b. Antianxiety e. Diuretic
		c. Antidepressant

SECTION P. SPECIAL TREATMENTS AND PROCEDURES

| 1. | SPECIAL TREAT-MENTS, PROCE-DURES, AND PROGRAMS | a. SPECIAL CARE-Check treatments or programs received during the last 14 days |

TREATMENTS		PROGRAMS	
		Ventilator or respirator	l.
Chemotherapy	a.	Alcohol/drug treat-ment program	m.
Dialysis	b.		
IV medication	c.	Alzheimer's/dementia special care unit	n.
Intake/output	d.	Hospice care	o.
Monitoring acute medical condition	e.	Pediatric unit	p.
Ostomy care	f.	Respite care	q.
Oxygen therapy	g.	Training in skills required to return to the community (e.g., taking medications, house work, shopping, transportation, ADLs)	r.
Radiation	h.		
Suctioning	i.		
Tracheostomy care	j.		
Transfusions	k.	NONE OF ABOVE	s.

b. THERAPIES-Record the number of days and total minutes each of the following therapies was administered (for at least 15 minutes a day) in the last 7 calendar days (Enter 0 if none or less than 15 minutes daily) [Note-count only post admission therapies]

(A) = # of days administered for 15 minutes or more
(B) = total # of minutes provided in last 7 days

	DAYS (A)	MIN (B)
a. Speech-language pathology and audiology services		
b. Occupational therapy		
c. Physical therapy		
d. Respiratory therapy		
e. Psychological therapy (by any licensed mental health professional)		

2.	INTERVEN-TION PROGRAMS FOR MOOD, BEHAVIOR, COGNITIVE LOSS	(Check all interventions or strategies used in last 7 days-no matter where received)	
		Special behavior symptom evaluation program	a.
		Evaluation by licensed mental health specialist in last 90 days	b.
		Group therapy	c.
		Resident-specific deliberate changes in the environment to address mood/behavior patterns-e.g., providing bureau in which to rummage	d.
		Reorientation-e.g., cueing	e.
		NONE OF ABOVE	f.

| 3. | NURSING REHABILI-TATION/ RESTOR-ATIVE CARE | Record the NUMBER OF DAYS each of the following rehabilitation or restorative techniques or practices was provided to the resident for more than or equal to 15 minutes per day in the last 7 days (Enter 0 if none or less than 15 min. daily.) |

a. Range of motion (passive)		f. Walking	
b. Range of motion (active)		g. Dressing or grooming	
c. Splint or brace assistance		h. Eating or swallowing	
TRAINING AND SKILL PRACTICE IN:		i. Amputation/prosthesis care	
d. Bed mobility		j. Communication	
e. Transfer		k. Other	

4.	DEVICES AND RESTRAINTS	(Use the following codes for last 7 days:)
		0. Not used
		1. Used less than daily
		2. Used daily
		Bed rails
		a. -Full bed rails on all open sides of bed
		b. -Other types of side rails used (e.g., half rail, one side)
		c. Trunk restraint
		d. Limb restraint
		e. Chair prevents rising
5.	HOSPITAL STAY(S)	Record number of times resident was admitted to hospital with an overnight stay in last 90 days (or since last assessment if less than 90 days). (Enter 0 if no hospital admissions)
6.	EMERGENCY ROOM(ER) VISIT(S)	Record number of times resident visited ER without an overnight stay in last 90 days (or since last assessment if less than 90 days). (Enter 0 if no ER visits)
7.	PHYSICIAN VISITS	In the LAST 14 DAYS (or since admission if less than 14 days in facility) how many days has the physician (or authorized assistant or practitioner) examined the resident? (Enter 0 if none)
8.	PHYSICIAN ORDERS	In the LAST 14 DAYS (or since admission if less than 14 days in facility) how many days has the physician (or authorized assistant or practitioner) changed the resident's orders? Do not include order renewals without change. (Enter 0 if none)
9.	ABNORMAL LAB VALUES	Has the resident had any abnormal lab values during the last 90 days (or since admission)?
		0. No 1. Yes

SECTION Q. DISCHARGE POTENTIAL AND OVERALL STATUS

1.	DISCHARGE POTENTIAL	a. Resident expresses/indicates preference to return to the community
		0. No 1. Yes
		b. Resident has a support person who is positive toward discharge
		0. No 1. Yes
		c. Stay projected to be of a short duration- discharge projected within 90 days (do not include expected discharge due to death)
		0. No 2. Within 31-90 days
		1. Within 30 days 3. Discharge status uncertain
2.	OVERALL CHANGE IN CARE NEEDS	Resident's overall self sufficiency has changed significantly as compared to status of 90 days ago (or since last assessment if less than 90 days)
		0. No change
		1. Improved-receives fewer supports, needs less restrictive level of care
		2. Deteriorated-receives more support

SECTION R. ASSESSMENT INFORMATION

1.	PARTICI-PATION IN ASSESSMENT	a. Resident: 0. No 1. Yes	
		b. Family: 0. No 1. Yes 2. No family
		c. Significant other: 0. No 1. Yes 2. None

2. SIGNATURE OF PERSON COORDINATING THE ASSESSMENT:

a. Signature of RN Assessment Coordinator (sign on above line)

b. Date RN Assessment Coordinator signed as complete

	Month		Day		Year

Along with specified dates to complete the initial assessment, nurses must systematically monitor a resident's status at specified intervals. Quarterly reviews help nurses detect changes in a resident's status. CMS designates these as minimum quarterly assessments. Therefore, the plan of care must be reviewed at least once every 90 days and revised as necessary. The plan of care does not have to be rewritten; however, the nurse should indicate if a problem has been resolved, is continuing, or requires different care and the revisions that are to be made. Quarterly reviews and summaries of the resident's status and plan of care must be date-specific to the completion date of the MDS. Careful documentation of the steps, and especially of an interdisciplinary conference, is very important. An annual MDS should be completed every 365 days. Table 10-13 lists a summary of the interdisciplinary assessment and plan of care process.

If a significant change occurs in a resident's status within 1 month, it is necessary to complete a new MDS. The schedule for reassessment is changed to correspond to the second MDS. The annual MDS assessment is also based on the second MDS.

Long-term care liability issues have greatly increased over the past 15 years. Settlements are likely to be less than they are for other lawsuits; however, the rapid increase in the number of LTC-related cases is overwhelming. Nursing home plaintiffs are being awarded money at a rate four times that of other personal injury suits. Numerous factors have contributed to this increase in nursing home litigation. Some of these factors are listed in Table 10-14 on page 214.

When an incident occurs, it is important that a facility investigate and determine which steps are working and which steps are not. A resident's plan of care may require revisions or addition of new interventions. Effective quality assurance programs and continual auditing are vital. As always, providing a documentation trail creates the evidence necessary to defend a case (see Figure 10-20 on pages 215-223 for other LTC forms).

The increasing frequency with which nurses are being named in lawsuits places emphasis on the delivery of quality care and documentation of that care. Medical records are closely reviewed when an incident occurs. Documentation should establish a defense that care was provided according to standards of care. Once again, concise, complete, timely, and frequent documentation of all facts can help nurses defend the care provided.

CONCLUSION

A patient's medical record is composed of a variety of forms, and specific settings may add

TABLE 10-13: INTERDISCIPLINARY ASSESSMENT AND PLAN OF CARE PROCESS

- At admission, assessments and plan of care completed
  - Nursing assessment completed in 24 to 48 hours
  - Other disciplines' assessments completed within 7 days
- MDS completed no later than 14 days after admission
- Interdisciplinary resident plan of care completed within 7 days of completion of MDS
- Interdisciplinary conference scheduled between days 14 and 21
- Amendments to MDS made within 21 days after admission if:
  - additional information becomes available
  - additional observations provide a different picture of the resident
  - factual data need correction
- Ongoing progress notes

(Burnett, Cavanagh, & Shearer, 2002; Cavallaro et al., 1999)

TABLE 10-14: FACTORS CONTRIBUTING TO LTC LAWSUITS

- Standards of care have been more precisely defined.

- MDS and RAPs provide a uniform method to establish priority needs.

- Health care has shifted from hospitals to LTC settings.

- Tort reform has caused attorneys to investigate LTC facilities.

- Baby boomers are more likely to file suits if a parent or relative is harmed in an LTC facility.

- Legal issues in LTC facilities have become more publicized by the media.

- Recruiting and hiring high-quality staff is a challenge.

- All assessments, plans of care, interventions, and evaluations not documented pose a problem.

- Staff reactions to an incident can mean the difference between litigation and no litigation.

(Cavallaro et al., 1999; Williams, 2002)

additional forms to facilitate documentation of care. Regardless of the method or forms used, the medical record is a formal, legal document that paints a picture of a patient's assessment, plan of care, interventions, evaluations, and progress. This chapter addressed many specific settings that are commonly seen in health care institutions and presented and discussed some of the specific forms required in each of those areas. Regardless of the forms used, careful, complete, and timely documentation can help defend a nurse's actions during litigation.

FIGURE 10-20: OTHER LTC FORMS (1 OF 7): PATIENT TRANSFER FORM (A)

PATIENT TRANSFER FORM
(INTER-AGENCY REFERRAL)

| 1. PATIENT'S LAST NAME | FIRST NAME | MI | 2. SEX ☐ M ☐ F | 3. SOCIAL SECURITY NUMBER |

| 4. PATIENT'S ADDRESS (Street, City, State, Zip Code) | 5. DATE OF BIRTH | 6. RELIGION |

| 7. DATE OF THIS TRANSFER | 8. FACILITY NAME AND ADDRESS TRANSFERRING TO | 9. PHYSICIAN IN CHARGE AT TIME OF TRANSFER |

Will this physician care for patient after admission to new facility? ☐ YES ☐ NO

10. DATES OF STAY AT FACILITY TRANSFERRING FROM

ADMISSION   DISCHARGE

11. PAYMENT SOURCE FOR CHARGES TO PATIENT

A. ☐ SELF OR FAMILY
B. ☐ PRIVATE INSURANCE
C. ☐ BLUE CROSS BLUE SHIELD
D. ☐ EMPLOYER OR UNION
E. ☐ PUBLIC AGENCY (Give name)
F. ☐ OTHER (Explain)

12-A. NAME AND ADDRESS OF FACILITY TRANSFERRING FROM

12-B. NAME AND ADDRESSES OF ALL HOSPITALS AND EXTENDED CARE FACILITIES FROM WHICH PATIENT WAS DISCHARGED IN PAST 60 DAYS.

| 13. CLINIC APPOINTMENT | DATE | TIME | ☐ CLINIC APPOINTMENT CARD ATTACHED | 14. DATE OF LAST PHYSICAL EXAMINATION |

15. RELATIVE OR GUARDIAN: Name   Address   Phone Number

16. DIAGNOSES AT TIME OF TRANSFER   EMPLOYMENT RELATED: ☐ YES ☐ NO

(a) Primary

(b) Secondary

VITALS AT TIME OF TRANSFER

T_____ P_____ R_____ B/P_____

CHECK ALL THAT APPLY

Disabilities
☐ Amputation
☐ Paralysis
☐ Contracture
☐ Pressure Ulcer

Incontinence
☐ Bladder
☐ Bowel
☐ Saliva

Activity Tolerance Limitations
☐ None ☐ Moderate ☐ Severe

Impairments
☐ Mental
☐ Speech
☐ Hearing
☐ Vision
☐ Sensation

Patient knows diagnosis?
☐ Yes ☐ No

Potential for Rehabilitation
☐ Good ☐ Fair ☐ Poor

IMPORTANT MEDICAL INFORMATION
(State allergies if any)

ADVANCE DIRECTIVES
☐ Yes ☐ No ☐ Copy Attached
CODE STATUS

DIET, DRUGS, AND OTHER THERAPY
at Time of Discharge

(Physician, please sign below)

Date of Last B.M. _____
TB Test   Date_____ Type_____ Result_____
Chest X-Ray   Date_____ Result_____
C.B.C.   Date_____ Result_____
Serology   Date_____ Result_____
Urinalysis   Date_____ Result_____

SUGGESTIONS FOR ACTIVE CARE

BED
Position in good body alignment and change position every_____ hrs.
Avoid_____ position
Prone position_____ times/day as tolerated.

SITTING
_____hrs. _____times/day.

WEIGHT BEARING
☐ Full ☐ Partial ☐ None
on_____ Leg

EXERCISES
Range of motion_____ times/day.
to_____ by
☐ patient ☐ nurse ☐ family
Stand_____ Min._____ times/day.

LOCOMOTION
Walk_____ times/day.

SOCIAL ACTIVITIES
Encourage (☐ Group ☐ Individual) activities
(☐ within ☐ outside) home.

Transportation: ☐ Ambulance ☐ Car
☐ Car for handicapped ☐ Bus

Signature of Physician or Nurse_____   Date_____ / _____

PATIENT TRANSFER FORM

FIGURE 10-20: OTHER LTC FORMS (2 OF 7): PATIENT TRANSFER FORM (B)

PATIENT INFORMATION

SELF CARE STATUS

(Check level of ability. Write S in space if needs supervision only. Draw line across if inapplicable.)

		Independent	Needs Assistance	Unable To Do
Bed Activity	Turns			
	Sits			
Personal Hygiene	Face, Hair, Arms			
	Trunk & Perineum			
	Lower Extremities			
	Bladder Program			
	Bowel Program			
Dressing	Upper Extremities			
	Trunk			
	Lower Extremities			
	Appliance, Splint			
Feeding				
Transfer	Sitting			
	Standing			
	Tub			
	Toilet			
Loco-motion	Wheelchair			
	Walking			
	Stairs			

BED ☐ Low   **Mattress:** ☐ Firm ☐ Reg.

Other _____

Side Rails: ☐ Yes ☐ No

BEHAVIOR ☐ Cooperative ☐ Oriented X _____

☐ Disruptive ☐ Belligerent ☐ Combative

☐ Senile ☐ Suspicious ☐ Withdrawn

MENTAL STATUS

☐ Alert ☐ Forgetful ☐ Confused

COMMUNICATION ABILITY	Yes	No
Able to make needs known		
Can speak		
Can hear		
Can write		
Understands speaking		
Understands writing		
Understands gestures		
Understands English		

If no, state language spoken or understood: _____
_____

DIET

☐ Regular ☐ Low Salt ☐ Diabetic ☐ Bland

☐ Low Residue ☐ Other _____

☐ Feeds Self ☐ Needs Help

☐ Partial Assist ☐ Total Assist

RESIDENT USES

☐ Appliance

☐ Catheter (date of last change ___ / ___ / ___

☐ Colostomy ☐ Cane ☐ Crutches ☐ Prosthesis

☐ Walker ☐ Chair ☐ Hearing Aid

☐ Dentures (Specify _____)

OTHER EQUIPMENT

ADDITIONAL PERTINENT INFORMATION

(Explain necessary details of care, diagnosis, medications, treatments, prognosis, teaching, habits, preferences, etc. Therapists and social workers add signature and title to notes.)

SOCIAL INFORMATION

(Adjustment to disability, emotional support from family, motivation for self-care, socializing ability, financial plan, family health problem, etc.)

FIGURE 10-20: OTHER LTC FORMS (3 OF 7): NURSING ADMISSION ASSESSMENT (A)

NURSING ADMISSION ASSESSMENT

Name:_____Admitting Physician_____

Admit time:_____a.m./p.m. Room_____From_____

Accompanied by:_____

Diagnosis:_____Allergies_____

History of TB? Y/N   Last TB Test_____ Last tetanus vaccination_____Last flu vaccination_____

Last Pneumonia vaccination_____

Medical History (Circle if present) CHF   COPD   Heart Disease   HTN

      Irregular Heartbeat Parkinson's Diabetes Arthritis CVA date_____

      Other_____

  I.   **COGNITIVE STATUS:**   Alert Y/N   Oriented X____Behavior Appropriate to situation Y/N
Comotose? Y/N

      A.   **Memory:**
Short term memory: Identified current season: Y/N   Name: Y/N Place: Y/N
Long term memory: DOB:_____ Place of Birth____Spouse:_____The name of any
past U.S. President: Y/N

      B.   Mood: Calm? Y/N   Sad? Y/N   Anxious? Y/N

      C.   Psychotropics: Y/N (if yes, initiate behavior record) Medication(s_____

           length of use:_____Diagnosis:_____

           Comments:_____

  II.   **COMMUNICATION:**

      A.   **Understands:** (circle answer) Always   Usually   Some   Rarely

      B.   **Able to be understood:**   Always   Usually   Some   Rarely

      C.   **Hearing:** Adequate   Minimal difficulty   Special situationsHighly impaired

      D.   **Wears hearing aide:** Y/N   Is hearing aide present? Y/N   R L

      E.   **Vision:** Able to read regular newspaper   Reads large print only   Only able to identify
objects   Legally Blind   Wears glasses
Comments:_____

  III.   **PHYSICAL FUNCTIONING:** (I=independent; LA=limited assistance:
EX=extensive assistance; D=dependent)

Bed mobility: I LA EX D   Locomotion: I LA EX D   Dressing: I LA EX D
Grooming: I LA EX D   Transfers: I LA EX D   Toileting: I LA EX D
Eating: I LA EX D   Bathing: I LA EX D

DEVICES USED (Circle)   Walker   Wheelchair   Cane   Prosthesis

      A.   **Weight bearing restrictions?** Y/N Activity limitations? Y/NParalysis? Y/N
Describe_____

      B.   **Need for Physical Therapy?** Y/N   Occupational Therapy? Y/N   Speech Therapy? Y/N
Orders present?

      C.   **Describe prior level of functioning** (Pre admission to hospital)_____

FIGURE 10-20: OTHER LTC FORMS (4 OF 7): NURSING ADMISSION ASSESSMENT (B)

ADMISSION ASSESMENT Pg 2

IV. ELIMINATION:
Is the resident continent of bowel and bladder without assistive devices? Y/N (If yes, skip to IV,C)

   A.   Bladder: indwelling catheter: Y/N Other_____
           Incontinence pattern: Never   Stress   Occasional   Frequently   Always
   B.   Bowel: Incontinence pattern: Never   Stress Occasioal Frequently   Always
           Length of time incontinence present?_____ Colostomy?Y/N
   C.   Last BM_____History of laxative use? Y/N Enema use? Y/N
   D.   History of UTI? Y/N

V. SAFETY:
   A.   Understands how to use call light?   Y/N
   B.   Fall History_____
   C.   Restraints: Y/N Type_____When used?_____(If yes, Consent form must be signed
           by resident/family and order must be noted from Physician)
   D.   Side rails: Resident preference? Up Down   Unable to determine

V. NUTRITION/HYDRATION:

   A.   Diet order_____ Supplement Order_____
           Height_____Current weight_____Usual weight_____
           History of recent wt loss? Y/N
   B.   Swallowing Problems? Y/N Mouth Pain Y/N   Dentures Y/N Chewing Problems Y/N
           Feeding tube Y/N   Type_____Date tube placed_____Diagnosis for
           tube_____Formula orders_____Flush orders_____---_____

VI. PHYSICAL ASSESSMENT:

   A.   Temp_____P(radial)_____(apical)_____Resp_____ B/P_____
   B.   Eyes:_____ Ears:_____Mucous Membranes _____
   C.   Respiratory status/lung sounds_____
   D.   Neurological status (pupils, extremeity grips, movement)_____

         _____
   E.   Cardiovascular assessment (Heart sounds, edema, nail beds)_____

         _____
   F.   Skin assessment (Complete the skin assessment form)
   G.   Abdominal assessment_____
   H.   Pain? Y/N Describe None (0) Mild (1-2) Moderate (3-4) Severe (5)
           Intermittant_____Constant_____Dull_____Sharp_____
           Does pain interfere with functioning? Y/N   Is medication Effective? Y/N   Does pain
           interfere with therapy? Y/N
           Comments:_____

Resident name_____ Nurse Signature_____

FIGURE 10-20: OTHER LTC FORMS (5 OF 7): QUARTERLY ASSESSMENT FORM (A)

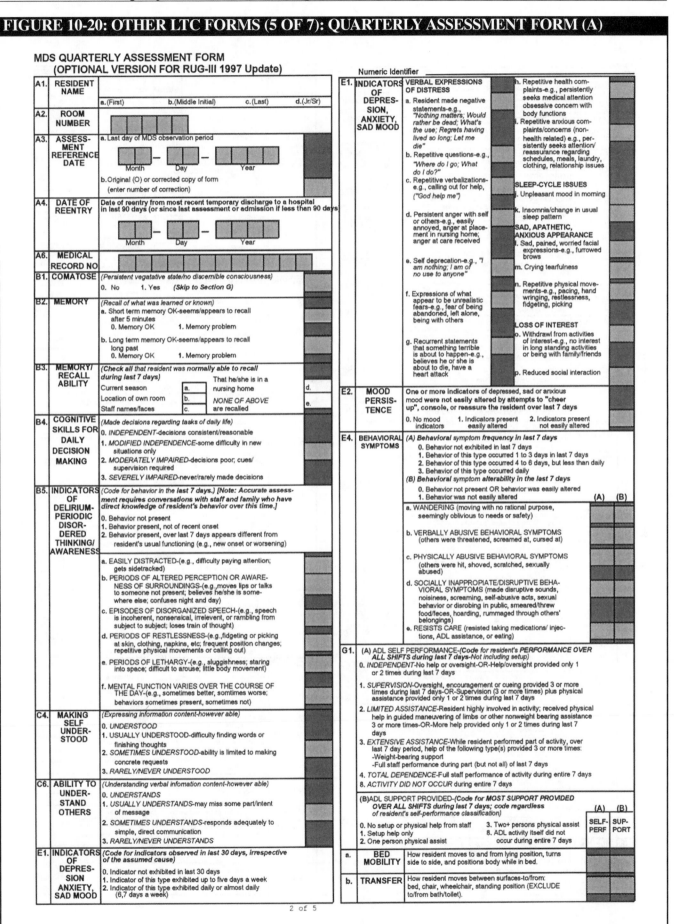

FIGURE 10-20: OTHER LTC FORMS (6 OF 7): QUARTERLY ASSESSMENT FORM (B)

Resident _____   Numeric Identifier _____

G1.

			(A)	(B)
c.	WALK IN ROOM	How resident walks between locations in his/her room		
d.	WALK IN CORRIDOR	How resident walks in corridor on unit		
e.	LOCOMO-TION ON UNIT	How resident moves between locations in his/her room and adjacent corridor on same floor. If in wheelchair, self-sufficiency once in chair		
f.	LOCOMO-TION OFF UNIT	How resident moves to and returns from off unit locations (e.g., areas set aside for dining, activities, or treatments). If facility has only one floor, how resident moves to and from distant areas on the floor. If in wheelchair, self-sufficiency once in chair		
g.	DRESSING	How resident puts on, fastens, and takes off all items of street clothing, including donning/removing prosthesis		
h.	EATING	How resident eats and drinks (regardless of skill). Includes intake of nourishment by other means (e.g., tube feeding, total parenteral nutrition)		
I.	TOILET USE	How resident uses the toilet room (or commode, bedpan,urinal);transfers on/off toilet, cleanses, changes pad, manages ostomy or catheter, adjusts clothes		
j.	PERSONAL HYGIENE	How resident maintains personal hygiene, including combing hair, brushing teeth, shaving, applying makeup, washing/drying face, hands, and perineum (EXCLUDE baths and showers)		

G2. BATHING

How resident takes full-body bath/shower, sponge bath, and transfers in/out of tub/shower (EXCLUDE washing of back and hair.) *Code for most dependent in self performance.*

(A) BATHING SELF-PERFORMANCE codes appear below

	(A)
0. Independent-No help provided	
1. Supervision-Oversight help only	
2. Physical help limited to transfer only	
3. Physical help in part of bathing activity	
4. Total dependence	
8. Activity itself did not occur during entire 7 days	

G3. TEST FOR BALANCE

(see training manual)

(Code for ability during test in the last 7 days)

0. Maintained position as required in test
1. Unsteady, but able to rebalance self without physical support
2. Partial physical support during test, or stands (sits) but does not follow directions for test
3. Not able to attempt test without physical help

a. Balance while standing	
b. Balance while sitting-position, trunk control	

G4. FUNCTIONAL LIMITATION IN RANGE OF MOTION

(Code for limitations during last 7 days that interfered with daily functions or placed residents at risk of injury)

(A) RANGE OF MOTION	(B) VOLUNTARY MOVEMENT
0. No limitation	0. No loss
1. Limitation on one side	1 Partial loss
2. Limitation on both sides	2. Full loss

	(A)	(B)
a Neck		
b. Arm-Including shoulder or elbow		
c. Hand-Including wrist or fingers		
d. Leg-Including hip or knee		
e. Foot-Including ankle or toes		
f. Other limitations or loss		

G6. MODES OF TRANSFER

(Check all that apply during last 7 days)

Bedfast all or most of time	a.	NONE OF ABOVE	f.
Bed rails used for bed mobility or transfer	b.		

G7. TASK SEGMENTA-TION

Some or all of ADL activities were broken into subtasks during last 7 days so that resident could perform them

0. No   1. Yes

H1. CONTINENCE SELF-CONTROL CATEGORIES

(Code for resident's PERFORMANCE OVER ALL SHIFTS)

0. *CONTINENT*-Complete control [includes use of indwelling urinary catheter or ostomy device that does not leak urine or stool]

1. *USUALLY CONTINENT*-BLADDER, incontinent episodes once a week or less; BOWEL, less than weekly

2. *OCCASIONALLY INCONTINENT*-BLADDER, 2 or more times a week, but not daily; BOWEL, once a week

3. *FREQUENTLY INCONTINENT*-BLADDER, tended to be incontinent daily, but some control present (e.g., on day shift); BOWEL, 2-3 times a week

4. *INCONTINENT*-Had inadequate control;BLADDER,multiple daily episodes; BOWEL, all (or almost all) of the time

a.	BOWEL CON-TINENCE	Control of bowel movement, with appliance or bowel continence programs, if employed	
b.	BLADDER CONTI-NENCE	Control of urinary bladder function (if dribbles, volume insuf-ficient to soak through underpants), with appliances (e.g., foley) or continence programs, if employed	

H2. BOWEL ELIMINATION PATTERN

Diarrhea		c.	NONE OF ABOVE	e.
Fecal Impaction		d.		

H3. APPLIANCES AND PROGRAMS

Any scheduled toileting plan	a.	Indwelling catheter	d.
Bladder retraining program	b.	Ostomy present	i.
		NONE OF ABOVE	j.
External (condom) catheter	c.		

Check only those diseases that have a relationship to current ADL status, cognitive status, mood and behavior status, medical treatments, nursing monitoring, or risk of death. (Do not list inactive diagnoses)

I1. DISEASES

(If none apply, CHECK the NONE OF ABOVE box)

ENDOCRINE/METABOLIC/NUTRITIONAL				
Diabetes mellitus	a.	Hemiplegia/Hemiparesis	v.
MUSCULOSKELETAL		Multiple sclerosis	w.
Hip fracture	m.	Quadriplegia	z.
NEUROLOGICAL		**PSYCHIATRIC/MOOD**	
Aphasia	r.	Depression	ee.
Cerebral palsy	s.	Manic depressive (bipolar disease)	ff.
Cerebrovascular acci-dent (stroke)	t.	**OTHER**	
		NONE OF ABOVE	rr.

I2. INFECTIONS

(If none apply, CHECK the NONE OF ABOVE box)

		Septicemia	g.
Antibiotic resistant infection (e.g., Methi-cillin resistant staph)	a.	Sexually transmitted diseases	h.
Clostridium difficile (c. diff.)	b.	Tuberculosis	i.
Conjuctivitis	c.	Urinary tract infection in last 30 days	j.
HIV infection	d.	Viral hepatitis	k.
Pneumonia	e.	Wound infection	l.
Respiratory infection	f.	NONE OF ABOVE	m.

I3. OTHER CURRENT DIAGNOSES AND ICD-9 CODES

(Include only those diseases diagnosed in the last 90 days that have a relationship to current ADL status, cognitive status, behavior status, medical treatments, nursing monitoring, or risk of death)

a. _____ | | | | . | |
b. _____ | | | | . | |

J1. PROBLEM CONDITIONS

(Check all problems present in last 7 days unless other time frame is indicated)

INDICATORS OF FLUID STATUS		OTHER	
		Delusions	e.
		Edema	g.
Weight gain or loss of 3 or more pounds within a 7 day period	a.	Fever	h.
		Hallucinations	i.
Inability to lie flat due to shortness of breath	b.	Internal bleeding	j.
		Recurrent lung aspirations in last 90 days	k.
Dehydrated; output exceeds input	c.	Shortness of breath	l.
		Unsteady gait	n.
Insufficient fluid; did NOT consume all/almost all liquids provided during last 3 days	d.	Vomiting	o.
		NONE OF ABOVE	p.

J2. PAIN SYMPTOMS

(Code the highest level of pain present in the last 7 days

a. FREQUENCY with which resident complains or shows evidence of pain	b. INTENSITY of pain
0. No pain (skip to J4)	1. Mild pain
1. Pain less than daily	2. Moderate pain
2. Pain daily	3. Times when pain is horrible or excruciating

J4. ACCIDENTS

(Check all that apply)

Fell in past 30 days	a.	Hip fracture last 180 days	c.
Fell in past 31-180 days	b.	Other fracture in last 180 days	d.
		NONE OF ABOVE	e.

J5. STABILITY OF CONDITIONS

Conditions/diseases make resident's cognitive, ADL, mood or behavior status unstable-(fluctuating,precarious, or deteriorating)	a.
Resident experiencing an acute episode or a flare-up of a recurrent or chronic problem	b.
End-stage disease, 6 or fewer months to live	c.
NONE OF ABOVE	d.

K1. ORAL PROBLEMS

Chewing problem	a.
Swallowing problem	b.
NONE OF ABOVE	d.

K2. HEIGHT AND WEIGHT

Record (a.)height in inches and (b.)weight in pounds. Base weight on most recent measure in last 30 days; measure weight consistently in accord with standard facility practice-e.g., in a.m. after voiding, before meal, with shoes off, and in nightclothes

a. HT (in.) _____   b. WT (lb.) _____

K3. WEIGHT CHANGE

a. Weight loss-5% or more in last 30 days; or 10% or more in last 180 days

0. No   1. Yes

FIGURE 10-20: OTHER LTC FORMS (7 OF 7): QUARTERLY ASSESSMENT FORM (C)

Resident _____   Numeric Identifier _____

K3.	**WEIGHT CHANGE**	b. Weight gain–5% or more in last 30 days; or 10% or more in last 180 days 0. No 1. Yes
K5.	**NUTRITIONAL APPROACHES**	*(Check all that apply in last 7 days)* Parenteral/IV ___a. On a planned weight change program ___h. Feeding tube ___b. NONE OF ABOVE ___i.
K6.	**PARENTERAL OR ENTERAL INTAKE**	*(Skip to Section M if neither 5a nor 5b is checked)* a. Code the proportion of total calories the resident received through parenteral or tube feedings in the last 7 days 0. None 3. 51% to 75% 1. 1% to 25% 4. 76% to 100% 2. 26% to 50% b. Code the average fluid intake per day by IV or tube in last 7 days 0. None 3. 1001 to 1500 cc/day 1. 1 to 500 cc/day 4. 1501 to 2000 cc/day 2. 501 to 1000 cc/day 5. 2001 or more cc/day

			Number at Stage
M1.	**ULCERS** (Due to any cause)	*(Record the number of ulcers at each ulcer stage—regardless of cause. If none present at a stage, record "0" (zero). Code all that apply during last 7 days, Code 9 = 9 or more.) [Requires full body exam.]*	
		a. Stage 1. A persistent area of skin redness (without a break in the skin) that does not disappear when pressure is relieved.	
		b. Stage 2. A partial thickness loss of skin layers that presents clinically as an abrasion, blister, or shallow crater.	
		c. Stage 3. A full thickness of skin is lost, exposing the subcutaneous tissues-presents as a deep crater with or without undermining adjacent tissue.	
		d. Stage 4. A full thickness of skin and subcutaneous tissue is lost, exposing muscle or bone.	
M2.	**TYPE OF ULCER**	*(For each type of ulcer, code for the highest stage in the last 7 days using scale in item M1-i.e., 0=none; stages 1, 2, 3, 4)*	
		a. Pressure ulcer-any lesion caused by pressure resulting in damage of underlying tissue	
		b. Stasis ulcer-open lesion caused by poor circulation in the lower extremities	

M4.	**OTHER SKIN PROBLEMS OR LESIONS PRESENT** (Check all that apply during last 7 days)	*(Check all that apply during last 7 days)* Abrasions, bruises	a.
		Burns (second or third degree)	b.
		Open lesions other than ulcers, rashes, cuts (e.g., cancer lesions)	c.
		Rashes-e.g., intertrigo, eczema, drug rash, heat rash, herpes zoster	d.
		Skin desensitized to pain or pressure	e.
		Skin tears or cuts (other than surgery)	f.
		Surgical wounds	g.
		NONE OF ABOVE	h.
M5.	**SKIN TREATMENTS** (Check all that apply during last 7 days)	*(Check all that apply during last 7 days)* Pressure relieving device(s) for chair	a.
		Pressure relieving device(s) for bed	b.
		Turning/repositioning program	c.
		Nutrition or hydration intervention to manage skin problems	d.
		Ulcer care	e.
		Surgical wound care	f.
		Application of dressings (with or without topical medications) other than to feet	g.
		Application of ointments/medications (other than to feet)	h.
		Other preventative or protective skin care (other than to feet)	i.
		NONE OF ABOVE	j.
M6.	**FOOT PROBLEMS AND CARE** (Check all that apply during last 7 days)	*(Check all that apply during last 7 days)* Resident has one or more foot problems–e.g., corns, calluses, bunions, hammer toes, overlapping toes, pain, structural problems	a.
		Infection of the foot-e.g., cellulitis, purulent drainage	b.
		Open lesions on the foot	c.
		Nails/calluses trimmed during last 90 days	d.
		Received preventative or protective foot care (e.g., used special shoes, inserts, pads, toe separators)	e.
		Application of dressings (with or without topical medications)	f.
		NONE OF ABOVE	g.

N1.	**TIME AWAKE**	*(Check appropriate time periods over last 7 days)* Resident awake all or most of time (i.e., naps no more than one hour per time period) in the: Morning ___a. Evening ___c. Afternoon ___b. NONE OF ABOVE ___d.
		(If resident is comatose, skip to Section O)
N2.	**AVERAGE TIME INVOLVED IN ACTIVITIES**	*(When awake and not receiving treatments or ADL care)* 0. Most-more than 2/3 of time 2. Little-less than 1/3 of time 1. Some from 1/3 to 2/3 of time 3. None

O1.	**NUMBER OF MEDICATIONS**	*(Record the number of different medications used in the last 7 days; enter "0" if none used)*
O3.	**INJECTIONS**	*(Record the number of DAYS injections of any type received during the last 7 days; enter "0" if none used)*
O4.	**DAYS RECEIVED THE FOLLOWING MEDICATION**	*(Record the number of DAYS during last 7 days; enter "0" if not used. Note--enter "1" for long-acting meds used less than weekly)* a. Antipsychotic c. Antidepressant b. Antianxiety d. Hypnotic e. Diuretic

P1.	**SPECIAL TREATMENTS, PROCEDURES, AND PROGRAMS**	**a. SPECIAL CARE-***Check treatments or programs received during the last 14 days* **TREATMENTS** Ventilator or respirator ___l. Chemotherapy ___a. **PROGRAMS** Dialysis ___b. Alcohol/drug treatment program ___m. IV medication ___c. Alzheimer's/dementia special care unit ___n. Intake/output ___d. Monitoring acute medical condition ___e. Hospice care ___o. Ostomy care ___f. Pediatric unit ___p. Oxygen therapy ___g. Respite care ___q. Radiation ___h. Training in skills required to return to the community (e.g., taking medications, house work, shopping, transportation, ADLs) ___r. Suctioning ___i. Tracheostomy care ___j. Transfusions ___k. NONE OF ABOVE ___s.	

b. THERAPIES-*Record the number of days and total minutes each of the following therapies was administered (for at least 15 minutes a day) in the last 7 calendar days (Enter 0 if none or less than 15 min. daily) [Note-count only post admission therapies]*

(A)=# of days administered for 15 minutes or more
(B)=total # of minutes provided in last 7 days

	DAYS (A)	MIN (B)
a. Speech-language pathology and audiology services		
b. Occupational therapy		
c. Physical therapy		
d. Respiratory therapy		
e. Psychological therapy (by any licensed mental health professional)		

P3.	**NURSING REHABILITATION/ RESTORATIVE CARE**	*Record the NUMBER OF DAYS each of the following rehabilitation or restorative techniques or practices was provided to the resident for more than or equal to 15 minutes per day in the last 7 days (Enter 0 if none or less than 15 min. daily)* a. Range of motion (passive) f. Walking b. Range of motion (active) g. Dressing or grooming c. Splint or brace assistance h. Eating or swallowing **TRAINING AND SKILL PRACTICE IN:** i. Amputation/prosthesis care d. Bed mobility j. Communication e. Transfer k. Other	

P4.	**DEVICES AND RESTRAINTS**	*Use the following codes for last 7 days:* 0. Not used 1. Used less than daily 2. Used daily **Bed rails** a. -Full bed rails on all open sides of bed b. -Other types of side rails used (e.g., half rail, one side) c. Trunk restraint d. Limb restraint e. Chair prevents rising
P7.	**PHYSICIAN VISITS**	In the **LAST 14 DAYS** (or since admission if less than 14 days in facility) how many days has the physician (or authorized assistant or practitioner) examined the resident? *(Enter 0 if none)*
P8.	**PHYSICIAN ORDERS**	In the **LAST 14 DAYS** (or since admission if less than 14 days in facility) how many days has the physician (or authorized assistant or practitioner) changed the resident's orders? *Do not include order renewals without change.* *(Enter 0 if none)*
Q2.	**OVERALL CHANGE IN CARE NEEDS**	Resident's overall level of self sufficiency has changed significantly as compared to status of 90 days ago (or since last assessment if less than 90 days) 0. No change 1. Improved-receives fewer supports, needs less restrictive level of care 2. Deteriorated-receives more support

R2. SIGNATURE OF PERSON COORDINATING THE ASSESSMENT:

a. Signature of RN Assessment Coordinator (sign on above line)

b. Date RN Assessment Coordinator signed as complete

☐☐ – ☐☐ – ☐☐☐☐
Month   Day   Year

4 of 5

Reprinted with the permission of Sears Methodist Retirement System, Inc.

EXAM QUESTIONS

CHAPTER 10
Questions 72-79

72. Documentation in specific departments may require

    a. all the same forms needed on any unit and no additional forms.

    b. block form narrative notes and no additional forms.

    c. special forms for documenting nursing hours worked.

    d. additional forms based on requirements for that specific department.

73. Some specific forms that might be used include

    a. MDS form in the pediatric unit.

    b. labor record in L&D and seclusion record in psychiatry.

    c. discharge summary forms only on medical-surgical units.

    d. insurance claim forms.

74. Specific departments commonly develop guidelines, procedures, standards, and forms based on

    a. institutional policies only.

    b. patient's needs and requests.

    c. specialty organizations' standards and guidelines.

    d. nurses' ideas about simplifying documentation and disregarding regulations.

75. EMTALA requires hospitals to

    a. immediately transfer preterm labor patients to hospitals with high-level NICUs.

    b. only treat patients with the ability to pay for the care provided.

    c. provide medical screening, determination of labor, and stabilization of a woman prior to transfer or discharge.

    d. do nothing before sending a patient to another hospital.

76. The Hollister Labor Progress Chart® is specifically designed for

    a. a critical care patient.

    b. a patient in labor.

    c. a pediatric patient.

    d. determining staffing needs.

77. When Junior, age 6, is admitted to a pediatric unit for a medical problem, a nurse should expect to find in his medical record

    a. an L&D record.

    b. an anesthesia record.

    c. a seclusion record.

    d. a growth and development form.

78. The key to receiving proper reimbursement for home health services is

    a. daily skilled nursing visits provided by a registered nurse.

    b. accurate submission of billing claims for home services every 2 weeks.

    c. clear and accurate documentation of the clinical services provided.

    d. documentation from the physician that the patient is better cared for at home than in an institution.

79. The RAI is composed of

    a. OBRA, CMS, and EMTALA regulations.

    b. MDS, RAPs, and utilization guidelines.

    c. AMA form, MDS, and CMS.

    d. AMA form, DNR order, and RAPs.

CHAPTER 11

CONSENT FORMS

CHAPTER OBJECTIVE

After completing this chapter, the reader will be able to discuss the legal importance of and nursing responsibilities involved with informed consent and describe the importance of the Patient's Bill of Rights.

LEARNING OBJECTIVES

After studying this chapter, the reader will be able to

1. identify the reason for informed consent.

2. indicate the basic elements of informed consent.

3. indicate a nurses' professional responsibility in informed consent.

4. identify the concept of *capacity* as it relates to a patient's right to accept or refuse medical treatment.

5. identify proper documentation of informed consent.

6. specify types of advanced directives.

7. identify two components of the Patient's Bill of Rights.

8. indicate the duty imposed on health care institutions by the 1990 Patient Self-Determination Act.

INTRODUCTION

Informed consent provides legal protection of a patient's right to personal autonomy. The concept of informed consent is one that has come to mean that patients are given the opportunity to choose a course of action in regard to care and to choose from available therapeutic alternatives. The concept of informed consent did not appear until the late 1950s and early 1960s. Prior to that time, it was believed that patients should not be informed of anything. It is necessary to obtain informed consent whenever a patient is faced with treatment choices and the need to make an informed decision.

Health care providers now accept a patient's right to know all relevant facts prior to consenting to a procedure or treatment. Therefore, it is a health care provider's duty is to secure informed consent, but the provider cannot make the decision for the patient. Even if the patient's decision is detrimental to the patient, the decision remains the patient's. Informed consent is a complex issue for nurses because of the differences in the laws between states, variations in what constitutes valid informed consent, exceptions to informed consent, and the liability associated with nurses' role in informed consent. This chapter discusses the nurse's professional responsibility involved in consent forms, what the nurse should document, advance directives, and the Patient Care Partnership (previously the "Patient's Bill of Rights").

INFORMED CONSENT

Informed consent is an agreement by a patient to accept a course of treatment or a procedure after complete information, including the risk of treatment and facts relating to it, has been provided by a health care provider (usually the physician performing the treatment or procedure). Normally, institutions have standardized forms with "fill-in-the-blank" areas that the health care provider completes. Generally, adequate informed consent contains the information found in Table 11-1.

TABLE 11-1: INFORMED CONSENT INFORMATION

- Patient's diagnosis or suspected diagnosis
- Nature and purpose of the proposed treatment or procedure
- Expected outcome
- Expected benefits
- Who will perform the proposed treatment or procedure
- The potential complications, risks, or side effects of the treatment or procedure
- Any reasonable alternatives
- If applicable, possible prognoses, if the treatment or procedure is not performed

(Brent, 2001; Mackay, 2001)

After the treatment or procedure is explained to the patient and the patient has asked all pertinent questions and received complete answers, the patient signs the form. The form becomes a legal part of the patient's medical record. If a health care provider proceeds without some form of consent, he or she could be charged with battery.

PROFESSIONAL RESPONSIBILITY

Obtaining informed consent for specific medical or surgical treatments is the responsibility of the physician or advanced practice nurse practitioner (NP) or other person performing the procedure. The responsibility is commonly delegated to nurses, an undesirable practice. However, no laws prohibit nurses from being part of the information-giving process. The nurse's main legal responsibility is to witness the giving of informed consent. This responsibility involves the items listed in Table 11-2.

TABLE 11-2: NURSE'S RESPONSIBILITY IN INFORMED CONSENT

- Witnessing the exchange between the patient and the health care provider who will perform the treatment or procedure
- Determining that the patient understood and was completely informed
- Witnessing the patient's signature

(Blais, Hayes, Kozier, & Erb, 2002; Burkhardt & Nathaniel, 2002; Schaffer, 1992)

In many cases, the patient is informed about the procedure in the health care provider's office and the institution nurse does not witness the information being given. If a nurse in an institution is required to obtain signatures on an informed consent form and has not witnessed the information being given to the patient, the nurse should write "witnessing signature only" on the form. If the patient does not understand what the health care provider plans to do, the nurse must notify the health care provider and ask the provider to re-explain the treatment or procedure to the patient.

Sometimes an informed consent form is completed and signed in the health care provider's office and then sent with the patient to the hospital. The consent form should be reviewed for completeness and signatures and placed in the patient's medical record. The nurse can inquire what the patient knows about the treatment or procedure. Once again, if the nurse believes that the patient does not understand the treatment or procedure, the health care provider should be notified.

To give informed consent, a patient must be mentally competent, must voluntarily give consent, and must not feel coerced. Patients should be encouraged to ask questions about anything they do not understand. Three major elements of informed consent are presented in Table 11-3.

TABLE 11-3: MAJOR ELEMENTS OF INFORMED CONSENT
• Consent must be given by a patient who has the capacity and competence to understand.
• Consent by the patient must be given voluntarily.
• The patient must be given enough information to understand the procedure and to be the ultimate decision maker.
(Blais et al., 2002; Kavaler & Spiegel, 1997)

Before informed consent is given, the patient must receive adequate and thorough information. The information provided must include a description of the procedure, the benefits, the risks, and any alternative procedures that could be tried. Technical words should be carefully explained in simple lay language. If a patient cannot read, the informed consent form should be read to her or him before it is signed. An interpreter may be necessary to provide information if the patient does not speak the same language as the health care provider.

After adequate information has been provided, the patient can then make an informed decision about the treatment or procedure to be performed. The patient must be a competent adult in order to provide informed consent. A competent adult is a person age 18 or older who is conscious, oriented, and capable of understanding information about a treatment or procedure. A patient who is confused, disoriented, or sedated is not considered functionally competent to give consent at that time (see Table 11-4).

A person who is younger than age 18 may give consent if he or she is considered an emancipated minor. An emancipated minor is defined as a minor who is financially independent, who lives apart from his or her parents, who is married, who is pregnant, or who is in the military services of the United

TABLE 11-4: PEOPLE WHO CANNOT GIVE CONSENT
• Minors, unless declared emancipated
• Unconscious, or sedated patients
• Confused or disoriented patients
• Incompetent patients
• Some mentally ill patients
• Some prisoners or other incarcerated individuals

States. Emancipated minors are considered to have the same legal capacity as adults. Pregnant minors may give consent for themselves and their fetuses. However, once a fetus is born, a minor mother usually retains the right to provide consent for her child but not for herself unless she fits into one of the other exceptions. Some states allow minors to give consent for blood donations, drug-dependence treatment, treatment for sexually transmitted diseases, birth control, and obstetric care. Each state defines emancipated minors differently and laws vary; therefore, it is advisable for nurses to check their state laws and definitions of emancipated minors.

It is normal for parents or guardians to act in the best interest of a minor and to provide consent before treatment is given. If parents are unavailable in a given situation, certain others, usually the next of kin in a hierarchical fashion, may be authorized to give consent. An advocate, a person with power-of-attorney, or a legal guardian can also give consent for adults who are not competent to do so. However, health care providers who communicate medical information to a third person who is not authorized by the patient to make health care decisions expose themselves to liability for breach of statutory privileges, invasion of privacy, or breach of contract.

For patients who are unconscious or sedated, consent is normally obtained from the closest adult relative if state statutes allow. When a life-threatening emergency occurs and consent cannot be obtained or the parents, guardians, or relatives cannot be reached, the law usually agrees that consent is assumed and implied.

Terminally ill people who participate in research or medical procedures can seldom expect to benefit personally from the research or procedure. Therefore, the cost/benefit needs to be carefully considered. If the terminally ill patient participates, the health care and comfort of these patients must not be compromised. It may be necessary to obtain informed consent from the spouse or legal guardian if the patient is physically or mentally incapacitated.

EXCEPTIONS TO INFORMED CONSENT

In some health care situations, the law waives the need to obtain consent. In relation to informed consent, the nature of the exception and the facts and circumstances of the situation must be clearly evaluated and documented. Exceptions to obtaining consent include true emergencies, patient waivers, and lack of decision-making capacity.

As previously discussed, in a true emergency, the life or well being of a person is threatened. If the next-of-kin or surrogate cannot be found, a lack or delay in treatment might compromise the person's life. In such situations, health care providers are able to provide necessary care. The nurse should document attempts to locate the next-of-kin or surrogate.

Patient waiver of the right to give informed consent is another exception recognized by the law. Sometimes patients do not wish to be given information about a procedure or treatment. When a patient expresses a desire not to be informed, this right should be honored. The nurse should document that the patient did not want to know about the procedure.

The last exception is made when decision making capacity does not exist. The health care provider is required to discuss the condition of the patient and the needed treatment or procedure with the parent, guardian, surrogate, or proxy decision-maker. Therefore, this is considered an exception in the fact that the information is not given directly to the patient but to someone else who is legally recognized as being able to provide or refuse authorization for the patient.

State and local legislative bodies have mental health acts that define mental incompetence. Patients who are mentally incompetent as determined by a court, intoxicated, under the influence of drugs, in shock, or unconscious are not considered capable of providing informed consent. If a patient is incompetent, the policies of the institution and the laws of the state specify what steps need to be taken to ensure legal consent and who can give consent for the patient. The nurse is advised to learn the institution's policy and the state laws in regard to obtaining consent from a person other than the patient.

DOCUMENTING INFORMED CONSENT

Regardless of the setting, a nurse who works with patients will be involved in some way with obtaining informed consent. Remember, nurses who sign as witnesses are not obtaining informed consent; they are only witnessing the person signing the informed consent form. The nurse may reinforce the information given by the primary health care provider but may not assume the primary health care provider's legal duty to inform the patient. In all cases, when informed consent is required, it should be documented in the nurse's notes that such consent was in fact obtained from the person who is required to provide the information.

The signed consent form should be a part of the patient's permanent medical record (see Figure 11-1). In the event of a lawsuit, proper documentation supports the health care practitioner's testimony regarding informed consent. Documentation includes the signed consent form and the nurse's note of the discussion and the patient's consent. The type and amount of documentation required depends on state

FIGURE 11-1: SAMPLE INFORMED CONSENT FORM

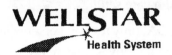

CONSENT FOR TREATMENT: I do hereby consent to medical or hospital care encompassing diagnostic procedures and medical treatments including without limitation to diagnostic x-rays, drugs, blood transfusions, etc, as may be ordered by physicians, employees, or agents responsible for such medical or hospital care. I further consent to treatment by authorized employees or agents of WellStar Health System who are assigned to my (or their) care. I am aware that the practice of medicine and surgery is not an exact science, and I acknowledge that no guarantees have been made to me as to the results of treatments, examinations or hospital care at WellStar Health System. I acknowledge that I can ask questions about my medical care. **I understand there are some physicians and their employees on the medical staff of WellStar Health System providing medical care who are not employees or agents of WellStar Health System but to the contrary, are independent medical practitioners exercising independent medical judgements at facilities provided by WellStar Health System.** I acknowledge that I have been provided a copy of my Patient Rights. **I certify that the personal information provided is correct and accurate.**

WITNESS	DATE	SIGNATURE OF PATIENT OR DESIGNEE

I. FINANCIAL AGREEMENT AND ASSIGNMENT OF BENEFITS: I, the undersigned, hereby authorize payment directly to WellStar Health System and treating physicians of the insurance benefits otherwise payable or due to become payable. I understand and agree that I am financially responsible for any charges not covered by this assignment of insurance benefits. In addition, I hereby assign to the hospital my rights under Georgia Law to have any insurance claim processed and/or paid within 15 working days of the receipt of the claim by the insurance company. It is further agreed that any credit balance resulting from insurance payments or other sources that are refundable to the responsible party will be applied to any other account owed to WellStar Health System by my family or me.

II. ASSIGNMENT OF MEDICARE AND MEDICAID BENEFITS, PATIENT CERTIFICATION AND PAYMENT REQUEST: I hereby certify that the information given by me in applying for payment under title XVII and XIX of the Social Security Act is correct. I request that payment of the authorized benefits be made and assigned the benefits payable for services rendered during this admission to the physician or organization furnishing the services. The undersigned if other than the patient and the patient are responsible for and agree to pay charges not covered by this assignment, including any Medicare deductibles.

III. POTENTIAL LIABILITY: The health insurance option you have selected may require prior authorization for coverage of each hospital inpatient admission and certification of hospital days beyond your established length of stay. If coverage for the services have been requested in this case and are not approved by your insurance company based upon medical information provided by the physician and/or WellStar Health System, you will be liable for total charges or a portion of the charges in accordance with your insurance program.

IV. PERSONAL VALUABLES: WellStar Health System shall not be liable for the loss or damage of any personal belongings, including but not limited to money, jewelry, hearing aids, or dentures, unless placed within a WellStar Health System safe.

V. MATERNITY PATIENT: The above consents are applicable to any series of in or outpatient services necessary prior to and associated with the prenatal course of treatment.

VI. CONTINUOUS CONSENTS: The above consents are applicable to all outpatient services provided hereafter for the term of one (1) year from this date.

SIGNATURE OF PATIENT OR DESIGNEE	RELATION	DATE

WITNESS	DATE

Form # WS0484 Item # 2238

(REV. 5/03)

laws. Some states have statutes that spell out requirements for written consent forms. The form is considered valid unless the plaintiff can prove that consent was obtained in bad faith, by fraud, or from a patient who could not understand English. Documentation should include a summary of the information given to the patient, a statement indicating all the patient's questions were answered, and any response by the patient acknowledging understanding of the information provided (see Table 11-5).

PATIENT SELF-DETERMINATION ACT

The Patient Self-Determination Act (PSDA) was passed in 1990 by the U.S. Congress and became effective in 1991 as part of the Omnibus Budget Reconciliation Act (OBRA). The PSDA requires all health care providers and institutions to inform patients of their rights to execute advance directives and to determine which lifesaving or life-prolonging actions they want to have carried out on their behalf. Nurses have a responsibility to facilitate informed decision-making with patients, particularly regarding end-of-life care and, therefore, nurses

have a critical role in the implementation of the PSDA within all health care settings.

In spite of the PSDA, only a small percentage of patients have advance directives, and many family members are not aware of seriously ill patients' wishes. Developing advance directives must be part of the ongoing process of communication between patients, family members, and health care providers. Open discussion of end-of-life decisions should occur routinely within health care settings, before the physical and emotional stress of serious illness or institutionalization.

ADVANCE DIRECTIVES

Advance directives allow individuals to choose in advance of physical or mental incapacity what health care treatments or life-sustaining measures are to be carried out or withdrawn and who may assist in making those decisions when the individual becomes incapacitated. An advance directive is a legal document that sets out the wishes of an individual in regard to health care in situations in which the individual is no longer capable of giving informed consent. It includes oral statements by the

TABLE 11-5: INFORMED CONSENT DOCUMENTATION

- If the nurse was present during the time the information was presented to the patient, document who was present (by name), the condition of the patient, the questions asked by the patient, and any other pertinent information.

- Make sure the signed consent form is for the exact treatment or procedure to be performed and is placed in the patient's medical record.

- Document any concerns about the patient's response, change of condition, or the patient's understanding of the procedure.

- Document communication of concerns with the physician, the NP, or the nursing supervisor.

- Document in the nursing notes and on the consent form the presence of an interpreter by name and address, if necessary; time; and others present during the informed consent process.

- Clearly document any exceptions to obtaining informed consent. Provide detailed information as to the circumstances, attempts to obtain consent, and any known waiver.

- If the patient withdraws consent, clearly document the reason, notification of the physician, time called, the patient's statement, individuals present, and any actions taken.

(Anderson, 2003; Brent, 2001; Mackay, 2001)

patient or a written document, possibly including a living will or durable power of attorney.

Advance directives as identified under the Uniform Health Care Decisions Act of 1994 include the following documents or instructions: living will, do-not-resuscitate (DNR) order, assisted suicide, and "right to die" versus "right to live."

Living Will

A living will is a legal document that gives directions to health care providers related to withholding or withdrawing life support if certain conditions exist. Statutes regulating living wills vary from state to state, and a living will written in one state usually cannot be enforced in another state. Therefore, nurses must be familiar with their own state laws.

Durable Power of Attorney for Health Care

A durable power of attorney for health care allows a competent person to designate another person as a surrogate or proxy to act on his or her behalf in making health care decisions in the event of the loss of decision-making capacity. The designation must be written, signed, and dated by the person making the designation and have two witnesses other than the designated surrogate. The authority of the surrogate does not become effective until it has been determined that the person has lost decision-making capacity.

The presence of a living will or durable health care power of attorney and designated surrogate should be documented in a patient's medical record. Nurses should ask patients if they have such documents. Likewise, nurses should be able to discuss the importance of such directives with patients and families. The ANA (1991a) recommends that nurses inquire about advance directives during the assessment process, including the location of the advance directive, the patient's desire to have one if he or she does not already, and if the patient has discussed end-of-life choices with family members.

Responses to these questions should be documented in the patient's medical record.

Do-Not-Resuscitate Order

A DNR order is a legal document that provides instructions to health care providers related to the patient's right to refuse specific life-saving treatments. Patients have the right to refuse treatment regardless of their health condition; however, the patient must have the capacity to refuse treatment. In order for a DNR order to be effective, the patient must be competent when the DNR order was made or the surrogate must agree to the order.

A physician is responsible for discussing the situation with the patient and family and must write the order in the patient's medical record. The DNR order must be periodically reviewed. Good communication is the most critical key factor in assuring that any DNR decision is acceptable to all persons involved. DNR orders should be documented, noting the reason the order was written, who gave the consent, who was involved in the discussion, whether the patient was competent to give consent or who was authorized to do so, and the time frame for the DNR order.

Assisted Suicide

In 1997, the U.S. Supreme Court ruled that state laws prohibiting assisted suicide were not constitutional. The act was amended in 1999 to clarify the language. Pharmacists were included as health care providers and immunity provisions were expanded. Active voluntary euthanasia is an act in which a health care provider provides the means for death and administers it, such as a lethal dose of a medication. With assisted suicide, the patient receives the means of death from someone but activates the process personally. The ANA (1994) defines assisted suicide as making a means of suicide available with knowledge of any physically and mentally capable patient's intention to end her or his own life. Because no national end-of-life standard exists, nurses must be familiar with the laws involving assisted suicide and euthanasia in their particular states. Within the parameters prescribed by law, dying patients and their families should be treated humanely and with dignity. Communication and documentation is vitally important at this time.

Right-to-Die versus Right-to-Live

Right-to-die or right-to-live documents include the patient's right to die with dignity, the right to receive the best treatment, and the right to refuse treatment versus the right to life-sustaining methods through use of ordinary medical treatment or heroic measures. Regardless of the method of treatment chosen, a multidisciplinary treatment team must provide analysis of the situation and follow a protocol for pain management. Orders should be clearly documented in regard to the procedures to be carried out. Nurses must be vigilant in documenting facts. Once again, communication and careful documentation is critical at this time.

PATIENT CARE PARTNERSHIP

In 1992, the American Hospital Association (AHA) revised the Patient's Bill of Rights, which guarantees certain rights and privileges to every patient. In 1998, the federal government undertook additional revisions to the act. In 2003 the American Hospital Association replaced the Patient's Bill of Rights with a plain language brochure which informs patients how they should expect to be treated and what is required of them during their hospital stay. *The Patient Care Partnership: Understanding Expectations, Rights and Responsibilities* is available in multiple languages on the American Hospital Association's website (www.aha.org).

A copy of *The Patient Care Partnership* should be given to every patient, in the patient's own language, upon entering a healthcare institution. Copies should be posted throughout the institution.

The institution must have a formal written plan addressing patient complaints, as well as documentation of any actions taken to resolve grievances.

The legal obligation of a registered nurse is to respect patients' rights to exercise personal autonomy by allowing them to take part in decision-making, respecting the privacy and dignity of patients, maintaining professional competence, and engaging in activities that establish and maintain quality patient care. Careful, complete, accurate, timely, and factual documentation assists nurses in meeting patient needs.

CONCLUSION

Nurses play a key role in the planning and implementation of informed consent, advance directives, and *The Patient Care Partnership* action. Nursing values promote and support the use of advance directives in health care. Because patients may be helpless and unable to speak for themselves, all health care providers should consider themselves patient advocates. Patient's rights provide the basis for advocacy in nursing care. Nurses should work toward excellent care of patients and the inclusion of patients' rights in nursing practice. Appropriate documentation serves as a record of such advocacy and provides a defense against any potential lawsuit. With the correct procedures and forms, the process of informed consent, advance directives, and patient advocacy can be fairly painless.

EXAM QUESTIONS

CHAPTER 11
Questions 80-89

80. The process of obtaining permission from a patient to perform a specific test or procedure by describing the risks, side effects, and benefits is known as

   a. informed consent.
   b. power of attorney.
   c. advance directives.
   d. assisted suicide.

81. Touching a patient or performing a procedure or treatment without authorization to do so could be considered

   a. touching.
   b. battery.
   c. assault.
   d. routine.

82. Obtaining informed consent for specific medical or surgical treatments is primarily the responsibility of the

   a. person witnessing the patient's signature on the consent form.
   b. health care provider performing the treatment or procedure.
   c. physician's surgical assistant.
   d. physician's office nurse.

83. In informed consent, the staff nurse working in an institution has the responsibility to

   a. witness the information given to the patient and the patient's signature.
   b. witness the physician's signature.
   c. determine the physician's understanding of the information.
   d. do nothing.

84. *Capacity* as it relates to a patient's rights to accept or refuse medical treatment means the patient is

   a. a competent adult age 18 or older who is conscious, oriented, and capable of understanding the information.
   b. a person who is younger than age 18 and is not an emancipated minor.
   c. a minor being cared for by a next-door neighbor.
   d. a patient who is institutionalized in a mental health facility who is incoherent and disoriented.

85. Some people, due to their cognitive status or age, cannot legally give consent. Informed consent *can* be obtained from a

   a. disoriented 88 year old male.
   b. heavily sedated 62 year old female.
   c. physically disabled 42 year old.
   d. 14 year old boy with diabetes.

86. An advance directive is a legal document of a competent person's health care wishes

    a. with regard to the person's health care in situations when he or she becomes unable to give consent.

    b. that are not identified under the Uniform Health Care Decisions Act as living wills and durable powers of attorney.

    c. that contains documents such as DNR orders, euthanasia wishes, and diet orders.

    d. that has to be completed when the patient is about to die.

87. A physician may enter a DNR order for a competent patient after a discussion of the patient's condition with and upon request of the

    a. patient.

    b. patient's spouse.

    c. patient's next of kin.

    d. patient's heirs.

88. The Patient Care Partnership establishes that the patient

    a. cannot ask for information about any diagnosis.

    b. has the right to considerate and respectful care.

    c. must always agree to any and all procedures or treatments.

    d. can expect to have private medical records made public.

89. The 1990 PSDA imposed the duty on health care institutions for

    a. obtaining informed consent.

    b. obtaining data for research and experimentation.

    c. informing patients of their right to advance directives.

    d. reprimanding patients who do not have advance directives.

CHAPTER 12

INCIDENT REPORTS

CHAPTER OBJECTIVE

After completing this chapter, the reader will be able to determine situations that require incident reports and explain the purpose of these reports.

LEARNING OBJECTIVES

After studying this chapter, the reader will be able to

1. select the definition of an incident report.

2. indicate two situations that require incident reports.

3. identify the proper documentation of an incident report.

4. specify how incident reports are used.

5. identify routing and location of the incident report.

INTRODUCTION

Also called accident, critical incident, or occurrence reports, incident reports describe an accident or a situation that could have resulted in an accident. Incident reports were developed in the late 1940s and early 1950s to identify events that were not consistent with routine operation of a hospital or routine care of patients or visitors, including but not limited to malfunctioning equipment or medication errors.

Incidents may lead to litigation, and a nurse may be named in the suit. Nursing negligence cases are beginning to appear with regularity in legal reports, legal journals, and insurance company publications. Although it is impossible to completely eliminate the risk of litigation, nurses must be aware of their actions. Nurses can prevent malpractice lawsuits if they pay careful attention to interpersonal relationships, use good communication techniques, and practice as any prudent nurse would in a similar situation. It is important for nurses to know and uphold institutional, professional, and legal standards of practice and work within their scope of practice. Attention to details helps improve patient outcomes and protect nurses against lawsuits.

Nurses can prevent litigation by providing safe, high-quality nursing care. Identifying potential problem areas, identifying risk areas in individual practice, and taking measures to minimize exposure to those risks may help nurses to avoid malpractice claims. Nursing actions that frequently end in malpractice cases tend to fall in four major categories: treatment; communication; medication; and monitoring, observing, and supervising. The 10 most common allegations in nursing malpractice cases that have been reported are listed in Table 12-1.

When an incident occurs, the nurse should first assess the patient for the extent of any injury that occurred and provide measures to prevent further injury. If a patient is injured, the nurse must take steps to protect the patient, himself or herself, and

TABLE 12-1: MALPRACTICE CLAIMS FOR ACCIDENTS

1. Patient falls
2. Failure to monitor
3. Failure to ensure patient safety
4. Improper performance of treatment
5. Failure to respond to patient
6. Medication error
7. Wrong dosage administered
8. Failure to follow hospital procedure
9. Improper technique
10. Failure to supervise treatment

(Aiken & Catalano, 1994)

the employer. Most agencies have policies regarding incidents. It is important to follow these policies and to not assume someone was negligent. Although negligence may be involved, incidents can and do happen even when every precaution has been taken to prevent them.

When an incident occurs, it is the legal responsibility of the nurse to document the facts in the patient's chart and to prepare an incident report. This chapter addresses the purpose and use of incident reports, situations that require incident reports, documentation in the medical record, and the proper routing and location of an incident report.

PURPOSE AND USE OF INCIDENT REPORTS

Incident reports are used to make all the facts about an unusual occurrence available to agency personnel, to contribute to statistical data about incidents, and to help health personnel prevent future incidents. The risk management department handles incident reports. Institutions that provide health care have risk management departments and programs to prevent, assess, and handle accidents when they occur. The purpose of these departments and programs is to identify potential risks, reduce the number of patient and staff injuries, and minimize the exposure of the institution to lawsuits.

An effective risk-management program includes monitoring and identifying potential risks to patients and staff and improving patient care and treatment practices. Risk management involves systematic screening with early detection of potential problems so changes can be made in an institution to prevent injuries or accidents. Staff education is a critical part of risk management. Not only must staff be educated in ways to avoid accidents, they also should be educated about what to do when an incident occurs. The staff must know also how to complete an incident report and where to send the form.

For a comprehensive risk management program to work, especially in relation to screening and reporting, the institution's employees must be encouraged to make reports without fear of retribution, loss of job, or other negative results. Only when staff, risk management, quality assurance, and peer review representatives work closely together in an atmosphere of trust and cooperation can patient care monitoring and evaluation work successfully.

As stated before, incident reports must be completed in the event of an unusual occurrence. There are numerous other reasons for reporting incidents; some are displayed in Table 12-2.

The incident reporting system relies on nurses and other staff members to recognize and report an incident. However, estimates vary from 5% to 30% on the accuracy of numbers of reports filed. Staff may not report incidents for several reasons, including but not limited to lack of understanding of the process, fear of punitive action, concern that the report exposes them to personal liability, reluctance to report incidents involving physicians, lack of time for paperwork, and lack of knowledge about results that may be achieved. Administrative actions that may result in reluctance to report incidents include withholding promotions, raises and disciplinary action, or firing employees who report incidents. Even though some situations do require these

TABLE 12-2: REASONS FOR REPORTING INCIDENTS
1. Federal, national, and state accrediting bodies require documentation and analysis of incidents as part of risk-management efforts.
2. The American Nurses Association Code for Nursing states that a nurse is expected to safeguard the patient and public when health and safety are affected by incompetent, unethical, or illegal practice of any person.
3. All health care institutions have a duty to inform the patient or his or her supervisors of a known deviation from the standard of care that caused an injury. Treating a patient with dignity means being honest about what happened during treatment.
4. Many lawsuits can be avoided if the institution takes prompt action following an incident. Strategies to use to reduce the incidence of lawsuits include showing concern, writing off a bill, providing no cost for future services, apologizing, or letting the family know a full investigation will be made.
5. The incident should trigger an investigation of the circumstances and the changes necessary to prevent recurrences. Employees may need referral for mental or substance abuse treatment.
6. Incident reports may be helpful in identifying situations that expose an institution to liability and indicate deficiencies in the institution. Recognition of these problems may result in improvements.
(Iyer & Camp, 1999; Kavaler & Spiegel, 1997; Pozgar, 2002)

actions, their routine use following an incident may prevent appropriate reporting.

When an incident is not reported, the health care institution is deprived of the opportunity to investigate the situation. The institution's attorney, risk manager, and insurance carrier review incident reports in order to determine how situations should be handled. Serious incidents should be reported to the risk manager immediately, and an incident report must be filled out. Failure to fill out an incident report or properly document an unusual event in the medical record can be considered a cover-up if and when an incident is revealed.

SITUATIONS THAT REQUIRE INCIDENT REPORTS

The Joint Commission for Accreditation of Healthcare Organizations (JCAHO) and the American Society for Healthcare Risk Management changed policies in 1997 and identified incidents that need to be reported. They also defined incidents as sentinel events. A sentinel event is any unexpected occurrence involving death or serious physical or psychological injury. Serious injury includes loss of

limb or function. The report signals the need for immediate investigation and follow-up. Incidents or sentinel events that should be reported are listed in Table 12-3. Various states, by law, require that certain incidents be reported within 24 hours of occurrence. Incidents that must be reported within 24 hours are found in Table 12-4.

Incidents on the lists in Tables 12-3 and 12-4 are reported to the health department by the institution's risk management department. Likewise, JCAHO encourages that a voluntary report of the event be submitted to JCAHO within 30 days. If corrective actions have not been taken in regard to the incident, JCAHO may make site visits, and the institution's accreditation could be in jeopardy.

Although it may not always be clear when an incident report should be filed, appropriate institutional procedures should be in place addressing how questionable events should be handled. When in doubt, it is wise to complete an incident report and send it through the proper channels.

TABLE 12-3: SENTINEL EVENTS THAT NEED TO BE REPORTED

- Treatment or procedural errors
- Medication, intravenous, and blood errors
- Hemolytic transfusion reactions
- Infections
- Falls
- Burns
- Equipment malfunctions and problems
- Rape (by another patient or staff member)
- Surgery on the wrong patient or wrong body part
- Patient death, paralysis, coma, or other major permanent loss of function associated with a medication error
- Suicide of a patient in an around-the-clock facility
- Suicide of a patient following elopement from a facility
- Any elopement that results in death or major permanent loss of function
- Any intrapartum maternal death
- Any perinatal death unrelated to a congenital condition in an infant weighing more than 2500 g
- Birth injuries
- Infant abduction
- Infant discharged to the wrong family
- Assault, homicide, or other crime resulting in a patient death or major permanent loss of function
- A patient fall that results in death or major permanent loss of function as a direct result of the injuries sustained in the fall

(Iyer & Camp, 1999; Kavaler & Spiegel, 1997)

TABLE 12-4: INCIDENTS REQUIRING REPORTS WITHIN 24 HOURS

- Patient deaths in circumstances other than those related to the natural course of illness
- Fires or internal disasters in an institution
- Equipment malfunction or equipment user error during treatment or diagnosis
- Poisoning occurring within the institution
- Reportable infection outbreaks
- Patient elopements and kidnappings
- Strikes by personnel
- Disasters or other emergency situations external to the institution's environment that affect operations
- Unscheduled termination of any services vital to the continued safe operation of the facility

(Kavaler & Spiegel, 1997; Pozgar, 2002)

INCIDENT REPORT DOCUMENTATION

The incident form is a formal document that requires objective information about the incident. Forms may vary greatly in format, size, shape, and comprehensiveness. Generally, they request information concerning the patient, a factual description of the incident, any injuries sustained, and the outcome of the situation. Lately, incident reports have changed from handwritten narrative reports to computerized reports. The computerized form facilitates the institution's ability to maintain statistics and analyze all incidents annually or more frequently. Overall, the form should be easy to use, objective, pertinent, and designed to be processed quickly. The nurse should become familiar with the employing institution's policies about how and when to complete an incident report.

A nurse with major concerns about the staffing of a unit may want to complete an incident form. This allows the nurse to express concerns about the potential inability to meet all patient needs. By filing an incident report, the nurse is making the supervisor and risk management department aware of a potentially dangerous situation.

Only the person who witnessed an incident or first discovered it should file and sign an incident report. Anyone else with firsthand knowledge should file a separate report. Anyone filling out an incident report should keep in mind that the written report will be available to lawyers, and any admissions or accusations could be damaging to the reporting individual as well as to the institution. Therefore, it is necessary to write only the facts about the incident. The plaintiff's attorney must subpoena the report to obtain a copy. There are some ways that an incident report may be protected from discovery. Some institutions have specific forms to complete for an inci-

dent, whereas others require narrative notes to be written. Following an incident, the nurse should either complete the form or write detailed narrative notes. Inquire about the incident reporting method at the institution in which you work.

If an incident report is directed to the legal department of the institution, it may be nondiscoverable because the institution can argue that the report was made in anticipation of litigation. Such documents are considered "work product," which are generally not discoverable.

When an incident occurs, the nurse should complete the incident report in accordance with institution rules and guidelines. There are several do's and don'ts regarding completing an incident report, as presented in Table 12-5. When writing an incident report, the nurse should remember to use the rules for good documentation. Use your senses—what you see, hear, smell, feel, taste—and document only facts. It is very critical to not place any blame or add any subjective information. Never admit a mistake or include explanations as to how the incident could have been avoided. Make sure to document the data and time of the incident and the names of the physician, supervisor, and family members who were notified. Complete the incident report as soon as possible, preferably on the same day that the incident occurred. If additional

TABLE 12-5: TIPS FOR REPORTING INCIDENTS

DO record the details in objective terms, describing exactly what was seen and nothing else. For example, Nurse Jones writes that she found Mrs. Smith sitting on the floor beside the bed, not that Mrs. Jones fell out of bed.

DO describe what actions were taken at the scene (for example, "helped patient back to bed"); assessment findings; and any instructions given to the patient.

DO document the time of the incident, the name of the doctor notified, and the time notified and have the supervisor review the report.

DON'T include names and addresses of witnesses, even if the form requests such information. Such data makes it easier for attorneys to sue the institution. Check with the supervisor about supplying this information.

DON'T file the incident report with the patient's chart and do not chart that an incident report was completed and filed. Send the incident report to the institution's designated person who collects and reviews such matters.

DON'T admit liability or blame or identify others as responsible. Any incrimination could be harmful to an institution if a lawsuit occurs.

(Kavaler & Spiegel, 1997; Tiller, 1994)

information is obtained after filling out an incident report, write an amendment and attach it to the report rather than crossing out, altering, or destroying the original report. Once the form is completed, the nurse should follow the chain of command in terms of submitting the report. This way, everyone necessary to the process will be informed.

DOCUMENTING IN THE MEDICAL RECORD

Communication of the facts of an incident is the most critical component for avoiding a lawsuit. Clear, concise, meaningful communication is essential, especially when an incident occurs. In today's health care environment, where downsizing, changes in staffing mix, and increased patient acuity are the norm, nurses must use effective and efficient communication to provide adequate care.

The patient's medical record should contain a factual, honest, and objective description of the incident. The nurse should clearly describe the patient assessment, intervention, follow-up care, and patient response. Directly quote the patient's description of what happened. Clearly indicate the date and time as well as the name of the physician notified, along with what the physician was told, and note any orders received. All follow-up assessments made need to be clearly documented. Close follow-up indicates that the patient's condition was closely monitored after the incident. Clear, concise documentation provides information about the appropriate care provided following an incident.

Never write in the chart that an incident report was completed. This prevents drawing attention to the report. Physicians should not write orders for incident reports to be written. The nurse may verbally remind the physician that doing so would prompt an attorney to request a copy of the incident report. The information documented in the medical record should provide adequate information to the plaintiff's attorney.

It is important to document any statement made by the patient, family members, and visitors. These statements sometimes demonstrate actions of the patient, family, or visitor that contributed to the incident. For example, "Patient stated she went to the bathroom and fell even though the nurse told her to call for help." The defense attorney can use this documentation to prove the patient, family, or visitor was guilty of contributory or comparative negligence. *Contributory negligence* refers to actions by the patient, family, visitor that contribute to the patient's injuries. In this case, the patient may not have a claim and would be unable to receive any compensation for the injury.

Known as *comparative negligence*, some states have adopted a policy so that a jury decides the percentage of the injury the patient caused and the percentage the nurse caused. Compensation is then based on the percentages. For example, a jury may find the patient 80% responsible and the nurse 20% responsible. Therefore, the patient would be compensated for only 20% of the requested damages.

When a patient or family member makes a comment about actions they will or may take against the institution, physician, or nurses, it is wise to document these comments. Once again, document the exact statement, place the statement in quotation marks, and describe it objectively. For an example, see Table 12-6.

TABLE 12-6: CHARTING FAMILY COMMENTS
Patient's husband stated very loudly, "I will have the physician's head for this and everyone else involved." Patient's husband then threw a book at the door.

Such comments help the defense attorney evaluate the tone of the situation, and the jury can evaluate the situation more completely.

If a nurse believes a certain situation might end up in a lawsuit, he or she should write an accurate description of the incident as a chronological listing of events. All factual details about the incident should be recorded. This information may be helpful if a case develops. Attach the list to the incident report and send it to the supervisor or the quality assurance department. It is not advisable for a nurse or anyone else to make a copy of an incident report or any other notes about an incident.

Even though factually documenting the incident in the medical record and completing an incident report may seem like duplication of effort, both are important. The information in the patient's record provides an accurate account of the incident and how it was handled and resolved. The incident report is critical so that everyone in the chain of command is informed and the incident can be analyzed for trends and needed changes in policy, if necessary.

Once an incident has occurred, the physician has been notified, and the incident report has been completed, the report is sent to the supervisor and then on to the risk manager. The nurse completing an incident report should clearly think through the situation and consult with other nurses, particularly the head or charge nurse. In critical or volatile situations, it is important that the head or charge nurse and the nursing supervisor be well informed of the situation. If the nurse believes that he or she knows what is going on with the patient, he or she should not be afraid to speak up, even if he or she uses a medical diagnosis. It is critical that a nurse inform the charge or head nurse with gathered facts so that instantaneous lifesaving interventions can be started in a timely manner to prevent the patients' condition from progressing into respiratory or cardiac arrest. Documenting the use of the chain of command is very important in difficult patient situations. It is critical that a nurse inform the charge or head nurse with gathered facts so that lifesaving interventions can be started in a timely manner to prevent a patient's condition from progressing into a poor outcome.

The scenario presented in Table 12-7 did not require an incident report, however, it demonstrates proper documentation and use of the chain of command. However, the baby was born severely depressed and eventually died. The documented information will be helpful to the defense attorney to demonstrate that the patient's actions contributed to the damages caused to the fetus, if litigation results.

How the nurse responds in a given situation depends on the emergent status of the patient. All persons notified should be fully informed of the situation. Each phase of activation of the chain of command should be clearly documented. The focus is always patient safety. Clear, concise communication is a powerful tool in assuring quality patient care. It is essential for a nurse, whose major responsibility is to advocate for the patient. In addition, effective documentation of the events provides legal protection for nurses and the institution.

ROUTING AND STORAGE OF INCIDENT REPORTS

Depending on the institution's organization, a nursing supervisor is likely to be responsible for getting an incident report to the risk manager. The risk manager may initiate an investigation of the incident. The incident report may be directed to the institution's legal department; then the institution's attorney retains the information. One example of the routing of an incident report is displayed in Table 12-8 on page 243. Copies of all incident reports are normally retained in the risk management office.

Incident reports should be kept for approximately 5 years, unless dictated otherwise by state law or the institution's record retention policy. The longest retention policy should be followed. Records that are subject to potential litigation, as well as all records requested by an attorney or administrative agency, should be retained until the case is completely resolved.

An institution's insurance company works closely with the legal department and risk management in the prevention and evaluation of incidents. Consultation between insurance company representatives and institutional risk management personnel

TABLE 12-7: DOCUMENTING CHAIN OF COMMAND

	08-14-03 FHTs 85-95 bpm after baseline of 130-142. Contractions q 5-6 min, mild.
13:00	Turned pt. to left side. O2 via nasal cannula at 8 L. Dr. Barnes notified of above findings. _____C. Crow, RN
13:30	Dr. Barnes (on call for Dr. Alph) at bedside. Talked with pt. re: need for C-section. Pt. refusing C-section. FHT 95-100, no variability, no accelerations. Contractions q 5-6 min., mild. Dr. Barnes telephoned Dr. Alph. Dr. Alph to come in. _____C. Crow, RN
13:35	J. Jones, RN, head nurse and C. Smith, RN, supervisor, at bedside. Both explained situation and need for C-section. Pt. refused to consent to C-section. Pt. stated, "wanted to wait for mother and Dr. Alph." See fetal monitor strip. _____C. Crow, RN
13:40	Mother at bedside. C. Smith, RN, supervisor, talked to pt. and mother. Mother encouraged pt. to have C-section. Pt stated, "I want to wait for Dr. Alph." Pt. turned to right side. O2 on, scalp stimulation, FHT 75-85 after stimulation. _____C. Crow, RN
13:45	C. Smith, RN, supervisor, at bedside. Dr. Alph arrived and advised of situation. Dr. Alph at bedside, repeated need for C-section. _____C. Crow, RN
13:47	Consent for C-section signed. Abdominal prep, Foley catheter inserted, NICU and pediatrician notified. Dr. Barnes notified to assist. _____C. Crow, RN
13:50	Patient transferred to surgery room for C-section. _____C. Crow, RN

aims to help the institution minimize the risk of malpractice claims. Insurance companies, the institution's legal counsel, and risk managers continuously evaluate claims against an institution. This is done to analyze and identify ways to prevent future claims or to correct situations that lead to claims. The computer program incident form mentioned earlier assists in the analysis process. Computer programs assist risk managers in identifing areas needing change, reducing preventable adverse events, and minimizing financial loss to an institution in the event of lawsuits.

CONCLUSION

Prompt identification of injuries and accidents to patients, family members, visitors, and staff members is a primary concern of a risk management program. Identification requires a nurse or other health care provider to complete an incident report. Incident reports help institutions address potential problems and correct their causes before they reoccur.

Incident reports are used to provide communication about and analysis of incidents. Specific forms are available for reporting an incident. Forms may vary from institution to institution as well as by state. It is important for a nurse witnessing the incident to complete an incident form, present it to the head nurse, and follow the chain of command so that all necessary personnel are informed. The report is then retained in the risk management department. Nurses must complete an incident report for any unusual event not consistent with the routine operation of an institution or the routine care of a patient. It is the legal and professional responsibility of a nurse to follow through with this process as part of the documentation process.

TABLE 12-8: OVERVIEW OF INCIDENT REPORT ROUTING

Patient incident occurs.

↓

Report significant medical and nursing facts in the patient's medical record.

↓

Write incident report during the shift on which the incident took place.

↓

Give incident report to supervisor.

↓

Unit supervisor forwards report to appropriate administrator within 24 hours.

↓

Administrator reviews report.

↓

Administrator forwards pertinent information from the report to
the appropriate department for follow-up action.

↓

Incident reports are collected and summarized to detect patterns and trends and highlight trouble spots.

↓

Administrator reviews patterns and trends and decides whether incidents are result of poor policies
or from nursing errors.

↓	↓
If incidents result from policy problems, the institution makes appropriate policy changes.	If incidents result from nursing errors, the appropriate personnel review nursing records to detect trends.
	↓
	If the records indicate a pattern of errors or if the error being reviewed is grievous, the institution offers appropriate remediation, such as counseling, a refresher course or, rarely, probation or suspension.

EXAM QUESTIONS

CHAPTER 12
Questions 90-94

90. An incident report is

    a. a report that is kept in the patient's record.

    b. completed by the supervisor involved in the incident.

    c. a report of an unusual event not consistent with routine operations or routine patient care.

    d. written so that recommendations on how to prevent further incidents are clearly spelled out.

91. Occurrences that could require an incident report include

    a. equipment malfunctions and patient falls.

    b. safety precautions in place and universal precautions being used.

    c. equipment sent for repair and use of the five rights of medication administration.

    d. education of staff in regard to infant abduction and infant discharged to wrong family.

92. When an incident report is completed, the nurse documents in the patient's record

    a. that an incident report was made and sent to the risk management department.

    b. that the physician was requested to write an order for an incident report.

    c. the facts of the incident, interventions, physician notification, and follow-up.

    d. all recommendations about how to prevent the incident in the future.

93. Incident reports are used because

    a. regulating bodies require documentation and analysis of incidents.

    b. institutions do not have a duty to inform patients of known deviations.

    c. an incident should trigger an investigation so necessary changes may be made to cover up the incident.

    d. incidents do not really need to be reported other than to the physician.

94. A nurse completing an incident report should

    a. place the report in the patient's medical record.

    b. give the report to the nursing supervisor.

    c. give a copy of the report to the patient.

    d. not bother to write a report, since it is too time consuming.

CHAPTER 13

DOCUMENTATION FOR ADVANCED PRACTICE NURSES

CHAPTER OBJECTIVE

After completing this chapter, the reader will be able to discuss how advanced practitioners differ from other nurses and how nurse practitioners document management of patient care.

LEARNING OBJECTIVES

After studying this chapter, the reader will be able to

1. indicate the definition of advanced practice nursing.

2. identify the laws that control advanced practice nursing.

3. specify four clinical areas in which advanced practice nurses specialize.

4. identify advanced practice nursing standards and clinical practice.

5. indicate legal issues that have an impact on the scope of practice of an advanced practice nurse.

6. identify situations in the advanced practice nurse's practice that may have potential legal liability.

INTRODUCTION

The advanced practice nurse (APN) role grew out of a need to increase access to primary care and a shortage of primary care physicians. The first APN program began in 1965 to prepare pediatric APNs with a focus on health and wellness. Federal legislation in the mid-1960s provided funding to support the development of primary care providers. In 1971, the Secretary of Health, Education, and Welfare issued primary care initiatives supporting APNs as primary care providers, with recommendations that nurses and physicians should work together and share responsibilities.

By the mid-1970s, more than 500 APN programs existed across the United States. Most of these programs were certificate-granting programs. By the 1980s, most APN programs had become incorporated into master's degree programs because accrediting bodies were requiring a higher level of education. In response to health care reform in the 1990s, APN programs proliferated. A National Sample Survey of Registered Nurses, conducted in 2000, (Spratley, Johnson, Sochalski, Fritz, & Spencer, 2002) found that an estimated 196,279 RNs or 7.3% of the RN population were practicing as APNs. Advanced Practice Nurses have been providing primary and preventative health care for over 35 years. They work in all 50 states, in a variety of settings, including hospitals, nursing homes, businesses, private practices, HMOs, schools, and community centers. Some APNs have their own practices, but most work in collaboration with a physician. Many APNs can prescribe medications, order and evaluate laboratory, x-ray and other diagnostic tests. They can refer to specialists and other community resources. Nurse-managed health care centers are often run by APNs and are frequently located in neighborhood and community settings. This chapter defines the APN, presents information about the differences between registered nurses (RNs) and APNs, and covers areas of specialization, governance, standards of practice, legal issues, and documentation requirements. An undergraduate nurse seeking information about the advanced nursing role may find this chapter helpful.

DEFINITION OF ADVANCED PRACTICE NURSE

The APN is a skilled RN who has successfully completed an additional course of study in a master's level nursing specialty that provides knowledge and skills to function in an expanded role. APNs use critical judgment in the performance of comprehensive health assessments, differential diagnosis, and the prescription of pharmacologic and nonpharmacologic treatments in the direct management of patients with acute and chronic illnesses and disease. APNs act independently or in collaboration with other health care professionals to deliver health care services.

APNs conduct comprehensive health assessments aimed at health promotion and disease prevention. They can diagnose and manage common acute illnesses, with appropriate referrals, and manage stable chronic conditions in a variety of settings. APNs are qualified to resolve unmet needs in primary health care by serving as patients' initial contact with the health care system. The focus of care is on promotion and maintenance of wellness as well as diagnosis and management of acute and stable chronic illnesses.

The overlap of functions performed by APNs and physicians is recognized within the medical-legal community. APNs who are functioning within their scope of practice provide quality care. An APN focuses on prevention, wellness, and education. Today the number of APNs equals the number of practicing family practice physicians. The growth in numbers of APNs has a significant impact in the delivery of timely, cost-effective, quality health care, especially to chronically underserved populations such as the elderly, the poor, and those in rural areas. With an emphasis on health promotion, disease prevention, and a proven record of providing excellent primary care in diverse settings, APNs form a critical link in the solution to America's health care crisis. Studies indicate that APNs provide safe, cost-effective, quality primary care and they also provide care equivalent to or better than that of physicians (American Nurses Association, 2005; Sherwood Brown, Fay, & Wardell, 1997).

The expanded role of the APN involves advanced education in an area of specialization with increased responsibility, both professionally and legally. The APN's focus is on providing quality nursing care in the promotion of health and the prevention of illness. An APN's goals are to be able to legally practice to the fullest extent of his or her education, skills, and training.

AREAS OF SPECIALIZATION

RNs who are academically prepared to function in an expanded role generally fall into four categories: certified RN anesthetists (CRNAs), certified nurse-midwives (CNMs), nurse practitioners (NPs), and clinical nurse specialists (CNSs). APNs practice in a variety of specialty areas, as displayed in Table 13-1.

A CRNA is a professional RN who is licensed to practice nursing and has become an anesthesia specialist by successfully completing an approved and accredited graduate nurse-anesthetist program. A CRNA has also passed a national qualifying exam and maintains certification through continuing education requirements. For more than 100 years, nurse-

TABLE 13-1: APN SPECIALTY AREAS
• Acute care
• Pediatrics
• Geriatrics
• Emergency medicine
• Family practice
• Obstetrics-gynecology
• Neonatology
• Adult medicine
• Psychiatry
• School health
• Women's health
(Berry & Mackay, 2001; Sherwood, et al. 1997)

anesthetists have been providing anesthesia in a safe, cost-effective, and highly competent manner.

A CNM is an RN with additional education in the independent management of women in the areas of pregnancy, childbirth, postpartum care, care of the newborn, and gynecology, including family planning. A CNM has advanced education and has successfully passed a certification exam. CNMs provide maternal-fetal services in traditional clinical and hospital settings as well as in birthing centers and patient's homes. Nurse-midwives have demonstrated that collaborative practice can exist in health care practice.

A CNS is an RN with a graduate level education and supervised practice who has become an expert in a defined area of knowledge and practices in that specific area of clinical nursing. There are more than 13,000 CNSs providing care to patients in a variety of practice areas, including but not limited to cardiology, pulmonology, oncology, rheumatology, medical-surgical, pediatrics, lactation, and psychiatry. A CNS is involved with case management and education of patients with specific diseases and conditions. Although role identification separates CNSs from APNs, they are still recognized as APNs; however, they have the least involvement with the legal system.

All APNs have some authority to prescribe certain medications according to established protocols and individual state laws. California was the first state to grant prescriptive authority to nurses. Since 1991, APNs in several states have received limited authority to prescribe medications.

Currently, Georgia is the only state in the U.S. that prohibits APNs from writing prescriptions. APNs are authorized to phone a prescription in under a physician's name, but only the physician can sign a medication order.

The battle continues today in regard to prescriptive authority. Regardless of the practice setting, all APNs provide direct care and all are capable of functioning independently or interdependently in a highly competent and cost-effective manner.

APN GOVERNANCE AND STANDARDS

Each state has a nurse practice act that was established by the legislature and is enforced by the executive branch of the government through the state's regulatory agencies. Some states regulate APNs through the state nursing board, some through the state medical board, and others use a combination of nursing and medical boards. In order to administer the state's statutory law regarding APNs, the designated regulatory board issues rules and regulations that govern specific acts performed by APNs. Regulatory agencies are also responsible for establishing licensure application requirements, the requirements for maintaining licensure, and disciplinary actions. Safe practice requires APNs to be familiar with the regulatory board's rules and regulations regarding practice as well as with the state's licensing and practice acts.

No uniform sources of law govern APNs. Most states have nurse practice acts that authorize APNs within statutory frameworks. Most rules and regulations govern the scope of practice of APNs; however, eight states do not recognize CNSs as APNs.

Many states rely on national standards developed by each specialty when defining the scope of practice. A licensed RN completes an additional state APN licensing form and pays an additional fee in order to be recognized as an APN within the state.

An APN must apply for recognition as an APN in each state. However, the National Council of State Boards of Nursing has recently released a draft for an Advanced Practice Registered Nurse Compact, similar to the RN intrastate compact. One of the general purposes of the APN compact is to encourage the cooperation of party states in the areas of APN licensure and authority to adopt regulations, including uniform licensure requirements. The draft indicates that to participate in the APN compact, the state must also participate in the RN compact.

Having successfully completed advanced education, a nurse may become licensed to practice as an advanced practitioner. Some states require APNs to have certification through the state board of nurse examiners or another certifying organization. Examples of some of the certifying organizations are listed in Table 13-2.

Credentialing refers to the validation of required education, licensure, and certification. Credentialing of APNs is necessary not only to assure the public of safe health care provided by qualified individuals but also to ensure compliance with federal and state laws relating to nursing practice. Legal regulations provide clear authority for qualified APNs to provide advanced nursing care. Credentialing acknowledges an APN's advanced scope of practice and mandates accountability. Credentialing allows the profession to be accountable to the public and its members by enforcing professional standards of practice.

In 1993, the American Academy of Nurse Practitioners (AANP) developed standards for practice that specify activities within the APN scope of practice and govern the services provided. The standards cover qualifications, the process of care, environment, collaborative responsibilities, documentation, patient advocacy, quality assurance, supporting roles, and research. APNs provide primary health care services to individuals, families, groups of patients, and communities. The general scope of services provided by APNs falls into three categories: assessment of health status, diagnosis, and case management. The National Organization of Nurse Practitioner Faculties (NONPF, 2002) provides detailed domains and competencies required for the education of APNs.

APNs with a designated clinical focus or specialty may add specific activities to their scope of practice that reflects the needs of the target population served. Specialty organizations provide standards and guidelines for APNs functioning within that specialty area. Some APNs seek additional training and experience to be able to perform additional advanced clinical procedures (such as colposcopy) that further expand their scope of practice. These procedures should be geared toward prior experience, additional education and training, and the practice restrictions of individual state nurse practice acts.

TABLE 13-2: APN CERTIFYING ORGANIZATIONS

American Academy of Nurse Practitioners (AANP)

American Nurses Association (ANA)

American Nurses Credentialing Center (ANCC)

National Association of Nurse Practitioners in Women's Health (NPWH)

National Certification Corporation for the Obstetric, Gynecological, and Neonatal Nursing Specialties (NCC)

Pediatric Nursing Certification Board (PNCB)

(Berry & Mackay, 2001; Sherwood et al., 1997)

APNs are held legally accountable for their own actions and are responsible for using independent and rational judgments based on competent assessments. The most important legal principle that an APN should understand is that each and every APN is responsible for any personal wrongful actions or omissions that may cause harm to another person. Statutory law has established that an APN has the legal authority to practice under the individual nurse's license; authority does not flow from a physician's or any other health care provider's license. These statutes include each state's nurse practice act, specific statutory rules and regulations, professional standards, and case law. APNs must have knowledge of the laws that affect their practice and know the legal parameters in which they may provide health care services.

LEGAL ISSUES

Barriers to APN practice remain, even though there have been changes in many states' nurse practice acts. The three major barriers to practice include lack of third-party reimbursement, prescriptive authority, and hospital admission privileges.

APNs working with specialty organizations and legislative powers are advocating for full reimbursement for all treatments provided. Medicare has changed over the past years, and some APNs may now be reimbursed 100%. Many insurance companies follow Medicare's lead about reimbursement; however, most insurance companies do not reimburse APNs completely. Federal and state legislative sessions involve efforts to support total reimbursement for APNs.

Nursing organizations are actively involved with various state legislative groups to obtain full prescriptive authority for APNs. States vary in their control over this issue. APNs argue that limiting prescriptive authority limits the care they can provide.

When APNs are not allowed to admit their patients to the hospital, follow them during their stay, or obtain referral information when discharged, the concept of continuity of primary care is altered. Depending on state regulations, some APNs are now able to apply for hospital privileges. Each APN must know state laws and hospital regulations in order to apply for privileges.

Relatively few lawsuits have been filed against APNs, despite an increase of the expanded role. The majority of reported cases filed against APNs involve allegations of negligence. Nurse-anesthetists have the longest history of practice and also have the greatest number of reported cases.

The best action to prevent malpractice is for an APN to become familiar with the laws, statutes, rules, regulations, standards, and practice guidelines that govern the boundaries of his or her practice. APNs should not extend their practice beyond those boundaries. Likewise, APNs should refer patients when the required care exceeds their abilities.

APNs must stay current in their practice to avoid lawsuits. Just like any other nurse, reading professional journals, attending conferences, and maintaining certification is important. It would also be beneficial for APNs to take an active role in state or national organizations and legislature to promote APN practice.

APN DOCUMENTATION

Documentation of an APN's management of care for a patient is very important because the impact of inadequate or poor documentation may result in the appearance of malpractice, negligence, fraud, or abuse. Proper documentation of each patient encounter is critical for professional practice.

All documentation standards, regulations, and suggestions previously discussed for RNs also apply to APNs. An APN's documentation may appear somewhat different because of the emphasis on the assessment and the medical diagnosis; however, most APNs use a form of a SOAP note. The purposes of documentation are to record the patient's report of symptoms, past medical history, lifestyle and family factors, positive and negative findings on physical exam, and the APN's conclusions and actions. An accurate record is essential to remind the practitioner of findings and actions for the next follow-up visit. Once again, it is very important that an APN's documentation be complete, accurate, and timely and that it clearly state the facts. An example of an APN's SOAP note is found in Table 13-3.

APNs are responsible for billing for services using current procedural terminology (CPT) codes. The CPT manual and the documentation guidelines for evaluation and management services are updated annually and can be accessed at the CMS website. Correct CPT coding can have a significant impact on reimbursement. An APN must stay up-to-date on changes to the codes and guidelines in order to prevent fraud or abuse concerns. *Fraud* refers to intentional deception of billing health care services to payers. Inadequate documentation of the code used for the service places an APN at risk for being charged with medical fraud. Substantiated charges of fraud may result in loss of provider status, loss of employment, loss of or restrictions on the APN's license by the board of nursing, a monetary fine, and a possible prison sentence. APN documentation is reviewed very closely. The APN role requires expert knowledge of the coding rules and regulations as well as appropriate documentation in order to prevent billing errors. APNs who document completely, accurately, and timely can minimize the risk of liability and avoid charges of fraud and abuse. Correct coding allows APNs to be properly reimbursed for their work.

CONCLUSION

The role of the APN continues to evolve in response to changing societal and health care needs as consumers in all settings seek increasing services. APNs have additional education and practices independently or interdependently with physicians. APNs are accountable for their actions, practice, and documentation. Following standards of practice as well as federal and state rules and regulations, APNs must clearly document management of patient care to prevent allegations of fraud or abuse and to be properly reimbursed.

TABLE 13-3: SAMPLE APN SOAP NOTE (1 OF 2)

September 30, 2004

HP: 31 y/o B.F.

CC: "My boyfriend has gonorrhea and he brought me in here to be tested."

S: Denies dysuria, frequency, urgency, or vaginal discharge. Afebrile. No OTC medications used. LMP 8/23/03. Last intercourse 2 days ago. PMH: None, denies previous STD. CHH: NKDA, does not smoke, alcohol occasionally, denies illicit drug use. Sexually active since age 14, several partners but in monogamous relationship last 8 months. G4T1P1A2L1. BTL in 2000. Uses condoms regularly. Routinely does SBE. Normal Pap smear 1 year ago. FH: Mother has HTN; father deceased, gunshot wounds. 4 sisters, 2 brothers, all healthy. P/S: Lives with boyfriend, daughter lives with patient's mother; Student at K Business College. ROS: Noncontributory.

O: Wt. 118 lbs., Temp. 97.8, BP 110/56, P. 74, R 18.

        Skin warm, pink, dry. HEENT: Benign. Neck supple, no adenopathy. Chest: CTA, respirations even and unlabored, symmetrical expansion. Heart: RRR, no murmurs, gallops, rubs, S3 or S4. ABD: Flat, soft, no tenderness, +BS X 4 quadrants, No organomegaly, bruit or CVAT. Genitalia exam: Labia clean, pink, moist; no discharge or erythema; BUS negative; no urethral discharge. Pelvic exam: Vagina pink and moist, without erythema or discharge. Cervix pink, no discharge, lesions, erosion, vesicles or CMT. Uterus not enlarged, ovaries barely palpable. No rectal bleeding or discharge. Labs: Wet-prep, minimal white cells present, otherwise noncontributory.

A: Diagnosis: Probable gonorrhea

        Differential Diagnosis: Chlamydia, BV, *Trichomonas, Candida,* UTI, PID

        Risk Identification: At risk for STD

P: **Medications:**

        Ceftriaxone (Rocephin) 250 mg IM X 1 dose now (in Rt. hip)

        Doxycycline 100 mg BID X 7 days

        Nonpharmacologic Measures:

        No sexual intercourse while on meds

        Report sexual contacts for treatment

        Labs:

        GC and *Chlamydia* cultures; Pap smear, blood for syphilis screen.

        Education and Interventions:

        1. Discuss with patient and partner the nature of the infectious process.

        2. Praise patient for using condoms and reemphasize continued use to protect herself from reinfection and spread of disease.

        3. Instruct about medications, including dosage, frequency, interactions, and need to complete amount given.

        4. Advise patient and partner to abstain from intercourse for 1 week and to always use condoms.

        5. Encourage patient to express concerns regarding condition to help alleviate anxiety. Provide emotional support.

TABLE 13-3: SAMPLE APN SOAP NOTE (2 OF 2)

Follow up:

Return in 1 week to review lab reports and repeat cultures for test of cure if previous cultures positive.

Consultation and Referral:

1. Failure to improve or recurrence or positive follow-up culture

2. Pharyngitis

3. Acute abdominal disorders or salpingitis

4. Tender, swollen adnexa

5. Disseminated gonococcal infection with skin lesions

6. Endocarditis

Contact and Reporting:

Report case and treatment to health department in patient's county of residence.

EXAM QUESTIONS

CHAPTER 13
Questions 95-100

95. A nurse who is educated in the delivery of primary health care and the assessment of psychosocial and physical health problems such as the performance of routine examinations and the ordering of routine diagnostic tests is

    a. a nursing supervisor.

    b. a student nurse.

    c. an APN.

    d. a CNS.

96. The APN's practice is governed by standards that have been developed by the

    a. AMA.

    b. NCC.

    c. AANP.

    d. JCAHO.

97. An advanced practice nurse who specializes in the management of pregnant women is best known as a

    a. CRNA.

    b. MDD.

    c. CNM.

    d. CNS.

98. An APN may specialize in a specific area such as

    a. pediatrics, adult medicine, or women's health.

    b. diet, telemetry, or surgery.

    c. women's health, labor and delivery, or postanesthesia care.

    d. family practice, surgery scrub nurse, or diet.

99. A legal issue that has impacted the scope of practice of APNs is

    a. lack of third-party reimbursement.

    b. collaboration with physicians.

    c. assessment of health status and diagnosis and treatment of common and chronic diseases.

    d. assurance of safe health care practices and compliance with federal and state laws.

100. Although relatively few lawsuits have been filed against APNs, the majority of the cases involved allegations of

    a. battery.

    b. fraud.

    c. negligence.

    d. conspiracy.

This concludes the final examination.

RESOURCES

ANA NURSING STANDARDS

(http://www.nursingworld.org/books/pdescr.cfm?CNum=15)

Scope and Standards for Nurse Administrators

Scope and Standards of Advanced Practice Registered Nursing

Scope and Standards of College Health Nursing Practice

Scope and Standards of Diabetes Nursing

Scope and Standards of Forensic Nursing Practice

Scope and Standards of Home Health Nursing Practice

Scope and Standards of Nursing Informatics Practice

Scope and Standards of Nursing Practice in Correctional Facilities

Scope and Standards of Parish Nursing Practice

Scope and Standards of Pediatric Oncology Nursing

Scope and Standards of Practice for Nursing Professional Development

Scope and Standards of Professional School Nursing Practice

Scope and Standards of Public Health Nursing Practice

Standards and Scope of Gerontological Nursing Practice

Standards of Addiction Nursing Practice with Selected Diagnoses and Criteria

Standards of Clinical Nursing Practice (2nd ed.)

Standards of Clinical Practice and Scope of Practice for the Acute Care Nurse Practitioner

Statement on the Scope and Standards for the Nurse Who Specializes in Development Disabilities and/or Mental Retardation

Statement on the Scope and Standards of Genetics Clinical Nursing Practice

Statement on the Scope and Standards of Oncology Nursing Practice

Statement on the Scope and Standards of Otorhinolaryngology Clinical Nursing

Statement on the Scope and Standards of Pediatric Clinical Nursing Practice

BOOKS

American Nurses Association. (2003) *Principles for Documentation*. Washington, DC: Author. Single copies of the *Principles for Documentation* (item PD-1) are available free to constituent nurses association members only by calling 1-800-274-4ANA.

Burke, L.J. & Murphy, J.A. (1995). *Charting by exception applications: Making it work in clinical settings*. New York: Delmar.

Carpenito, L.J. (2003). *Nursing care plans and documentation (4th ed.)*. Philadelphia: Lippincott Williams & Wilkins.

ChartSmart: *The A-to-Z guide to better nursing documentation*. (2001). Philadelphia: Lippincott Williams, & Wilkins.

Fuzy, J. (2000). *The importance of observation and documentation*. Albuquerque, NM: Hartman.

Iyer, P.W. & Camp, N.H. (1999). *Nursing documentation: A nursing process approach.* St. Louis: Mosby.

Joint Commission on Accreditation. (2002). *A Practical Guide to Documentation in Behavioral Health Care*, 2nd ed. To order call 1-877-223-6866 or go to http://www.jcrinc.com/ publications

Marrelli, T.M. (2000). *Nursing documentation handbook (3rd ed.).* St. Louis: Mosby.

Meiner, S.E. (Ed.). (1999). *Nursing documentation: Legal focus across practice settings.* Thousand Oaks, CA: Sage.

Richmond, J. (1997). *Nursing documentation. Writing what we do.* Melbourne, Australia: Ausmed Publications.

Surefire documentation: How, what, and when nurses need to document. (1999) St. Louis: Mosby.

White, L. (2003). *Documentation & the nursing process: A review.* Albany, NY: Delmar.

JOURNAL ARTICLES

Andrus, S., Dubois, J., Jansen, C., Kuttner, V., Lansberry, N., & Lukowski, L. (2003). Teaching documentation tool: Building a successful discharge. *Critical Care Nurse, 23*(2), 39-48.

Anonymous. (1999). Charting tips. Using SOAP, SOAPIE, & SOAPIER formats. *Nursing, 29*(9), 75.

Anonymous. (1999). How to document patient education effectively: Records prove teaching and communication. *Hospital Case Management, 7*(5), 94-95.

Anonymous. (2000). Recommended practices for documentation of perioperative nursing care. *AORN Journal, 71*(1), 247-246, 250.

Benitez, O., Devaux, D., & Dausset, J. (2002.) Audiovisual documentation of oral consent: A new method of informed consent for illiterate populations. *Lancet, 359*(9315), 1406-1407.

Beyea, S.C. (2001). The ideal state for perioperative nursing. *AORN Journal, 73*(5), 897-901.

Boroughs, D.S. (1999). Documentation in the long-term care setting. *Journal of Nursing Administration, 29*(12), 46-49.

Cagliuso, N.V. (2000). Take note! Thorough documentation of patient care may prevent legal wranglings. *Emergency Medical Services, 29*(2), 30-32.

Chalmers, J., & Muir, R. (2003). Patient privacy and confidentiality. *British Medical Journal,* 326(7392), 725-726.

Chapman, G. F. (1999). Charting tips. Documenting an adverse incident. *Nursing, 29*(2), 17.

Cudmore, J. (2000). Write it down, for everyone's sake. *Nursing Times, 96*(10), 26.

Dumpel, H., James, M., & Phillips, T. (1999). Charting by exception. *California Nurse, 95*(5), 12-14, 23.

Heatherly, D. (1999). Home care 101: Focus on documentation: Excellence is in the details. *Home Care Nurse News, 6*(8), 1-2, 6.

Henley, D.E. (2003). Coding better for better reimbursement. *Family Practice Management, 10*(1), 29-35.

Hill, M. (2002). Are you aware? Are you prepared? *Dermatology Nursing, 14*(5), 302-303.

Jones, M.L., Day, S., Creely, J., Woodland, M.B., & Gerdes, J.B. (1999). Implementation of a clinical pathway system in maternal newborn care: A comprehensive documentation system for outcomes management. *Journal of Perinatal & Neonatal Nursing, 13*(3), 1-20.

Knight, S., Calvesbert, K., Clarke, J., & Williamson, J. (2002). Developing a nursing observation chart. *Emergency Nurse, 10*(3), 16-17.

Light, I., Immanuel, M.S., Augustine, A., & Seshadri, L. (2000). Flow sheet for better documentation in the labour room. *Nursing Journal of India, 91*(3), 70.

Lundberg, C.B. (2000). Nursing informatics: Using uniform language in patient care documentation. *Nursing Economic$, 18*(1), 38-39.

Martin, A., Hinds, C., & Felix, M. (1999). Documentation practices of nurses in long-term care. *Journal of Clinical Nursing, 8*(4), 345-352.

Minix, S. & Mercer, C. (2000). Review of old process uncovers better methods: Improving documentation step by step. *Patient Education Management, 7*(3), 32-34, 36, insert 4p.

Nelson, A. (2000). Accurate documentation. *Nursing Times, 96*(4 NT plus), 10-11.

Radcliffe, M. (1999). Don't let the notes grind you down. *Nursing Times, 95*(48), 27.

Rybak, S. & Bush, P. (1999). A guide to revising the postanesthesia care unit documentation record. *Journal of Perianesthesia Nursing, 14*(5), 251-259.

Salantera, S., Lauri, S., Salmi, T.T., & Aantaa, R. (1999). Nursing activities and outcomes of care in the assessment, management, and documentation of children's pain. *Journal of Pediatric Nursing, 14*(6), 408-415.

Schwoebel, A. & Jones, M.L. (1999). A clinical pathway system for the neonatal intensive care nursery. *Journal of Perinatal & Neonatal Nursing, 13*(3), 60-69.

Siddall, S. & Barnes, D. (1999). Collaborative care documentation. *Paediatric Nursing, 11*(4), 30-32.

Stelman, M.A. (2003). The integrated summary: A documentatin tool to improve patient care. *Family Practice Management, 10*(4) 33-39.

Tang, P.C., LaRose, M.P., & Gordon, S.M. (1999). Use of computer-based records, completeness of documentation, and appropriateness of documenting clinical decisions. *Journal of the American Medical Informatics Association, 6*(3), 245-251.

Teichman, P.G. (2000). Documentation tips for reducing malpractice risk. *Family Practice Management, 7*(3), 29-33.

Weintraub, M.I. (1999). Documentation and informed consent. *Neurologic Clinics, 17*(2), 371-381.

WORLD WIDE WEB SITES

Agency for Healthcare Research and Quality (AHRQ)
http://www.ahrq.gov/

American Nurses Association
http://www.nursingworld.org/

American Society for Healthcare Risk Management
http://www.ashrm.org/

Canadian Institute for Health Information
http://www.cihi.com

Centers for Disease Control and Prevention
http://www.cdc.gov/

Centers for Medicare & Medicaid Services
CPT guidelines can be ordered from
www.cms.gov/medlearn/emdoc.asp

HealthWorld Online
http://www.healthy.net

HIV InSite
http://hivinsite.ucsf.edu

Joint Commission on Accreditation of Healthcare Organizations
http://www.jcaho.org/

Journal of the American Medical Association
http://jama.ama-assn.org/

National Association of School Nurses
http://www.nasn.org/

National Council of State Boards of Nursing
http://www.ncsbn.org/

National Health Information Center
http://www.health.gov/nhic/

National Heart, Lung, and Blood Institute
http://www.nhlbi.nih.gov

National Institute for Occupational Safety and Health
http://www.cdc.gov/niosh/homepage.html

National Institutes of Health
http://www.nih.gov/

National League for Nursing
http://www.nln.org/

National Organization for Rare Disorders
http://www.rarediseases.org/

Occupational Safety & Health Administration
http://www.osha.gov/

Sigma Theta Tau International Honor Society of Nursing
http://www.nursingsociety.org/

Supreme Court of the United States
http://www.supremecourtus.gov/

U.S. Department of Health & Human Services
http://www.os.dhhs.gov/

U.S. Department of Health and Human Services Food and Drug Administration.
Guidance for Industry Part 11, Electronic Records; Electronic Signatures – Scope and Application.
http://www.fda.gov/cder/guidance/5667fnl.htm

U.S. Government Printing Office
http://www.access.gpo.gov/

U.S. House of Representatives
http://www.house.gov/

U.S. National Institute of Diabetes & Digestive & Kidney Diseases
http://www.niddk.nih.gov

U.S. Senate
http://www.senate.gov/

Women's Interactive Network
http://www.womens-health.com/

GLOSSARY

accountability: Reason for maintaining nursing standards of care.

active euthanasia: The facilitation of a patient's death by some direct intervention, such as with assisted suicide.

admissibility of evidence: Legal concept that refers to the issue of whether a court, applying the rule of evidence, is bound to receive or permit introduction of a particular piece of evidence.

advance directive: Written instruction expressing an individual's health care wishes in the event that he or she becomes unable to make decisions.

advanced practice nurse (APN): A registered professional nurse who is prepared for advanced nursing practice with knowledge and skills obtained through an advanced educational master's degree program to act independently or in collaboration with other health care professionals in the delivery of health care services.

against medical advice (AMA): A situation in which a patient decides to leave a health care institution against the advice of a health care provider.

American Nurses Association (ANA): Organization of professional nurses in the United States that focuses on standards of health care, nurses' professional development, and the economic and general welfare of nurses.

Americans with Disabilities Act (ADA): Federal act that bars employers from discriminating against disabled people in hiring, promotion, or other provisions of employment.

(A)PIE charting: A method of documentation that focuses on assessment, problem, intervention, and evaluation.

assisted suicide: A form of active euthanasia through which a person assists another person with her or his death.

beneficence: Ethical principle that provides that a nurse must "do good" for a patient.

benefits: Specific rights and duties obtained through an insurance policy. Under an individual insurance policy for nursing malpractice, additional advantages that may be obtained include legal fees and court costs, reimbursement of defense costs, and reimbursement to the nurse for lost work time.

block charting: Method of documentation that covers a broad time frame, frequently a whole shift.

Board of Nurse Examiners (BNE): An administrative agency that regulates nursing practice on the state level.

Board of Nursing: A state regulatory agency given the authority to prescribe educational requirements and admission standards for licensure of nurses and, sometimes, advanced practice nurses; delineate tasks a nurse or advanced practitioner is allowed to perform; and establish criteria and administrative processes for disciplining nurses.

borrowed servant: Refers to a situation in which an employee is temporarily under the control of someone other than the primary employer, such as when a nurse is employed by a hospital is "borrowed" and under the control of an attending surgeon in an operating room.

breach: Neglect or failure to fulfill in an appropriate and proper manner the duties of a job.

capacity: Possession of a set of values and goals; the ability to communicate and understand information; and the ability to reason and deliberate about one's choices.

captain of the ship: A doctrine making a physician responsible for the negligent acts of other professionals because he or she had the right to control and oversee the totality of care provided to a patient.

care map: A type of charting that is based on an integrated treatment plan, identified services, patient outcomes, and length of stay.

care plan: A statement of goals and objectives of nursing care provided for a patient and the interventions required for accomplishing the plan, including the criteria to be used to evaluate the effectiveness and appropriateness of the plan.

causation: A direct relationship between damages suffered and the negligence of a provider.

Centers for Medicare & Medicaid Services (CMS): Federal agency that coordinates participation in the federal government's Medicare and Medicaid programs; previously known as Health Care Financing Administration (HCFA).

certification: Examination developed by a professional organization that provides verification of a claim to competence at a certain level of practice.

certified nurse-anesthetist (CNA): An advanced practice nurse whose practice involves evaluating a patient's overall physical health in anticipation of anesthesia administration and providing anesthesia to patients, including selection and administration of drugs, intravenous fluids, and ventilator support.

certified nurse-midwife (CNM): Nurse who is educated in midwifery and possesses certification in accordance with criteria of the American College of Nurse-Midwives.

charitable immunity: Legal doctrine developed out of the English court system that holds charitable institutions blameless for their negligent acts.

charting by exception: A charting method in which data is entered only when there is an exception from what is normal or expected. Reduces time spent documenting.

civil law: Body of law that describes the private rights and responsibilities of individuals. It involves actions filed by one individual against another.

claims-made insurance: A type of insurance that provides coverage only for claims made during the time the policy is in force.

clinical nurse specialist (CNS): An advanced practice nurse with a master's degree in nursing and expertise in a specific area of practice, with a focus on education, consultation, and therapy.

clinical pathway: A series of sequential steps in a process that is required to ensure a satisfactory outcome.

clinical practice guidelines: The clinical steps for patient management.

clinical privileges: With qualifications, the diagnostic and therapeutic procedures that an institution allows a physician or an advanced practice nurse to perform on a specified patient population.

code of ethics: A set of values and standards regulating a profession.

comparative negligence: The legal theory of liability involving dividing the amount of each party's fault or responsibility in causation of injury.

competency: Presence of characteristics, such as legal age and mental capacity, that make a patient legally fit and qualified to make independent decisions, give testimony, or execute legal documents.

computerized documentation: The use of a computer for long-term collection of an individual's health care information over a lifetime; the electronic chart used to collect information about a specific patient in a health care institution; replacement for manual documentation.

confidentiality: Privacy; a nurse must maintain the confidentiality of information related to a patient's health care.

contributory negligence: A legal theory of liability whereby the amount of a plaintiff's fault or responsibility in causing an injury is considered in calculation of reduction of damages.

CORE charting: A method of documentation that focuses on the nursing process and consists of a data base, plan of action, and evaluation.

credentialing: Validation of the education, training, and experience of a provider; a voluntary form of self-regulation within a profession that requires a higher standard of education, experience, or testing than does licensure.

crime: Act against society in violation of the law that is prosecuted by and in the name of the state.

critical pathways: A multidisciplinary care plan through which diagnosis and interventions are sequenced on a timetable.

cross-examination: Period in a legal trial when the attorney asks the witness leading questions designed to elicit specific information, such as a "yes" or "no" answer, without opportunity to explain or qualify.

current procedural terminology (CPT) codes: Five-digit codes used in billing insurance companies by which services, treatments, and procedures are classified.

damages: Injuries of a physical, emotional, psychological, or economic nature.

deep pocket: The defendant who has the most money from which the plaintiff may recover damages.

defendant: In a criminal case, the person accused of committing a crime. In a civil suit, the party against whom a suit is brought, with a demand to pay the other party legal relief.

defense: Legal theory under which a defendant may prove that he or she is not liable for a plaintiff's claim.

delegation: The process of assigning another member of the health care team aspects of patient care, for example, assigning a nurse assistant to bathe a patient.

Department of Health and Human Services (DHHS): The federal agency in charge of Medicaid and Medicare programs.

deposition: A method of pretrial discovery that consists of statements of fact taken by a witness under oath in a question-and-answer format, as it would be in a court of law, with opportunity given to the adversary to be present for cross-examination. Such statements may be admitted into evidence if it is impossible for a witness to attend a trial in person.

diagnosis related groups (DRGs): Group of patients classified for measuring a hospital's delivery of care, with classification based on the following variables: primary and secondary diagnosis, primary and secondary procedures, age, and length of stay.

discharge summary: Part of a medical record that summarizes a patient's initial complaints, course of treatment, final diagnosis, and suggestions for follow-up care.

discovery: Pretrial investigation used to obtain facts and information about a case to assist with preparation for trial.

documentation: Act of authenticating events or activities by keeping written records.

do-not-resuscitate (DNR): Directive of a physician to withhold cardiopulmonary resuscitation in the event that a patient experiences cardiac or respiratory arrest.

downsizing: A reduction in the size of the workforce.

durable power of attorney for health care: A document that designates an agent or proxy to make health care decisions for a patient who is unable to do so.

duty: Acts or interactions required after the presumption of a relationship between a provider and a patient.

elopement: The term used when an institutionalized patient escapes or runs away from the treatment center.

emancipated minor: A minor who is financially independent; lives apart from his or her parents; is married or pregnant; or is in the military services of the U.S. and is considered to have the legal capacity of an adult.

Emergency Medical Treatment and Active Labor Act (EMTALA): Contains an antidumping provision under which hospitals must provide a medical screening examination and stabilize a patient before discharging or transferring her or him to another facility.

euthanasia: Act conducted for the purpose of causing the merciful death of a person who is suffering from an incurable condition.

evaluation: Category of nursing behavior in which a determination is made and recorded regarding the extent to which a patient's goals have been met.

evidence: Pertinent information surrounding the patient, the scene, or the suspect that might substantiate claims of innocence, guilt, or responsibility for outcomes.

expressed consent: Explicit acknowledgment of a health care provider's request to provide treatment; consent to medical treatment that takes the form of a verbal agreement or signed consent.

FACT charting: A method of documentation that focuses on flow sheets for specific services which include assessment; concise, integrated progress notes and flow sheets; and timely entries of care given.

feasibility: A legal concept that holds that, but for an act of negligence, an injury would not have occurred.

floating: A staffing arrangement in which one may be asked to work on any of several hospital units, depending on the immediate needs of the health care institution.

flow sheets: Form of documentation on which frequent observations or specific measurements are recorded.

focus charting: A charting method for structuring progress notes according to the focus of the note, such as symptoms and nursing diagnoses. Each note includes data, actions, and patient response.

Food & Drug Administration (FDA): Federal agency responsible for the enforcement of federal regulations regarding the manufacture and distribution of food, drugs, and cosmetics to ensure protection against the sale of impure or dangerous substances.

foreseeability: A legal requirement that the general danger, not the exact sequence of events that produced the harm, be foreseeable.

good Samaritan laws: Laws designed to protect those who stop to render aid in an emergency. These laws generally provide immunity for specified persons from any civil suit arising out of care rendered at the scene of an emergency, provided that the one rendering assistance has not done so in a grossly negligent manner.

graphic sheet: Record of repeated observations and measurements, such as vital signs, daily weight, and intake and output.

guardian: Person appointed by a court to protect the interests of and make decisions for a person who is incapable of making her or his own decisions.

guidelines: Recommended nursing practices designed to meet standards of care.

health care provider: A member of the multidisciplinary treatment team who renders health care to a patient, for example, a physician, an advanced practice nurse, or a nurse assistant.

health care proxy: Document that delegates the authority to make a person's health care decisions to another adult, known as the *health care agent*, when one has become incapacitated or is unable to make decisions.

Health Insurance Portability and Accountability Act (HIPAA): The 1996 act that establishes privacy and security standards to protect patient health care information. In December 2000, the U.S. Department of Health & Human Services issued final regulations governing privacy of this information under HIPAA.

Homan's sign: Discomfort behind the knee on forced dorsiflexion of the foot; a sign of thrombosis in the leg.

home health agency: Any public agency or private organization, or a subdivision of such an institution, that provides home health services. Home health care involves any services provided to patients in their homes because of acute illness, exacerbation of chronic illness, or disability.

home health care: Care provided daily, weekly, or even monthly to those who are unable to leave their homes or who need continued care following discharge from a health care institution. Such services include part-time or intermittent nursing care; physical, occupational, or speech therapy; medical social services; home health aid services; nutritional guidance; medical supplies other than drugs prescribed by a health care provider; and assistance with the use of medical appliances.

home state: Under the Nurse Multistate Licensure Compact, a nurse's state of residence and the state that grants license, sets licensure standards, and takes disciplinary action under that license.

host state: Under the Nurse Multistate Licensure Compact, the state in which the patient resides or in which telenursing care is provided.

immunity: Right to be free from any type of claim, including liability.

implementation: Category of nursing behavior in which the action necessary for achieving projected outcomes of a health care plan are initiated and completed.

implied consent: Nonverbal acknowledgement of a health care provider's request to provide treatment.

inadequate staffing: Staffing that is inadequate to provide services contracted for or that does not meet an acceptable standard.

incident: A broad term used to describe any occurrence that is not consistent with routine hospital activities.

incident report: A report of special, unusual, or unexpected occurrences or outcomes that may become the subject of litigation.

incompetent: Designation for a person who is unable to speak for herself or himself, comprehend, or make decisions as a result of some incapacity, including but not limited to medical condition, age, deformity, or retardation.

informed consent: Process of obtaining permission from a patient to perform a specific test or procedure after describing all risks, side effects, and benefits.

injury: The consequences or harm caused by an action or inaction.

insurance tails: The extension of a malpractice policy beyond the policy period that would be in effect until there is no longer any possibility of a claim being made against a nurse's professional practice.

Interstate Compact for the Mutual Recognition Model on Nursing Regulations: Developed by the National Council of State Boards of Nursing, compact that allows nurses to practice outside their states of licensure, as long as they adhere to the nurse practice act in the state of practice and the host state is a member of the compact.

interventions: Part of the nursing process involving all aspects of actual care provided to a patient, which requires full knowledge of the assessment and planning stages.

Joint Commission on Accreditation of Healthcare Organizations (JCAHO): A not-for-profit independent organization dedicated to improving the quality of health care in organized health care settings. Its major functions include developing organizational standards, awarding accreditation decisions, and providing education and consultation to health care institutions.

justice: An ethical principle that encompasses a nurse's duty to be fair and equitable and provide access to and appropriate care to all patients.

Kardex: Trade name for card-filing system that allows quick reference to the particular need of the patient for certain aspects of nursing care.

liability: As it relates to damages, an obligation one has incurred or might incur through a negligent act.

licensure: A legal process by which a designated authority grants permission to a qualified individual to perform designated skills and services in a given jurisdiction; mechanism by which a state establishes and unifies compliance with standards.

litigation: Adversarial contest in a court of justice for the purpose of enforcing a right, legal action, or process.

living will: Document in which an individual expresses wishes in advance regarding the use of life-sustaining treatment in the event he or she is incapable of doing so at some future date.

long-term care: Health care services, such as physical, psychological, spiritual, social, and economic services, provided on a long-term basis to help people attain, maintain, or regain their optimum level of functioning.

malpractice: Professional misconduct, improper discharge of professional duties, or failure to meet the standard of care of a professional that results in harm to another.

malpractice insurance: The type of insurance that protects professional people against claims of negligence or malpractice.

medical record: Documentation designed to provide a summary of all observations made regarding nursing and medical diagnosis and to accurately reflect measures taken to alleviate identified problems as well as a patient's response to interventions.

Medicaid: State medical assistance based on Title XIX of the Social Security Act. States receive 50% in matching federal funds to provide medical care and services to people meeting categorical and income requirements. Covers home health services based on Medicare guidelines. Medicaid can cover many innovative home health programs as long as they meet the recipient's needs and cost less than institutionalization. Called *Medi-Cal* in California.

medical diagnosis: Identification of a specific disease or pathological process.

Medicare: Federal government insurance coverage for persons over age 65 disabled and people who have paid into the Social Security or Railroad Retirement system. Covers inpatient hospital charges and some home health services.

medication administration record (MAR): A record listing the medication, amount, route, and time of administration.

minimum data set (MDS): A specific form used in long-term care to collect the minimum information needed for assessing a resident's needs in order to develop a plan of care.

multidisciplinary treatment team: A team of health care providers that monitors and determines all aspects of the security, diagnosis, treatment, and rights of a health care patient through a shared decision-making process.

narrative notes: Notes regarding a patient's status written in the nurse's own handwriting that provide an overview of patient care for a shift.

National Council of State Boards of Nursing (NCSBN): A nonprofit organization composed of boards of nursing from the 50 states, the District of Columbia, and the five territories of the United States; it is the organization through which boards of nursing act and develop licensing exams.

National League for Nursing (NLN): Organization of nurses and laypeople concerned with improving nursing education, nursing service, and the delivery of health care in the United States. The NLN is an official accrediting agency for some schools of nursing.

negligence: Careless act of omission or commission of an act that a reasonable person would or would not do under given circumstances that results in injury to another.

North American Nurses Diagnosis Association (NANDA): Organization involved in developing and promoting the use of nursing diagnoses.

Nursing Information and Data Set Evaluation Center (NIDSEC): Center established by the American Nurses Association to develop and disseminate standards pertaining to information systems that support documentation of nursing practice and to evaluate voluntarily submitted information systems against these standards.

nurse practice act: Statute enacted by the legislature of a state delineating the legal scope of the practice of nursing within the geographical boundaries of the jurisdiction.

nursing care plan: Written guidelines of nursing care that document specific nursing diagnoses, goals, interventions, and projected outcomes for a patient.

nursing code of ethics: The professional values and standards of nursing practice.

nursing diagnosis: A statement that describes a patient's actual or potential response to a health problem that a nurse is licensed and competent to treat.

nursing history form: Data collected about a patient's present level of wellness, changes in life patterns, sociocultural role, and mental and emotional reactions to illness.

nursing intervention: Any action by a nurse that implements the nursing care plan or any specific objective of the plan.

nursing process: Systematic problem-solving method by which nurses individualize care for a patient. The five steps of the nursing process are assessment, diagnosis, planning, implementation, and evaluation.

objective data: Data relating to a patient's health problem that are obtained through observation or diagnostic measurement.

obligation: Something owed to another.

occurrence: An incident; an event that is not consistent with routine operations of an institution or care of a patient.

occurrence-based insurance: Type of insurance policy that covers any occurrence of an injury or damage that occurred during the time the policy was in force.

Omnibus Budget Reconciliation Act (OBRA): A federal statute enforcing a standard and monitoring the disposition of patients arriving at emergency departments (1981, 1987, 1989, and 1990). The 1987 Act changed the standard of care in nursing homes by defining minimum standards.

ordinary negligence: Failure to meet the standard of conduct required of reasonably prudent people.

outcome indicators: Condition of a patient at the end of treatment, including the degree of wellness and the need for continuing care, medication, support, counseling, or education.

patient: A person who is receiving or has received health care, including the deceased.

patient medical record: Written form of communication that permanently documents information relevant to health care management.

patient rights: A guarantee of certain rights and privileges to every hospitalized patient.

Patient Self-Determination Act (PSDA): A federal law that mandates hospitals and other health care agencies to inform patients of their rights under state law to have living wills and durable powers of attorney for health care.

plaintiff: Party who brings a civil suit seeking damages or other legal relief.

premium: The amount of money paid to an insurer in return for insurance coverage.

prescriptive authority: Within the scope of professional practice, conditions under which an advanced practice nurse is given statutory permission to prescribe medications based on a medical diagnosis.

primary care provider: A provider who gives comprehensive care to an assigned group of patients or members; term usually reserved for physicians, nurse practitioners, and physician's assistants.

problem-oriented medical record (POMR): Method of recording data about the health status of a patient that fosters a collaborative problem-solving approach by all members of the health care team.

prognosis: Informed judgment regarding the likely course and probable outcome of a disease.

protocol: A set of rules governing a required process or procedure.

punitive damage: An amount of money awarded to a plaintiff, designed to punish the defendant, if a wrongful action or inaction is found to have been performed with malice.

quality assurance: Process by which the total health care services provided to a patient is monitored for compliance with standards of care.

registered care technologist (RCT): A health care position proposed by the American Medical Association that would provide direct patient care and report to a physician.

registered nurse (RN): Health care professional who has completed a course of study at an accredited school of professional nursing and has passed an examination administered by a state board of nursing or the Canadian Nurses Association Testing Service.

registration: The listing, or registering, of names of individuals on an official roster when they have met certain pre-established criteria.

reimbursement: Payment for services rendered to a patient by a third-party payer, such as Medicare, Medicaid, managed care organizations, or insurers; depends on individual fee schedules, laws, and policies of each third-party payer.

remote state: Under the compact, any state in which a nurse practices other than the home state.

respondeat superior: Legal concept by which an employer is responsible for the legal consequences of the acts of a servant or employee who is acting within the scope of employment; Literally, "Let the master answer."

responsibility: Carrying out duties associated with a particular role.

restraint: Device to aid in the immobilization of a patient or a patient's extremity.

review of systems (ROS): A systematic method for collecting data on all body systems.

rights: Something claimed by or owed to another by virtue of legal, moral, or ethical authority.

risk factor: Any internal or external variable that makes a person or group more vulnerable to illness or an unhealthy event.

risk management: Process used to monitor and improve the quality of health care through prevention of injuries; by monitoring health care equipment; and through early, prompt identification of negligent injuries by health care providers.

scope of practice: The nursing diagnosis and treatment of human responses to health and illness; defined by the knowledge base of the nurse, the role of the nurse, and the nature of the patient population within the practice environment.

SOAP(IER) notes: A method of charting that documents the subjective, objective, nursing assessment, and planned nursing interventions. In some cases, interventions, evaluations, and revisions are also included.

specialty organization: Local, state, national, or international organization focused on one area of medical or nursing specialty. Nurses may voluntarily join the organization for an annual fee. Many specialty organizations have developed standards used as guidelines for nurses practicing within a specialty area.

spoliation: Any action including destruction, alteration, or concealment of records, which deprives the court or parties to a dispute of evidence.

standard: Measure or guide that serves as a basis for comparison when evaluating similar phenomena or substances.

standards of care: The minimum level of care accepted to ensure high quality of care to patients. Standards of care define the types of therapies typically administered to patients with defined problems or needs. They represent the degree of care that a reasonably prudent person in that profession should exercise under the same or similar circumstances.

standards of practice: Serve as the framework for statements about competency levels and form the basis for outcomes for education and standards for the delivery of nursing care.

standardized care plan: Plan based on an institution's standards of nursing practice that is preprinted; established guidelines used to care for patients who have similar health problems.

standing orders: Written and approved document containing rules, policies, procedures, regulations, and orders for the conduct of patient care in various stipulated clinical settings.

State Board of Nursing: An official agency responsible for enforcing a state's nurse practice act and regulating nursing practice.

statute of limitations: Legal limits on the time allowed for filing suit in civil matters, usually measured from the time of the wrong or from the time when a reasonable person would have discovered the wrong.

statutory law: Of or related to laws enacted by a legislative branch of the government.

subjective data: Data relating to a patient's health problem described in the patient's own words.

suit: Court proceedings in which one person seeks damages or other legal remedies from another.

surrogate decision-maker: Individual who has been designated to make decisions on behalf of an individual determined incapable of making his or her own decisions.

testimony: Oral statement of a witness given under oath at a trial.

timely documentation: Documentation that is recorded shortly after observation, intervention, or evaluation of a patient.

tort: Act that causes injury for which the injured party can bring civil action.

triage: A process by which a group of patients is sorted according to their needs for care. The kind of illness or injury, the severity of the problem, and the facilities available govern the process.

trial court: Court in which evidence is presented to a judge or jury for a decision.

twenty-four-hour patient care record: A documentation method that consolidates the nursing record into a system that accommodates a 24-hour period.

unlicensed assistive personnel (UAP): Individuals who are trained to function in an assistive role to the registered professional nurse in the provision of patient care activities as delegated by and under the supervision of a registered nurse.

variance: An event that occurs during patient care and that is different from what is predicted. Variance or exceptions are interventions or outcomes that are not achieved as anticipated. Variance may be positive or negative.

VIPS charting: A method of documentation based on four key concepts: well-being, integrity, prevention, and safety, yielding the acronym VIPS in the Swedish spelling.

vulnerable population: Special group of people whose rights need special protection because of their inability to provide meaningful informed consent or because their circumstances place them at higher-than-average risk for adverse effects; examples include young children, mentally retarded people, and unconscious patients.

waive: To give up a legal right, such as the privilege of confidentiality of all health care information; for example, to refuse, relinquish, or forgo health care treatment.

witness: Person who is called to give testimony in a court of law.

Aiken, T.D. (2003). The law, standards of care, and liability issues. In P.W. Iyer (Ed.), *Legal nurse consulting: Principles and practice* (2nd ed., pp. 3-34). Boca Raton, FL: CRC Press.

Aiken, T.D. & Catalano, J.T. (1994). *Legal, ethical, and political issues in nursing.* Philadelphia, PA: F.A. Davis.

American Association of Critical Care Nurses. (1989). *Standards for nursing care of the critically ill.* Englewood, NJ: Prentice Hall.

American Association of Retired People (AARP). (July/August 2003). Your Health: *"Medical Privacy – What Are Your Rights."* Washington, DC: Author. Retrieved April 21, 2005 from http://www.aarp.org/bulletin/yourhealth/Articles/a2003-08-28-rights.html

American Federation of State, County and Municipal Employees. (2003). *Solving the nursing shortage — Worst practices: Mandatory overtime.* Retrieved August 31, 2003, from http://www.afscme.org/una/sns10.htm

American Hospital Association. (2003). *The Patient Care Partnership: Understanding expectations, rights and responsibilities.* Retrieved May 12, 2005 from http://www.aha.org/aha/ptcommunication/partnership/index.html

American Hospital Association, Special Member Briefing. (1992). *Emergency Medical Treatment and Active Labor Act requirements and investigations.* Chicago: Author.

American Nurses Association. (1980). *Nursing: A social policy statement.* Washington, DC: Author.

American Nurses Association. (1985). *Code for nurses with interpretive statements.* Washington, DC: Author.

American Nurses Association. (1986). *Standards for home health care.* Washington, DC: Author.

American Nurses Association. (1991a). *Position statement on nursing and the Patient Self-Determination Act.* Washington, DC: Author.

American Nurses Association. (1991b). *Standards of clinical nursing practice.* Washington, DC: Author.

American Nurses Association. (1992, April 2). *Position statement: Nursing care and do-not-resuscitate decisions.* Washington, DC: Author. Retrieved September 2, 2003, from http://www.nursingworld.org/readroom/position/ethics/etdnr.htm

American Nurses Association. (1994). *Ethics and Human Rights Position Statements: Assisted Suicide.* Retrieved May 27, 2005, from http://www.nursingworld.org/readroom/position/ethics/prtetsuic.htm

American Nurses Association. (1995). *The ANA basic guide to safe delegation.* Washington, DC: Author.

American Nurses Association. (1998a). *Multistate regulation of nurses.* Retrieved August 25, 2003, from http://nursingworld.org/gova/multibg.htm.

American Nurses Association. (1998b). *Standards of clinical nursing practice (2nd ed.).* Washington, DC: Author.

American Nurses Association. (2001). *Code of ethics for nurses with interpretive statements.* Washington, DC: Author.

American Nurses Association. (2003). *Principles for Documentation.* [Brochure]. Washington, DC: Author.

American Nurses Association. (2005). *Nursing Facts: A new age in health care.* Retrieved June 3, 2003, from http://nursingworld.org/readroom/fsadvprc.htm

Anast, D.G. (2002, October). FDA draft guidance on electronic records, signatures & maintenance release. *Medical Design Technology, 8.*

Anderson, J.C. (2003). Informed Consent. In P.W. Iyer (Ed.). *Legal nurse consulting. Principles and practices* (2nd ed., pp. 91-104). Boca Raton, FL: CRC Press.

Association of Operating Room Nurses. (1996.). Recommended practices for documentation of perioperative nursing care. *AORN Journal 63*(6), 1145, 1148, 1150.

Association of Operating Room Nurses. (2000). Recommended practices for documentation of perioperative nursing care. *AORN Journal, 71*(1), 247-250.

Association of Women's Health, Obstetric and Neonatal Nurses. (1998). *Standards and guidelines for professional nursing practice in the care of women and newborns* (5th ed.). Washington, DC: Author.

Basler, B. (2003, July/August). Your eyes only – mostly. *AARP Bulletin, 20.*

Berry, V. & Mackay, T.R. (2001). Advanced practice nursing. In M.E. O'Keefe (Ed.), *Nursing practice and the law: Avoiding malpractice and other legal risks* (pp. 301-315). Philadelphia: F.A. Davis.

Blais, K., Hayes, J.S., Kozier, B., & Erb, G. (2002). *Professional nursing practice: Concepts and perspectives* (4th ed.). Upper Saddle River, NJ: Prentice Hall.

Borchers, E.L. (1999). Improving nursing documentation for private-duty home health care. *Journal of Nursing Care Quality, 13*(5), 24-43.

Brent, N.J. (2001). *Nurses and the law: A guide to principles and applications* (2nd ed.). Philadelphia: W.B. Saunders.

Buppert, C. (2003a). HIPAA patient privacy. *Nurse Practitioner World News, 8*(1-2), 1, 4, 6.

Buppert, C. (2003b). HIPAA patient privacy. *The American Journal for Nurse Practitioners, 7*(1), 17-22.

Burkhardt, M.A., & Nathaniel, A.K. (2002). *Ethics & issues in contemporary nursing* (2nd ed.). Albany, NY: Delmar.

Burnett, V.W., Cavanagh, S., & Shearer, J. (2002). Multidisciplinary documentation in care of the elderly. *British Journal of Therapy and Rehabilitation, 9*(10), 382-385.

Cairone, D. (1999). Perioperative documentation. In P.W. Iyer & N.H. Camp (Eds.), *Nursing documentation. A nursing process approach* (3rd ed., pp. 256-274). St. Louis: Mosby.

Carelock, J. & Innerarity, S. (2001). Critical incidents: Effective communication and documentation. *Critical Care Nursing Quarterly, 23*(4), 59-66.

Catalano, A.M.K. (2001). The nurse-patient relationship. In M.E. O'Keefe (Ed.), *Nursing practice and the law: Avoiding malpractice and other legal risks* (pp. 177-188). Philadelphia: F.A. Davis.

Cavallaro, R., Newman, J.R., & Iyer, P. (1999). Long-term care documentation. In P.W. Iyer & N.H. Camp (Eds.), *Nursing documentation: A nursing process approach* (3rd ed., pp. 319-351). St. Louis: Mosby.

CBS News. (2003, January 17). Nursing Shortage in Critical Stage. 60 Minutes, Author.

Cutrona, A.K. (2001). Home health nursing. In M.E. O'Keefe (Ed.), *Nursing practice and the law: Avoiding malpractice and other legal risks* (pp. 317-335). Philadelphia: F.A. Davis.

Daniels, R. (1997). Documentation and reporting. In P.A. Potter & A.G. Perry (Eds.), *Fundamentals of nursing: Concepts, process, and practice* (4th ed., pp. 179-205). St. Louis: Mosby.

Demoro, R.A. (2000, December 27). A crisis in Nursing Threatens Patients. *Los Angeles Times.*

Eggland, E.T. (1995). Charting smarter: Using new mechanisms to organize your paperwork. *Nursing 95, 25*(9), 34-41.

Ehrenberg, A., Ehnfors, M., & Thorell-Ekstrand, I. (1996). Nursing documentation in patient records: Experience of the use of the VIPS model. *Journal of Advanced Nursing, 24*(4), 853-867.

Eldridge, C. (n.d.). *Nursing delegation to unlicensed assistive personnel.* Retrieved August 25, 2003, from http://www.e-quipping.com

Emergency Nurses Association and the Association of Women's Health, Obstetric, and Neonatal Nurses. (1991). Position statement. The obstetric patient in the ED. *AWHONN Voice, 2,* 13.

Georgia Board of Nursing. (n.d.) RN Assignment Decision Tree: Assignment to Unlicensed Assistive Personnel (UAP). Retrieved June 9, 2005, from http://www.sos.state.ga.us/plb/rn/decision_tree.htm

Georgia NPs rally for right to write. (2005). *Nurse Practitioner World News, 10*(2), 1, 5.

Grant, P., Skinner, H.G., Fleming, L.E., & Bean, J.A. (2002). Influence of structured encounter forms on documentation by community pediatricians. *Southern Medical Journal, 95*(9), 1026-1031.

Gudgell, K. (2003). Access to medical records. In P.W. Iyer (Ed.), *Legal nurse consulting: Principles and practice* (2nd ed., pp. 35-57). Boca Raton, FL: CRC Press.

GuideOne Insurance: The GuideOne Center for Risk Management® (2004). *SLC Checklist: Documentation.* Retrieved May 14, 2005, from http://www.guideonecenter.com/SLC/FreePDFs _SLC/checklist_doc02.pdf

Habel, M. (2003a). *Documenting patient care, Part I: Requirements, charting systems, and reimbursement.* Retrieved April 25, 2003, from http://www.nurseweek.com/ce/ce10a.html

Habel, M. (2003b). *Documenting patient care, Part 2: Limit liability, trends, and computer charting.* Retrieved April 25, 2003 from http://www .nurseweek.com/ce/ce10a.html

Hall, J.K. & Hall, D. (2001). Negligence specific to nursing. In M.E. O'Keefe (Ed.), *Nursing practice and the law: Avoiding malpractice and other legal risks* (pp. 132-149). Philadelphia: F.A. Davis.

Hamlin, J. & Coplein, G. (1999). Pediatric documentation. In P.W. Iyer & N.H. Camp (Eds.), *Nursing documentation: A nursing process approach* (3rd ed., pp. 176-199). St. Louis: Mosby.

Hickok, T.A. (n.d.). *Downsizing and organizational culture.* Retrieved August 31, 2003, from http://www.pamij.com/hickok.html.

Holly, J.L. (2003, August). Safeguarding patients with electronic medical records: Using technology to direct care. *Advance for Nurse Practitioners,* 69-71.

Iyer, P.W. & Camp, N.H. (Eds.). (1999). *Nursing documentation: A nursing process approach* (3rd ed.). St. Louis: Mosby.

Joint Commission on Accreditation of Healthcare Organizations. (1995). *Standards for the accreditation of home care.* Chicago: Author.

Joint Commission on Accreditation of Healthcare Organizations. (1996). *The 1997 comprehensive accreditation manual for hospitals: The official handbook.* Oakbrook Terrace, IL: Author.

Kavaler, R. & Spiegel, A.D. (1997). Risk management dynamics. In F. Kavaler & A.D. Spiegel (Eds.), *Risk management in health care institutions: A strategic approach* (pp. 3-25). Sudbury, MA: Jones & Bartlett.

Kuc, J.A. (1999). Postanesthesia care unit documentation. In P.W. Iyer & N.H. Camp (Eds.), *Nursing documentation: A nursing process approach* (3rd ed., pp. 274-286). St. Louis: Mosby.

Lewin, K. (1951). *Field theory in social science.* NY: Harper.

Lewis, K. (2002, July). Do the write thing: Document everything. *PT Magazine, 30-33.*

Lopez, Andrew. (January 29, 2002). Nurse Sued for "Too Many Sticks" How Many Attempts Is Too Many? Clinical Nursing Malpractice Case Studies. Retrieved April 29, 2005 from http://nursefriendly.com/nursing/clinical.cases/020129

Lopez, Andrew. (January 13, 2000a). *Cytomegalovirus Test Result, Misinterpreted By Nurse. Did Negligence Lead to Child With Birth Defects?* Clinical Case of The Week. Retrieved April 29, 2005 from http://www.nursefriendly.com/nursing/clinical.cases/011300.htm

Lopez, Andrew M. October 22, 2000b. Trauma Patient, In Shock And In Decline, ER Physician Does Not Transfer. Clinical Case of The Week. Retrieved April 29, 2005 from the World Wide Web: http://www.nursefriendly.com/nursing/clinical.cases/2000/102200.htm

Mackay, T.R. (2001). Informed consent. In M.E. O'Keefe (Ed.), *Nursing practice and the law: Avoiding malpractice and other legal risks* (pp. 199-213). Philadelphia: F.A. Davis.

Matthews, M.D. (2001). The nurse and the legal system. In M.E. O'Keefe (Ed.), *Nursing practice and the law: Avoiding malpractice an other legal risks* (pp. 42-57). Philadelphia: F.A. Davis.

McCartney, P.R. (2003). HIPAA and electronic health information security. *The American Journal of Maternal-Child Nursing, 28*(5), 333.

Mullin, R. (2002, April 24). FDA steps up enforcement of electronic documentation rules. *Chemical Week.* www.chemweek.com

National Council of State Boards of Nursing. (2003, April). Compact implementation. Retrieved August 25, 2003 from http://www.ncsbn.org/public/nurselicensurecompact/mutual_recognition_state.htm

National Organization of Nurse Practitioner Faculties. (2000). *Domains and competencies of nurse practitioner practice.* Washington, DC: Author.

Nevidjon, B., & Erickson, J.I. (2001, January 31). The nursing shortage: Solutions for the short and long term. *Online Journal of Issues in Nursing.* Retrieved May 7, 2005 from http://nursingworld.org/ojin/topic14/tpc14_4.htm

Oldham, R. & Meyer-Tulledge, P. (1999). Psychiatric documentation. In P.W. Iyer & N.H. Camp (Eds.), *Nursing documentation: A nursing process approach* (3rd ed., pp. 288-304). St. Louis: Mosby.

Perry, A.G. (1997). Acute care. In P.A. Potter & A.G. Perry (Eds.), *Fundamentals of nursing: Concepts, process, and practice* (pp. 61-78). St. Louis: Mosby.

Peters, D.A. (1999). Home care documentation. In P.W. Iyer, & N.H. Camp (Eds.), *Nursing documentation: A nursing process approach* (3rd ed., pp. 304-318). St. Louis: Mosby.

Peterson, C.A. (2001, January 31). Nursing shortage: Not a simple problem—No easy answers. *Online Journal of Issues in Nursing.* Retrieved May 7, 2005 from http://nursingworld.org/ojin/topic14/tpc14_4.htm

Philpott, M. (1986, August). 20 rules for good charting. *Nursing86, 16*(8), 63.

Pozgar, G.D. (2002). *Legal aspects of health care administration* (8th ed.). Gaithersburg, MD: Aspen.

Ramos, F., Jr. (2003). HIPAA's new privacy rules. *Advance for Nurse Practitioners, 11*(5), 24.

Santarelli-Kretovics, A.M. (1999). Intensive care documentation. In P.W. Iyer, & N.H. Camp (Eds.), *Nursing documentation: A nursing process approach* (3rd ed., pp. 231-255). St. Louis: Mosby.

Satarawala, R (2000). Confronting the Legal perils of I.V. Therapy. *Nursing2000, 30*(8), 44.

Schaffer, C.L. (1992, May). Documenting special legal situations. *Nursing 92,* 32C-32D.

Sheeler, C. (2003, January/February). Tips for depositions. *Chief Executive Group,* 6.

Sherwood, G.D., Brown, M., Fay, V., & Wardell, D. (1997). Defining nurse practitioner scope of practice: Expanding primary care services. *The Internet Journal of Advanced Nursing Practice, 1*(2), 12 pages. Retrieved August 24, 2003, from http://www.ispub.com/ostia/index.php?xml/filepath=journals/ijanp/vol1n2/scope.xml

Singleton, J.K. (1997). Identifying and controlling risks in long term care. In F. Kavaler & A.D. Spiegel (Eds.), *Risk management in health care institutions: A strategic approach* (2nd ed., pp. 245-268). Sudbury, MA: Jones & Bartlett.

Solomon, J. (1995). Career options: Retirement living = jobs for nurses. *RN, 58*(5), 52-55.

Starr, D.S. (2003). Tips for everyday clinical practice. Complying with HIPAA. *The Clinical Advisor, 6*(1), 77.

Spratley, E., Johnson, A., Sochalski, J., Fritz, M., & Spencer, W. (2002). The Registered Nurse Population. March 2000. Retrieved June 3, 2005, from http://www.nursingworld.org/readroom/fsdemogr.htm

State of Missouri, Department of Health and Senior Services. (n.d.). General documentation guidelines. Retrieved May 18, 2005 from http://www.health.state.mo.us/LPHA/PHNursing/Documentation_04.htm

Texas Department of Human Services. (2003). *The 10 most-often cited deficiencies in long-term care facilities.* Austin, TX: Author. Retrieved September 25, 2003, from http://www.dhs.state.tx.us

Tiller, C.M. (1994). *Everything you always wanted to know about nursing documentation in labor and delivery.* Workshop sponsored by American Healthcare Institute. Silver Spring, MD: American Healthcare Institute.

Tiller, C.M. (1999). Documentation & legalities. Presented at the Texas State Society of American Medical Technologists Meeting, Abilene, Texas, March 27, 1999.

Triplett, L. (2002). Electronic supportive documentation: Welcome to the future. *Nursing Homes: Long Term Care Management, 51*(12), 40-42.

U.S. Department of Labor (1991). *Americans with Disabilities Act of 1990.* 42 U. S. C.s 12101 et. seg. Public Law No. 101-336, 140 Stat.327.

White, C. & Hemby, C. (1997, February). Case in point: Automating the bedside. *Healthcare Informatics.*

Williams, L. (2002, August). Avoid liability. Let Will Rogers be your guide. *Nursing Homes: Long Term Care Management,* 6-8.

Wysoker, A. (1997). Risk management in psychiatry. In F. Kavaler & A.D. Spiegel (Eds.), *Risk management in health care institutions: A strategic approach* (2nd ed., pp. 225-244). Sudbury, MA: Jones & Bartlett.

Yocum, F. (1993). *Documentation skills for quality patient care.* Tipp City, OH: Awareness Productions.

Yocum, R.F. (2002). Documenting for quality patient care. *Nursing2002, 32*(8), 58-64.

INDEX

PRETEST KEY

Documentation for Nurses

1.	a	Chapter 1
2.	a	Chapter 1
3.	b	Chapter 2
4.	d	Chapter 2
5.	c	Chapter 3
6.	a	Chapter 3
7.	d	Chapter 4
8.	c	Chapter 5
9.	c	Chapter 5
10.	b	Chapter 6
11.	a	Chapter 7
12.	c	Chapter 7
13.	c	Chapter 8
14.	c	Chapter 9
15.	d	Chapter 9
16.	b	Chapter 10
17.	a	Chapter 11
18.	a	Chapter 12
19.	d	Chapter 12
20.	a	Chapter 13

Notes

Notes

Western Schools® offers over 2,000 hours to suit all your interests – and requirements!

Visit us online at westernschools.com for additional CE offerings!   REV 3/25/09